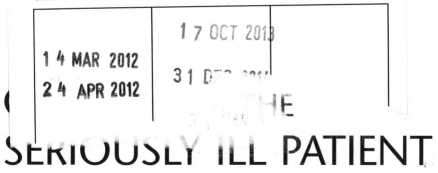

SERIOUSLY ILL PATIENT

CARING FOR THE SERIOUSLY ILL PATIENT

SECOND EDITION

Edited By

Mike Macintosh RGN, BA (HONS) MMEDSC

Lecturer, School of Nursing and Midwifery, University of Sheffield

Tracey Moore RGN, BSC(HONS) MSC PGDIP(ED)

Senior Lecturer, School of Nursing and Midwifery, University of Sheffield;
and Chair of the National Critical Care Outreach Forum (NORF)

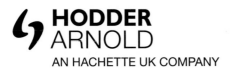

HODDER
ARNOLD
AN HACHETTE UK COMPANY

First published in Great Britain in 2000 Arnold

This second edition published in 2011 by
Hodder Arnold, an imprint of Hodder Education, an Hachette UK Company,
338 Euston Road, London NW1 3BH
www.hodderarnold.com

Hachette UK's policy is to use papers that are natural, renewable and recyclable products and made from wood grown in sustainable forests. The logging and manufacturing processes are expected to conform to the environmental regulations of the country of origin.

Whilst the advice and information in this book are believed to be true and accurate at the date of going to press, neither the author[s] nor the publisher can accept any legal responsibility or liability for any errors or omissions that may be made. In particular (but without limiting the generality of the preceding disclaimer) every effort has been made to check drug dosages; however it is still possible that errors have been missed. Furthermore, dosage schedules are constantly being revised and new side-effects recognized. For these reasons the reader is strongly urged to consult the drug companies' printed instructions before administering any of the drugs recommended in this book.

British Library Cataloguing in Publication Data
A catalogue record for this book is available from the British Library

Library of Congress Cataloging-in-Publication Data
A catalog record for this book is available from the Library of Congress

ISBN-13 978 0 340 967 577

1 2 3 4 5 6 7 8 9 10

Commissioning Editor:	Naomi Wilkinson
Project Editor:	Joanna Silman
Production Controller:	Jonathan Williams
Cover Designer:	Lynda King

Cover image © Jose Luis Pelaez Inc/Blend Images/Photolibrary.com

Typeset in 9.5pt Minion Pro by Phoenix Photosetting, Chatham, Kent ME4 4TZ
Printed and bound in Spain by Graphycems

What do you think about this book? Or any other Hodder Arnold title?
Please visit our website: www.hodderarnold.com

Contents

Contributors

Mick Ashman BSc (Hons), PG Cert Ed, MA, RGN

Lecturer. Programme Lead for BMed Sci Health and Human Sciences
School of Nursing and Midwifery
University of Sheffield

Robert Donald RGN, BA(Hons), MA, PG Cert Ed

Clinical Educator for Renal Unit
Sheffield Teaching Hospital
Sheffield

Derek Darling BA(Hons), RGN, BA(Hons) Nursing and Education, MMedSci in Palliative Care

Lecturer
School of Nursing & Midwifery
University of Sheffield

Nicola Morton RN, ADip, ENB 100, BSc (Hons) Critical Care

Critical Care Outreach Sister
Scunthorpe General Hospital
Northern Lincolnshire and Goole Hospitals NHS Foundation Trust

Sue Snelson RGN, ENB 100, BSc (Hons) Health Studies, PGCE

Critical Care Outreach Sister
Scunthorpe General Hospital
Northern Lincolnshire and Goole Hospitals NHS Foundation Trust

Paul Swainsbury BA(Hons), RGN, MMedSci Nursing

Senior Lecturer
Faculty of Health and Wellbeing
Sheffield Hallam University

Catharine Thomas BSc(Hons), MSc

Consultant Respiratory Physiotherapist
Tameside Hospital NHS Foundation Trust
Ashton-under-Lyne

Catheryne Waterhouse BA(Hons), PG Cert Ed, MSc, RGN

Clinical Educator for Regional Neuro ITU/HDU
Sheffield Teaching Hospital
Sheffield

Preface

The first edition of *Caring for the Seriously Ill Patient* published in 2000 and was written in response to the changing needs of hospital-based nurses and allied health professionals who found themselves routinely managing patients who were older and sicker than ever before. Patients who in previous years would have been cared for in intensive care and high dependency units were now being cared for in general medical and surgical wards. This created a need for all acute hospital staff to develop the knowledge and skills that would normally have been the preserve of a few specialists.

The situation today is one where this trend and need has not only continued but escalated[1]. In recent years there has also been an increasing recognition that the care of these acute seriously ill patients may be suboptimal[2], that patients at risk of deterioration regularly go unrecognised in hospital, and that there is an unacceptably high number of preventable deaths,[3] partly due to lack of knowledge, skills and appropriate responses among those caring for this group of patients.[4] In both the UK and the USA there has been a call for systems to be put in place to improve the detection and management of seriously ill patients and this includes improving the knowledge and skills of staff. This new edition aims to contribute to this by providing a readable, easy-to-understand text that will be accessible to a wide range of healthcare staff from those in training to qualified professionals.

The second edition has been thoroughly updated to take account of both therapeutic (for example the current management of acute coronary syndromes) and organisational (for example critical care outreach, early warning scoring systems) developments since the first edition, and includes material that was considered an omission from the first edition including pain assessment and management, and sepsis and infection control. In addition it makes more use of case studies and scenarios to bring the content to life. The material in the new edition is fully supported by current evidence, is comprehensively referenced, and linked to current guidelines wherever possible.

The depth of the material in this second edition is similar to the first edition; the book is not intended to be a 'critical care' textbook; rather it is aimed at a level of practice that extends from the general ward to high dependency beds. The text focuses on three ideas; firstly a solid understanding of the underlying physiology/pathophysiology presented in a manner that is accessible and concentrates on key principles and relationships; secondly assessment and the clinical relevance and importance of assessment findings; and thirdly management of patient-centred problems.

The approach is to some extent pragmatic and guided by what is useful to those involved in, or studying for, practice. For example: rare or obscure problems are not discussed in order to give more attention to problems that are more common and more likely to be encountered; and broadly applicable and usable principles are presented rather than pages of detail. Whilst not all possible clinical conditions are discussed, the underlying principles are presented in such a way as to make them transferable to a wide range of problems.

We would like to acknowledge the work and the vision of the editors of the first edition; and the original contributors whose work formed the foundation for the second edition. We would also like to thank the new contributors who have produced additional chapters for this edition and those contributors who have updated and revised their original chapters.

Mike Macintosh
Tracey Moore
2011

1   NICE (2007) *Acutely ill patients in hospital: recognition of and response to acute illness in hospital* NICE, London
2   NCEPOD (2005) *An Acute Problem* NCEPOD, London
3   NPSA (2007) *Safer care for the acutely ill patient: learning from serious incidents* NPSA, London
4   Sari AB *et al* (2007) Extent, nature and consequences of adverse events: results of a retrospective casenote review in a large NHS hospital *Quality and Safety in Health Care* 16 (**6**) 434–439

CHAPTER 1

CARDIOVASCULAR ASSESSMENT AND MANAGEMENT

Mike Macintosh

LEARNING OUTCOMES

On completion of this chapter the reader will:

1   have a good understanding of the underlying physiology and pathophysiology of the cardiovascular system

2   be able to discuss assessment of the cardiovascular system

3   have an understanding of the assessment and management of acute coronary syndromes

4   understand the underlying physiology, assessment and management of acute heart failure

5   be able to discuss the physiology, assessment and management of cardiogenic and hypovolaemic shock.

Introduction

An understanding of the cardiovascular system, including assessment and management of common cardiovascular problems, is at the core of safe, effective acute care. Most, if not all, serious illnesses will impact on the cardiovascular system in some way. More specifically, cardiovascular disease remains the most common cause of mortality in the developed world. This chapter explores normal and altered physiology, discusses cardiovascular assessment, and introduces common cardiovascular problems.

Anatomy and physiology

Oxygen delivery

The cardiovascular system is a transport system with continuous responsibility for the delivery of *oxygen*

and nutrients to the cells of the body, and for the removal of the *waste products* of metabolism. The quantity of oxygen that is supplied to the tissues depends on three factors:

* the arterial oxygen saturation;
* the haemoglobin content of the blood;
* the cardiac output.

Expressed as an equation, this is:

$$\text{oxygen delivery } (Do_2) = \text{oxygen saturation } (Sao_2) \times \text{haemoglobin (Hb)} \times \text{cardiac output.}$$

To maintain adequate delivery of oxygen to all the tissues of the body, and to be able to increase delivery when demands dictate, the body needs to be able to increase the value of one or all of these physiological parameters. For the cardiovascular system this means being able to increase cardiac output in relation to the resistance in the vessels to maintain perfusion. This section will focus on the maintenance of adequate cardiac output and tissue perfusion and go on to consider the conditions that may threaten effective cardiovascular function.

Parts of the cardiovascular system

The cardiovascular system (CVS) can be thought of as having three parts:

- a pump (the heart);
- volume (the blood);
- pipes (the veins and arteries).

Each of these three parts is constantly being adjusted in response to demand, and a problem with one of the three must be compensated for by one or both of the other two. The aim of the CVS in continually making these adjustments is to maintain *perfusion*. To ensure adequate delivery of oxygen to the cells there has to be adequate tissue perfusion. In other words, there needs to be an acceptable level of pressure maintained at the delivery end of the CVS. When this perfusion pressure falls, the delivery of oxygenated blood will fall.

Continuing with this simple model, the cardiovascular system can be likened to any system that delivers fluid under pressure, such as a garden hose. The purpose of a garden hose is to deliver a jet of water under sufficient pressure to supply the flowers with enough fluid to prevent them from dying.

Consider for a moment the pump (heart) to be represented by the tap. The tap can be turned up, or the hosepipe (the blood vessels) can be made to have a narrower diameter. Provided there is a sufficient and constant supply of water (the blood), then either of these measures will result in the jet of water at the end of the pipe increasing – that is, perfusion. If, however the pump starts to fail by the tap being turned down, the jet of water will fall. Similarly, if the hosepipe is changed for one that has a larger diameter, a fire hose for example, the jet of water will again fall. In each of these examples there must be compensation – either the tap is turned up to increase the pressure drop caused by the larger diameter hose, or the hose must be made smaller to increase the pressure drop caused by the turning down of the tap.

So it is with the cardiovascular system. However, this ability to compensate has limits. Just as the tap has a limit beyond which it cannot be increased, so the heart has a limit to its output. Just as the hose has a

limit to which it can be made to have a smaller diameter, so the blood vessels have a limit beyond which further constriction will not help. This, then, is the model of perfusion that will be used to describe the normal physiology and abnormal pathology, and to discuss assessment and management of the individual with an actual or potential problem with the CVS.

Chapter 3 explains how the oxygen saturation of haemoglobin may be compromised, and how it can be optimized by appropriate nursing and medical interventions. The aim of this chapter is to help the practitioner understand the factors that determine cardiac output and its role in oxygen delivery, to consider the possible situations that may contribute to failure of the cardiovascular system, and to help meet the needs of these seriously ill individuals.

Oxygenation of blood

The cardiovascular system is essentially a closed transport circuit, comprising a double pump and a network of blood vessels. The unidirectional flow of blood is ensured by *valves*, which are positioned at the entrance and exit to each ventricular chamber. Here the normal blood flow through this system is described (Fig. 1.1).

- The right atrium receives deoxygenated blood from the inferior and superior vena cava. This blood has drained from the systemic venous circulation and from the coronary sinus.
- This blood then flows through the tricuspid valve and into the right ventricle.
- From here it is pumped up through the pulmonary valve and into the pulmonary artery, which takes the blood to the lungs for oxygenation.
- The reoxygenated blood then flows back to the heart via the four pulmonary veins that empty into the left atrium.
- The blood then passes through the mitral valve into the left ventricle. From there it is pumped out through the aortic valve into the aorta, and so into the systemic arteries where it is distributed to the peripheral circulation.

This simple description follows the passage of blood around the system. It is also important to understand the events that comprise the cardiac cycle.

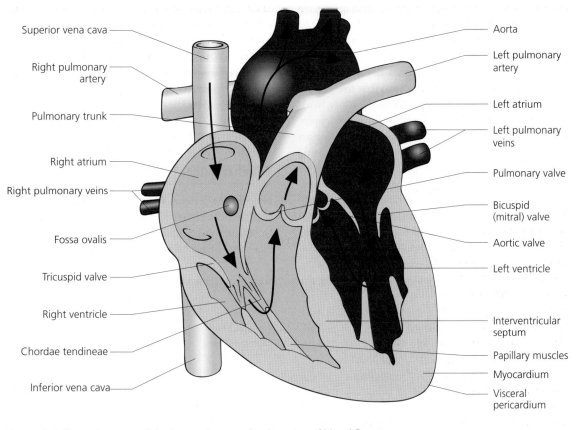

Figure 1.1 Frontal section of the heart, showing the direction of blood flow

The cardiac cycle

The following description of the stages of the cardiac cycle begins at the point immediately following ventricular contraction. Remember that the two sides of the heart operate simultaneously rather than in tandem (Fig. 1.2).

The heart has just emptied its contents into the two arteries that leave the ventricles. On the left is the aorta, taking oxygenated blood to the organs and peripheral circulation. On the right is the pulmonary artery, taking deoxygenated blood back to the lungs. The two ventricles then relax. This begins the phase of *diastole*. During this phase, blood flows into the atria and the ventricles, from the pulmonary veins on the left and the vena cava on the right; the atria now are resting and acting as passive conduits to the flow of blood. Between 60 and 70 per cent of ventricular

filling is achieved in this way, the blood flowing along its pressure gradient from the venous system into the relaxed ventricles.

Next is the phase of atrial contraction. Both atria contract and effectively 'top up' the ventricles, giving the volume that is in the ventricle at the end of the diastolic phase – the *end-diastolic volume*. This volume represents preload stress (discussed later) and plays an important part in the cardiac output. In the seriously ill patient the loss of the atrial component can reduce cardiac output, and this can be seen in atrial fibrillation or ventricular pacing.

At the end of the atrial contraction the phase of ventricular contraction or *systole* begins. Tension increases in the muscular walls of the ventricles and pressure within the ventricular chambers rises rapidly. The valves of the heart are at this point all closed. The rising pressure in the ventricles causes the atrioventricular valves to close against the relatively low pressure in the atria. The aortic and pulmonary valves are still shut at this point.

This phase is called isovolumetric contraction – that is, pressure is increasing but the volume has not yet changed. This phase consumes the most energy and therefore oxygen. It can be seen that the greater the pressure that has to be overcome the more work the heart must do. For example, a hypertensive patient with a high diastolic pressure will have an increase in myocardial oxygen demand during this phase because of the extra pressure that must be generated.

Once the pressure in the ventricles overcomes the pressure in the aorta and pulmonary artery, the valves will open and the contents of the ventricles will be ejected into the systemic and pulmonary circulation. This is the phase of ejection. About 70 per cent of the total end-diastolic volume will be ejected, leaving the remainder in the ventricle. The term that is used to describe the amount of blood ejected as a fraction of the total in the ventricle is the *ejection fraction*, and it is normally between 0.60 and 0.75. This represents about 70–80 mL of blood in the normal adult.

Once the ventricles have completed their contraction they relax to allow ventricular filling to begin again. An explanation of the electrical events will be given later.

Cardiac output

The heart is a demand-led pump: it will increase or decrease its output according to need. When demand increases, for example when running, the tissues – in this case the muscles of the legs – require more oxygen. This extra demand is met by increasing the output of the heart. In illness, such as when there is

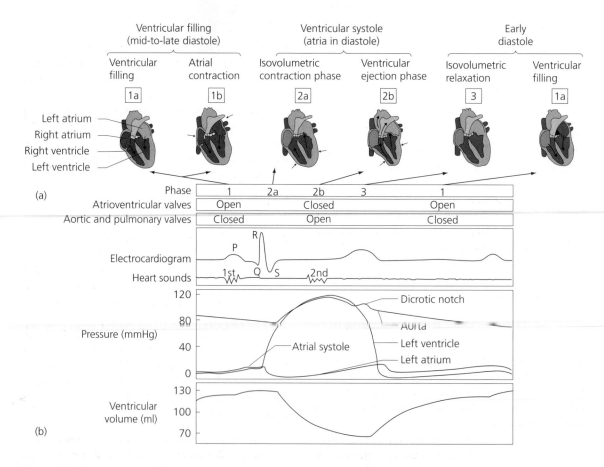

Figure 1.2 Mechanical events of the cardiac cycle

sepsis, there may be a mismatch between the demand for oxygen and the ability to meet this demand.

The output of the heart is called the *cardiac output*. This output can be defined as the volume of blood ejected by either ventricle per minute, and in a normal resting adult it is approximately 5–6 L. However, the true value for the output of the heart must be correlated with body mass, and for clinical use the body surface area is commonly used. Thus, in a normal healthy adult the mean cardiac output per minute is about 80 mL/kg, or about 3.2 L/m². When output is adjusted for body surface area, the term *cardiac index* is used. The figure of 5–6 L used above is arrived at by multiplying the heart rate by the *stroke volume*, this being the amount ejected per contraction.

For example, if at a heart rate of 70 beats per minute the stroke volume of a resting adult is approximately 80 mL, then:

$$\text{heart rate (70 bpm)} \times \text{stroke volume (80 mL)}$$
$$= \text{cardiac output} \left(5600 \frac{mL}{min}\right).$$

To understand cardiac output it is important to first understand the factors that will determine heart rate and stroke volume.

Heart rate

The rate at which the heart contracts is normally determined by the rate of impulse generation in the sinoatrial node – the 'pacemaker' of the heart. This in turn is regulated by autonomic control.

The regulatory centre for circulatory control via the autonomic nervous system is in the medulla of the brain. It is the cardiac centre in the medulla that is concerned with heart rate. This cardiac centre is divided into two discrete parts: the inhibitory part which slows down the heart rate via the vagus (parasympathetic) nerve, and the acceleratory part which speeds up the heart rate via the sympathetic nerve.

The cardiac centre responds to feedback from baroreceptors situated in the aortic and carotid arteries. Stimulation of these receptors, as occurs when the pressure in the arteries changes, leads to a change in heart rate.

The heart rate is also affected by direct chemical action. Adrenaline, produced by the adrenal medulla in response to sympathetic stimulation, will cause an increase in heart rate. An important reflex that affects the heart rate is the Bainbridge reflex. In this reflex the heart rate increases in response to increased atrial filling. This may be seen when administering a 'fluid challenge' (Hakumaki 1987).

Inappropriate heart rates may have a significant effect on the cardiac output in the seriously ill patient, as will be discussed later.

ACTIVITY ?

What are the causes for alterations in heart rate that you have seen in clinical practice?

Stroke volume

In the normal heart, stroke volume is principally determined by:

- preload;
- contractility.

A third factor, afterload, is most important in determining cardiac work and becomes particularly important as a factor in cardiac output in the failing heart.

These are key concepts to understand when caring for the acutely ill patient. Each concept will be examined separately, but it is important to recognize that they are interrelated and will affect, and be affected by, each other.

Preload

Preload is related to the volume of blood in the ventricle at the end of diastole, which is the end-diastolic volume. The volume of blood in the ventricle is important because of a key property of cardiac muscle. The strength with which cardiac muscle contracts is related to the degree of pre-contraction stretch. The more it is stretched the greater the force of contraction. Much like an elastic band, the more you stretch it the harder it springs back. In the heart this stretch is gained as a result of the volume of blood, pouring into the ventricle during diastole, stretching the ventricular wall. This is 'Starling's law of the heart', which states:

As the end diastolic volume increases, so does the strength of contraction, within physiological limits.

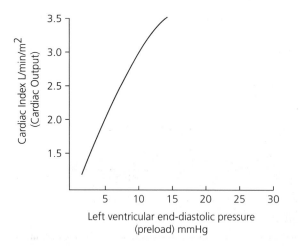

Figure 1.3 Left ventricular function curve

Therefore, the greater the venous return, the greater the subsequent contraction, as long as it remains within normal physiological parameters (Fig. 1.3). However, it is possible to overload the heart with volume when the heart is failing – this will be discussed in more detail later when reviewing the impact of cardiac failure.

If the venous return is low, as in hypovolaemia, then preload will fall, the force of contraction will be reduced, and subsequently cardiac output will drop. The main factors affecting preload are blood volume and the vasomotor tone.

In the healthy heart, increasing preload is one of the principal ways in which an increase in cardiac output is achieved. However, the failing heart responds poorly to increasing preload, with little or no increase in output (Lilly 2003).

ACTIVITY   ?

Consider the factors that might effect the preload in patients you have seen.

Contractility

The contractile (or 'inotropic') state of the myocardium is the ability of the myocardium to contract effectively. Factors that influence myocardial contractility include:

- neurohormonal effects – due to the influences of the sympathetic or parasympathetic nervous systems, either by direct innervation or through

circulating catecholamines (adrenaline, noradrenaline);
- chemical and pharmacological effects – for example, contractile changes due to alterations in blood potassium, acid–base balance or the effects of 'inotropic' drugs such as dobutamine;
- pathological effects – for example, ischaemia or infarction of the myocardium.

So, sympathetic stimulation will produce a positive effect; increased contractility will also result from injections of adrenaline or dobutamine. Conversely, myocardial ischaemia, and toxic and anaesthetic agents, will produce a negative effect.

Afterload

Whereas preload is a major determinant of myocardial contractile power, afterload is mainly a mechanical factor that determines the energy consumption of the myocardium. Afterload may be described as 'the resistance against which the ventricle must work'. In order to open the aortic valve and eject the blood into the systemic circulation, the ventricle must generate enough pressure to overcome the resistance in the circulation. Therefore, alteration of this resistance will produce important effects on cardiac function because of the resistance it imposes on ventricular emptying.

The healthy heart can overcome pressure increases well, and increases in afterload are quickly compensated by increases in preload and contractility, but result in greater energy consumption for the same output. A significant increase in afterload in the failing heart, however, can be devastating as it cannot overcome the added resistance. This resistance can be likened to any muscle trying to contract against a resistance, such as a biceps contracting to move a 1 kg dumb-bell. Consider the work/effort required to lift the dumb-bell if it increased to 2 kg. There is increased resistance to the contraction but it is easily overcome and the weight can be moved. This is like the healthy ventricles contracting against increasing afterload: more work is required but output is achieved. Now imagine contracting the biceps against the weight if the biceps has been torn or injured in some way. It may be able to move 1 kg but no longer be able to move the 2 kg weight as far. This is the situation in the heart when the ventricles are compromised: the output of the heart may fall because the ventricle cannot now overcome the resistance it faces.

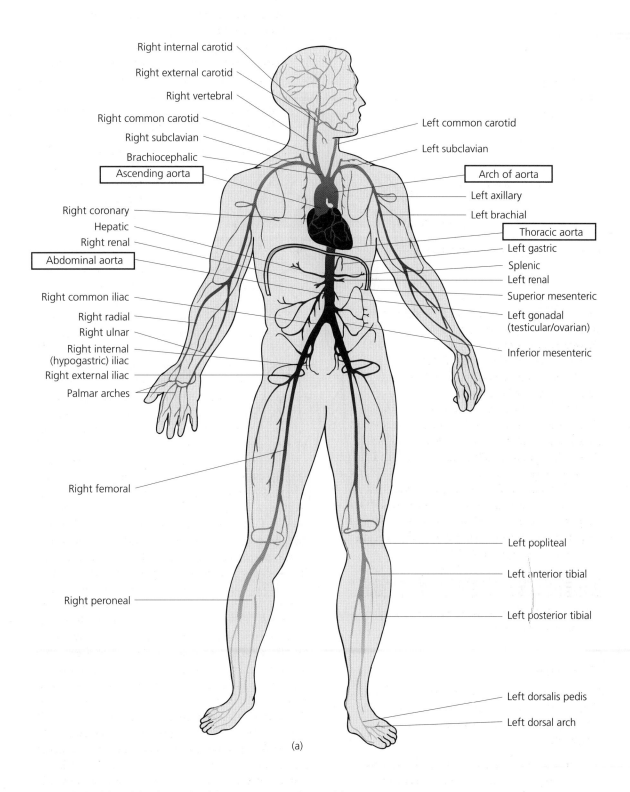

Figure 1.4a Major blood vessels of the systemic circulation: (a) arteries

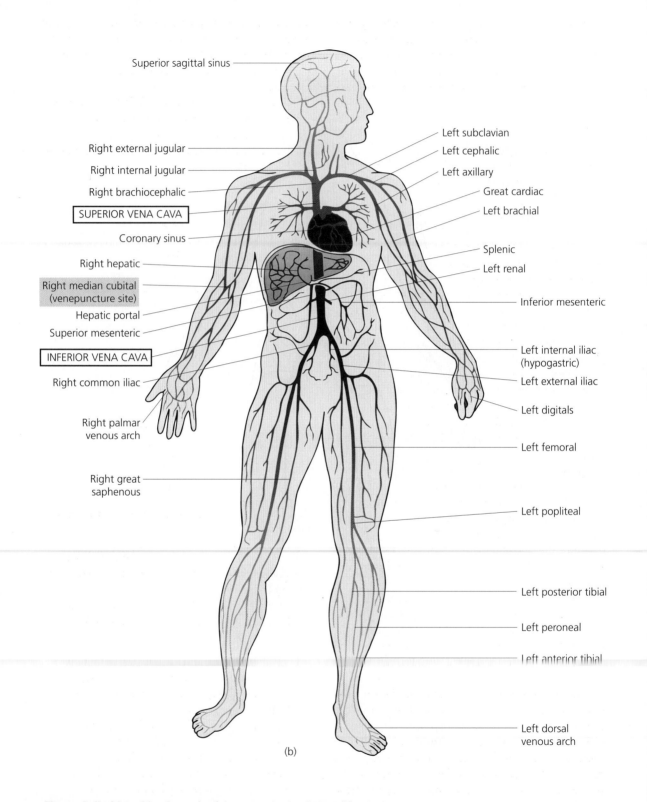

(b)

Figure 1.4b Major blood vessels of the systemic circulation: (b) veins

This resistance is determined largely by the vascular tone and is referred to as *vascular resistance* – 'systemic' on the left and 'pulmonary' on the right. While there are a number of determinants of resistance, it is the level of vasoconstriction or vasodilation that is most important clinically.

The blood vessels

The second part of the cardiovascular system to discuss is the 'pipes' (Fig. 1.4). The network of blood vessels that are the conduits by which the transport system operates are not passive tubes that simply carry the blood around the body; they are dynamic and interactive structures that are constantly responding to an ever-changing environment.

The vessels are usually described as arteries, veins and capillaries. Each of these has a different function within the circulatory system.

The large arteries that leave the heart are the pressure stores of the system. Their strong elastic walls allow them to recoil after expansion to aid the flow of blood and supplement the wave of pressure from the heart. The smaller arterioles are the pressure regulators. It is mainly these vessels that expand and contract to manipulate the total pressure within the system. In this way they are acting much like the nozzle on the end of the hosepipe in our garden hose model. The capillaries are where the exchange of oxygen, nutrients and waste products takes place. The veins are the volume store of the system; if one were to pour a litre of fluid into the cardiovascular system, 90 per cent of it would be stored in the venous side, so acting as a reserve for ventricular filling (Priebe and Skarvan 2000).

The purpose of regulation of the blood vessels is to maintain the required perfusion pressure within the system (the mean arterial pressure), and to provide local regulation for specific tissue needs – for example, to constrict vessels to an area that is haemorrhaging.

Central regulation lies predominately with the vasomotor centre in the medulla. The vasomotor centre is continually sending impulses to the arteriolar walls maintaining a degree of moderate vasoconstriction at all times. These impulses pass down the sympathetic nerves, maintaining the sympathetic tone. To vasoconstrict, sympathetic impulses are increased; to dilate they are decreased.

So, if sympathetic impulses are lost, vasodilation will occur, as for example in a spinal cord transection where the loss of sympathetic tone leads to profound vasodilatation, with the resulting drop of blood pressure.

The vasomotor centre responds to information received from the baroreceptors and chemoreceptors. The baroreceptors are situated in the carotid artery and the aorta and elicit a vasoconstrictive response to a fall in blood pressure (Fig. 1.5).

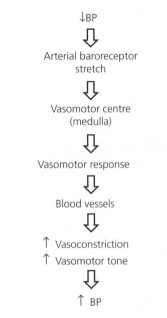

Figure 1.5 Vasoconstrictive response to a fall in blood pressure

Chemoreceptors respond to biochemical changes in the blood and are sensitive to changes in Po_2, Pco_2 and hydrogen ions.

As well as being under the influence of the medulla, the vascular pressure is also affected by direct chemical action:

- Adrenaline and noradrenaline cause dilation of cardiac and skeletal muscle arterioles and constriction of gut and skin arterioles in response to physiological stress.
- Histamine produced in the inflammatory response causes local vasodilatation.
- Antidiuretic hormone (ADH) causes vasoconstriction in response to severe bleeding.
- The renin–angiotensin pathway leads to vasoconstriction and water retention.

The blood

The third component in our model of the cardiovascular system is the volume, the blood. Blood essentially consists of two parts: cellular elements and a liquid medium, the plasma.

Cellular elements

The cellular elements are red cells (erythrocytes), white cells (leukocytes) and platelets. Red cells occupy about 40–45 per cent of the total volume of the blood and give the blood its characteristic colour through the presence of the pigment haemoglobin. In the healthy adult there are, per cubic millimetre (mm^3), some 4.5–6 million red blood cells, 5–10 thousand white cells and 150–300 thousand platelets.

Plasma

The plasma fraction of the blood normally occupies about 55 per cent of the normal volume. It carries a variety of substances, including plasma proteins, electrolytes, hormones, enzymes and blood gases. The normal concentrations of some of the most important constituents are given in Table 1.1.

Total blood volume in a normal adult is about 70 75 mL per kilogram of body weight, so a 70 kg adult may have a total blood volume of 5 L. The total amount of fluid in the human body is, however, much greater – about 40 L in our example. The physiological response to a low circulating volume is discussed later.

Table 1.1 Normal ranges of various organic and inorganic substances in plasma

	Concentration
Organic substances	
Glucose	
– fasting	3.3–5.5 mmol/L
– after a meal	≤ 10.0 mmol/L
– 2 hours after glucose	< 5.5 mmol/L
Urea	2.7–8.5 mmol/L
Uric acid (urate)	150–580 γmol/L
Creatinine	40–110 γmol/L
Bilirubin	3–21 γmol/L
Aspartate aminotransferase (AST)	5–30 iu/L
Alanine aminotransferase (ALT)	5–30 iu/L
Hydroxybutyrate dehydrogenase (HBD)	150–325 iu/L
Creatine kinase	< 130 iu/L
Amylase (AMS)	150–340 iu/L
Alkaline phosphatase (ALP)	21–100 iu/L
Acid phosphatase (ACP)	< 8.2 iu/L
Inorganic substances (ions)	
Sodium (Na^+)	135–146 mmol/L
Potassium (K^+)	3.5–5.2 mmol/L
Total calcium (Ca^{2+})	2.10–2.70 mmol/L
Chloride (Cl^-)	98–108 mmol/L
Hydrogen carbonate (HCO_3^-)	23–31 mmol/L
Phosphate (PO_4^{2-})	0.7–1.4 mmol/L

Coronary circulation

The blood supply to the myocardium is via the coronary arteries. The coronary arteries arise from the root of the aorta just above the aortic valve. Anatomically there are two coronary arteries, the left and the right. However, in clinical terms three arteries are described, the left being referred to by its two major divisions, the left anterior descending (LAD) and the circumflex (Cx) (Fig. 1.6).

As in other tissues, the balance between oxygen supply and demand in the myocardium is crucial. Myocardial oxygen demand (MVo_2) is determined by:

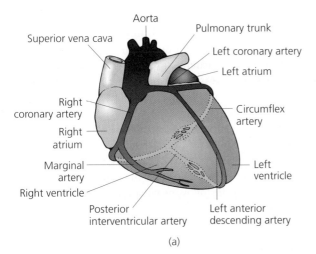

(a)

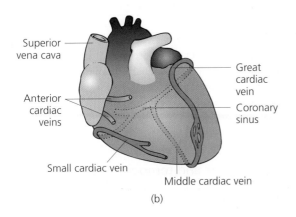

(b)

Figure 1.6 Coronary circulation: (a) arterial supply; (b) venous drainage

- myocardial contractility – the greater the strength of contraction, the greater the oxygen consumption;
- myocardial wall tension – which reflects the systolic blood pressure, the left ventricular end-diastolic volume and the left ventricular wall thickness (conditions such as hypertension and secondary hypertrophy will therefore increase oxygen demand);
- heart rate – which will increase MVo_2 as the rate increases.

Unlike skeletal muscle, the myocardium extracts 70–80 per cent of the available oxygen delivered. There is therefore little reserve and an increase in MVo_2 can be met only by an increase in coronary flow.

Coronary blood flow is dependent on diastolic blood pressure and diastolic time:

- The arterial diastolic pressure must be above 50 mmHg to maintain coronary artery perfusion.
- Coronary filling occurs primarily during diastole, so the diastolic time is important. There is an inverse relationship between diastolic time and the heart rate. As the heart rate increases, so the diastolic time (coronary filling time) reduces. This is one of the reasons why tachyarrhythmias are poorly tolerated in patients with coronary artery disease.

Assessment of the cardiovascular system

Cardiovascular assessment of the seriously ill patient begins with recognition of the system's role in adequate delivery of oxygen to tissues. Survival in severe illness often depends on the ability of the body to respond to the needs of adequate oxygen delivery (Leach and Treacher 2002). Having explored some of the factors that determine adequate cardiovascular function, this section will now consider how to apply this knowledge to patient assessment.

Heart rate and pulse

The heart rate can be an important early warning sign of circulatory failure. As stroke volume falls, the heart rate must rise to compensate. Thus, a steadily rising heart rate is often the first objective sign of falling stroke volume and can presage more obvious and serious clinical features.

Any situation that results in a fall in stroke volume will result in a rise in heart rate. A falling heart rate will usually be the result of either increased vagal tone slowing the pacemaker of the heart, or some type of conduction problem.

In addition to the pulse rate, its rhythm and volume should be checked, so it is important to palpate the pulse and not rely on averaged readings from automated equipment. An irregular pulse may be a sign of an arrhythmia such as atrial fibrillation or ectopic beats, and pauses may indicate conduction problems. If there are any concerns about the rate or rhythm of the pulse, then an ECG should be performed or a cardiac monitor attached to assess the rhythm (see page 16). A weak or thready pulse may be a sign of a poor cardiac output. A pulse volume that falls significantly with inspiration is called 'pulsus paradoxus' and may be a sign of pericardial effusion.

Blood pressure

The systemic arterial blood pressure is a reflection of the relationship between the ventricular function and the degree of vasomotor tone. Thus it is not a true reflection of cardiac output alone, but it is a widely used and reliable indicator of cardiovascular function.

Normal (or, more accurately, recommended) blood pressure is no more than 140/90 mmHg, with the optimum being 120/80 mmHg (Williams *et al.* 2004). With the seriously ill or deteriorating patient it is usually a low blood pressure that is of concern, but giving a figure below which blood pressure becomes 'abnormal' is difficult. As with many aspects of monitoring and assessment, it may be the *trend* that is as important as absolute values, and each must be assessed in the light of the patient's clinical status and history.

It is probably reasonable to suggest that a systolic blood pressure that is either less than 90 mmHg or has dropped 20 mmHg suddenly since the last reading is indicative of cardiovascular failure and suggests a situation in which tissue perfusion – and therefore oxygen delivery – may be compromised.

The diastolic pressure is also important, although it is harder to record by non-invasive means when it is low. Recall from the discussion on coronary blood flow that the coronary arteries will not properly perfuse if the diastolic pressure is less than 50 mmHg.

The *pulse pressure* is a useful tool in detecting falling cardiac output. Pulse pressure is the difference between the systolic pressure and the diastolic pressure. For example, if the systemic blood pressure is 120/70 then the pulse pressure will be 120 minus 70, that is 50 mmHg. When the cardiac output begins to fall, a steady fall in pulse pressure will be seen. This is because the vasoconstriction that occurs in an attempt to maintain perfusion pressure in the system (recall the garden hose analogy) keeps the diastolic pressure up while the systolic pressure, which is more an expression of cardiac ejection, is falling.

Consider this example of readings taken: 10pm, 120/70; 11pm, 110/70; 12pm, 100/65; 1am, 95/65; 2am, 90/65 mmHg. The pulse pressure has fallen thus: 50, 40, 35, 30 and 25 mmHg. This is a classic sign of falling cardiac output, whatever the cause. It is therefore important to recognize this trend early, rather than wait until the pressure reaches the point at which you may feel the systolic pressure is getting too low.

The *mean arterial pressure* (MAP) is often used in critical care and is the arterial pressure averaged during one cardiac cycle. The MAP gives a reasonable idea of perfusion pressure in the system and can be estimated by the following equation:

$$MAP = DP + \frac{SP - DP}{3}$$

where SP and DP stand for systolic and diastolic pressures. A MAP of 65 mmHg or less is indicative of severe circulatory failure.

It must be noted that, in situations of circulatory failure where there is significant peripheral vasoconstriction, indirect (non-invasive) blood pressure monitoring may be less reliable than direct (invasive) measurement via an arterial line (Stover *et al.* 2009), although non-invasive technology continues to evolve (Box 1.1).

Skin colour and temperature

The patient's skin can give a good indication of the state of cardiovascular function and therefore perfusion. When perfusion falls, the response is to begin to vasoconstrict to maintain the pressure in the system. This will be manifested in the patient by cool

Box 1.1 Manual versus automated blood pressure recording

There has been a call to re-examine the routine use of automated blood pressure devices and to consider a return to manual recording, particularly in vulnerable patients (Santry 2010). There are two aspects to this debate.

- There is some evidence of differences in the systolic pressure recorded by manual technique compared to automated devices. with some suggestion that manual has greater accuracy (Bern *et al.* 2007).
- Some have suggested that promoting manual recording also encourages the nurse to record the heart rate and rhythm with greater accuracy, and makes it more likely that the nurse will make physical contact with the patient, thereby increasing the detection of signs of low perfusion (Jeavon 2009).

and clammy skin owing to the increase in sympathetic stimulation causing peripheral vasoconstriction.

One important exception to this picture is the early stages of septic shock (see Chapter 5). Capillary refilling provides an estimation of the rate of peripheral blood flow to the skin. When the fingernail is depressed for a few seconds the nail bed blanches white, and on release it should regain its colour almost instantly. When perfusion is poor the colour returns much more slowly, giving an indication of the rate of perfusion. A capillary refilling time of more than two seconds may indicate poor perfusion.

Urine output

Twenty per cent of cardiac output perfuses the kidneys, which are very sensitive to a fall in perfusion pressure. The urine output should be monitored hourly in situations of circulatory failure because it gives a good indication of the extent of the failure of perfusion. A minimum of 0.5 mL/kg per hour of urine should be produced, so in a 70 kg person that would be 35 mL. Again, it is the *trend* that is as important as the absolute value of 35 mL, and a falling urine output should be addressed early rather than waiting for the output to reach any particular figure. The quality of

the urine as well as its quantity is also an important factor that will be affected, the longer the circulatory failure is left untreated (see Chapter 3).

Central venous pressure

Central venous pressure (CVP) is an expression of the pressure that is in the central venous system as it returns to the right side of the heart. The volume of fluid that is available to return, and the ability of the heart to deal with the fluid (to pump it forward), determine this pressure. It may also be referred to as the right atrial pressure or right ventricular end-diastolic pressure. The importance of the relationship between this pressure and cardiac output has already been discussed. Central venous pressure is measured using a central venous catheter attached to either a fluid manometer or a pressure transducer.

ACTIVITY   ?

Make lists of situations that may result in a high CVP and a low CVP.

Insertion of a CVP catheter

A central vein, usually the internal jugular or subclavian, is cannulated using a radio-opaque catheter to give access to the vena cava as it enters the right atrium. The catheter is sited with the patient in the head-down (Trendelenburg) position if possible, to minimize the risk of air embolus during insertion by ensuring a positive venous pressure. The catheter position should be checked by chest X-ray following insertion, as it is not uncommon for such catheters to double back on themselves, pass into the veins of the neck, or enter the right ventricle. As the dome of the pleura is close to the vessels being cannulated, the complication of a pneumothorax or haemothorax must also be looked for. Other complications associated with the insertion of these lines include:

- cardiac tamponade caused when the tip of the catheter pierces the wall of the right atrium and enters the pericardial sac;
- infection, either local around the site of entry or systemic, due to organisms introduced through the catheter;

- venous thrombosis;
- blockage due to kinking of the catheter or obstruction by a blood clot.

Measurement of CVP

Where possible, the CVP should be measured in the mid-axillary line on a level with the 4th intercostal space (the phlebostatic axis), as this is on a level with the right atrium. In this position, when measured with a fluid manometer, the normal range of CVP is 3–10 cmH$_2$O, or 0–5 cmH$_2$O when measured from the sternal angle.

To read the CVP using a simple fluid manometer, the following procedure is followed (Fig. 1.7).

1. Place the patient in a supine position or, if this is not possible, at a 45-degree angle. All future readings should be made in the same position so that the trend can be monitored.
2. Check that the fluid is running freely.
3. Turn the three-way tap to allow the fluid to run into the manometer and so that it is closed to the patient.
4. Fill the manometer to a level above the expected pressure.
5. Close the three-way tap to the infusion source so that the manometer is open to the patient.
6. Watch the fluid level in the manometer. It will fall until the pressure from the column of fluid is equal to the pressure at the tip of the catheter.

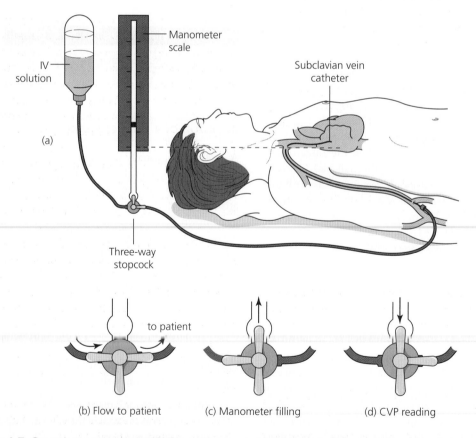

Figure 1.7 Central venous pressure (CVP) measurement. (a) Placement of the manometer in relation to the patient. The zero level of the manometer is at the phlebostatic axis. (b) The stopcock is turned for intravenous flow to the patient. (c) The stopcock is turned so that the manometer fills with fluid. (d) The stopcock is turned so that fluid in the manometer flows to the patient. A CVP reading is obtained when the fluid level stabilizes.

You should also see the fluid column rise and fall slightly when it has settled: this is due to changes in the intrathoracic pressure due to respiration.

7. When the fluid stops falling, read the figure on the manometer. This is the central venous pressure.

Increasingly CVP is being measured via an electronic pressure transducer and displayed as a figure on the monitoring system. This equipment may, however, be confined to intensive care units, high-dependency care units, coronary care units and operating departments. When CVP is measured in this way the units are millimetres of mercury (mmHg) and the normal range is 3–8.

Clinical value of the CVP measuement

When the CVP deviates from the normal range this may be due to a number of clinical scenarios. The two main factors that determine CVP are the volume of fluid and the cardiac function. Therefore changes to the CVP are likely to be caused by situations that affect one of these two factors.

High CVP

The possible causes of a high or rising CVP are mainly related to either an excess volume of fluid or an inability of the right side of the heart to pump the available fluid forward, and may include:

- over-transfusion;
- right heart failure (in acute right-sided failure it is important to recognize that the high CVP does not indicate a high volume of fluid);
- cardiac tamponade;
- pulmonary embolism.

Low CVP

The possible causes of a low or falling CVP are those that relate to a lack of fluid volume. Any significant cause of actual or relative hypovolaemia may lead to a fall in CVP, for example:

- haemorrhage;
- diuresis;
- a fluid shift out of the circulation such as in sepsis or following cardiopulmonary bypass.

When there is a loss of volume, the compensatory vasoconstriction that is trying to maintain perfusion pressure keeps the CVP from falling significantly until quite late. So, for example, in a patient who is haemorrhaging a low CVP indicates a considerable blood loss.

The pulmonary artery catheter

A key study showed little evidence of improved patient outcomes resulting from pulmonary artery (PA) catheter insertion (Connors et al. 1996). As a result, the PA catheter as a tool is used less frequently now, but it is likely to be seen occasionally in the intensive care setting and perhaps a little more frequently in cardiac settings.

The PA catheter gives more direct information about the left side of the heart than can the CVP, specifically left ventricular filling pressures. These pressures are measured by attaching a transducer to the catheter, which allows the pressure wave to be seen and the pressure to be displayed as a digital readout.

The PA catheter is a flexible, radio-opaque tube with a small inflatable balloon at its tip that is introduced via a large vein, usually the internal jugular vein. The catheter is advanced through the right atrium, the right ventricle and then floated up into the pulmonary artery by inflating the balloon. As the tip advances the changing pressure wave can be observed on the monitor. The tip of the catheter then has an unobstructed 'view' across the pulmonary capillary system to the left side of the heart, specifically the left atrium, and can give a figure called the *pulmonary capillary wedge pressure* (PCWP). This is essentially the left atrial pressure and is approximately the same as left ventricular end-diastolic pressure.

While not strictly true as the PA catheter measures pressure and not volume, it is reasonable to interpret this as the left ventricular preload. Where the pressures are low, this is mainly associated with volume depletion or vasodilatation. Both of these will result in a reduced volume of blood returning to the left side of the heart. So, a low PA pressure in a patient who has been bleeding postoperatively will indicate that more volume is required to allow the ventricle to fill adequately.

Situations that will raise the PA pressure are mainly those that cause left ventricular failure and therefore suggest an inability of the left side of the heart to deal with the volume that is returning to it. The PA will also be raised in mitral stenosis and cardiac tamponade.

In the critical care environment, the PA catheter will also allow a wide range of haemodynamic data to be collected, including the cardiac output and the systemic vascular resistance. It remains an important tool despite concerns over its value.

Mental state

If the patient has a low cardiac output then cerebral perfusion may be at risk. This will manifest itself as restlessness, confusion, agitation and sometimes aggression. If cerebral perfusion falls enough, stupor and coma will eventually result. It must also be recognized that a patient with compromised cardiac output may be exhibiting signs of anxiety and agitation that are not the result of low cardiac output, but are a result of the very real fear that may be present in a person who has in fact got a life-threatening condition. Objective assessment is difficult, but tools such as those used to measure cognitive impairment could be adopted. In reality it should be recognized that such changes are a late and worrying sign if related to poor perfusion.

Assessing the cardiac rhythm

The heart rate is a key factor in maintenance of adequate cardiac output. Therefore, a disturbance of cardiac rhythm has the potential to cause significant impact on the seriously ill patient and requires careful monitoring and assessment (Fig. 1.8).

Sinus rhythm

A normal heart rhythm is called sinus rhythm because it is generated by the natural pacemaker of the heart, the sinoatrial (SA) node. The impulse that is generated by the SA node spreads across the atria, causing the atrial cells to depolarize. This wave of depolarization is detected by the electrocardiograph (ECG) and shown as the P-wave. The impulse then passes through the atrioventricular node into the ventricles. There is a slight delay here to allow for the atria to contract and start to relax before the ventricular activation begins. This period is called the P–R interval. The impulse then passes down the bundle branches and activates the ventricular muscle; this ventricular part is the QRS complex. The S–T segment

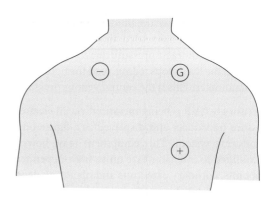

Figure 1.8 Monitor lead placement for three-lead monitoring (lead II)

immediately follows the QRS complex and should be isoelectric – that is, approximately level with the base line of the ECG. The S–T segment should curve gently into the proximal limb of the T-wave without forming sharp angles. The T-wave represents ventricular repolarization, a return to the resting state (Fig. 1.9).

The ECG criteria for normal sinus rhythm (Fig. 1.10) are as follows:

- rate – 60–100 beats/minute (determined by the QRS complex);
- rhythm – regular (does not vary by more than 0.12 seconds);
- P-waves – normally 0.11 s duration, height 2.5 mm;
- P–R interval – between 0.12 s and 0.20 s;
- QRS complex – between 0.08 s and 0.11 s (bundle branch block will increase the duration of the QRS without affecting the rhythm).

Identifying cardiac arrhythmias

Learning to interpret ECG rhythms is not easy. The vast range of possible abnormalities, combined with the considerable variation in the *normal* ECG, make ECG patterns difficult to learn. However, it is important to be able to respond quickly in emergency situations when a potentially life-threatening arrhythmia arises.

It is possible to analyse the ECG rhythm without a detailed knowledge of electrocardiography. If a logical process is used then it will be possible to describe accurately the arrhythmia that you see on the monitor or rhythm strip. An adaptation of an approach

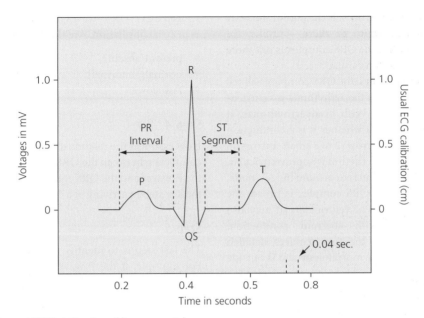

Figure 1.9 Normal ECG deflections (diagrammatic)

suggested originally by Henry Marriott (Wagner 1994) is described here as it gives a logical way of analysing the rhythm using the information available. If these steps are understood and applied consistently then most, if not all, rhythm disturbances should be correctly identified.

Step 1

The first step is to identify the type of disturbance that you see. What disturbance would draw your attention to the rhythm? These are some examples:

- There are early or extra beats.
- It is too fast (tachycardia).
- It is too slow (bradycardia).
- It is irregular.
- There are gaps or pauses.

Understanding the potential causes for each of the above allows you to identify the arrhythmia precisely once the features have been analysed. This first step starts you thinking about what type of problem you are facing.

Step 2

Next examine the QRS complex. The QRS complex gives the most information and represents the most important part of the cardiac cycle, namely,

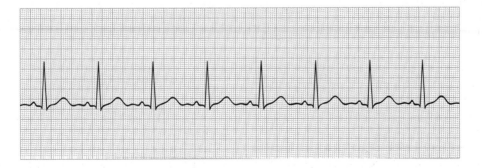

Figure 1.10 Sinus rhythm

ventricular contraction. Also, it is the part of the ECG that you can guarantee to be there – unlike, for example, the P-wave. If the QRS complex is not there then the patient may be in cardiac arrest!

With tachyarrhythmias, the QRS complex will tell you whether the origin of the arrhythmia is ventricular or supraventricular. With bradyarrhythmias, it will help you to work out whether it is a conduction problem or not. If it is narrow (2 to 3 small squares on the ECG paper), then the rhythm is supraventricular, namely, arising from the atria or around the AV node, not the ventricle. If the QRS complex is broad, the problem is most likely to be ventricular. (It may also be supraventricular with aberrant conduction. Distinguishing between the two requires detailed knowledge of the possible morphology and is outside the scope of this book. If in doubt, it is ventricular.)

Step 3

Next examine the P-wave. Finding the P-wave may be difficult, particularly in the tachycardias, and may require you to examine several leads if you have a 12-lead ECG. The P-waves may be completely absent, as in atrial fibrillation. Are the P-waves.

- present/absent?
- normal/abnormal?
- fast/slow?

Step 4

Now establish the relationships between the different complexes: between the QRS complexes, and between the P-waves and the QRS complexes. This may well be the key step in arriving at a diagnosis.

Step 5

The last step is to identify the primary disturbance. For example, if the P-waves stop then the primary disturbance is with the SA node. In other words, what is the root cause of the problem?

The above steps will now be applied to some of the common arrhythmias that may be encountered in the seriously ill patient.

Supraventricular arrhythmias

Atrial ectopic (premature atrial contraction).

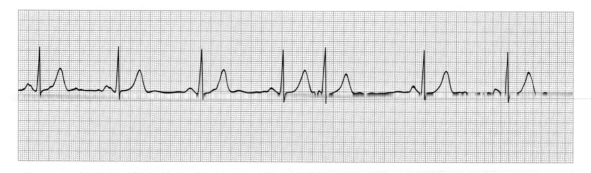

Figure 1.11 Atrial ectopic

Analysis. (1) The rhythm looks irregular because there is an extra beat. (2) The QRS of the extra beat (fifth complex) is narrow, therefore supraventricular. (3) The P-wave for the extra beat looks different from the normal beats. (4) The extra beat is early. (5) Therefore it is an atrial ectopic.

Atrial fibrillation

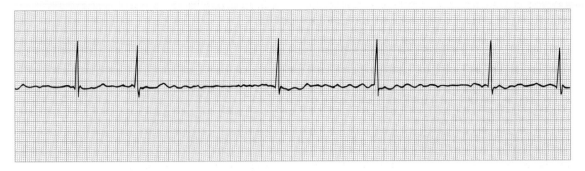

Figure 1.12 Atrial fibrillation

Analysis. (1) The rhythm is irregular. (2) The QRS is narrow, therefore supraventricular. (3) No P-waves, but a 'chaotic' base line. (4) The rhythm is 'irregularly irregular'. (5) No P-waves and irregular QRS make this atrial fibrillation (AF).

Atrial flutter

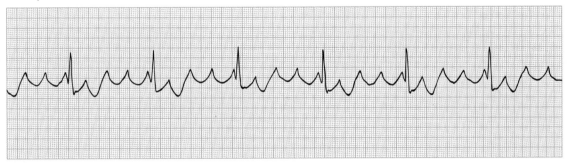

Figure 1.13 Atrial flutter

Analysis. (1) Normal QRS rate but rapid P-wave rate. (2) The QRS is narrow, therefore supraventricular. (3) Very rapid abnormal P-waves at a rate of 300/min; the atria are 'fluttering'. (4) There appears to be one QRS for every four flutter waves. (5) Therefore this is 4:1 atrial flutter.

Supraventricular tachycardia

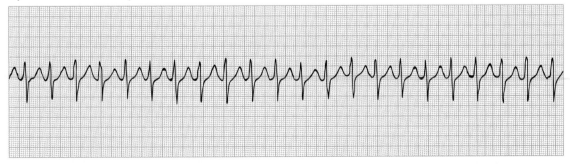

Figure 1.14 Supraventricular tachycardia

Analysis. (1) The rate is fast at 200/min. (2) The QRS is narrow, therefore supraventricular. (3) P-waves cannot be seen. (4) The QRS rhythm is regular. (5) A regular narrow complex tachycardia, therefore supraventricular tachycardia (SVT).

Ventricular arrhythmias

Ventricular ectopic (premature ventricular contraction)

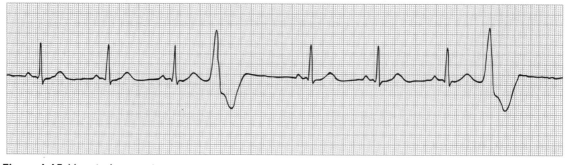

Figure 1.15 Ventricular ectopic

Analysis. (1) There are extra beats: 4 and 8. (2) The extra beats (QRS) are wide, therefore ventricular. (3) The extra beats have no P-wave. (4) The extra beats are early: premature. (5) Wide early beats, therefore ventricular ectopics.

Ventricular tachycardia

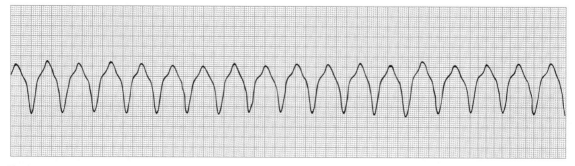

Figure 1.16 Ventricular tachycardia

Analysis. (1) There is a tachycardia: 160–170 beats/min. (2) The QRS are wide, therefore ventricular. (3) There are no P-waves. (4) The rhythm is regular. (5) A regular, broad, complex tachycardia, therefore ventricular tachycardia (VT).

Ventricular fibrillation

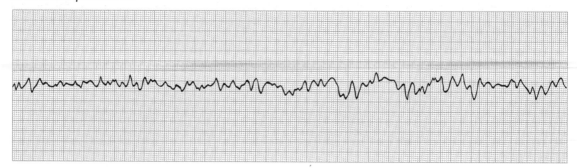

Figure 1.17 Ventricular fibrillation

Analysis. There is chaos: no real complexes. Check pulse and start cardiopulmonary resuscitation!

Disorders of conduction

First-degree AV block (delay in the AV node)

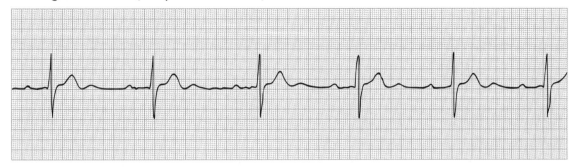

Figure 1.18 First-degree AV block

Analysis. (1) The rate is a little slow (50/min) and there is a pause between the P-wave and QRS. (2) The QRS complexes are narrow, therefore supraventricular (normal). (3) P-waves are regular and 1:1 with the QRS. (4) Relationship between the P-waves and the QRS complexes is wrong (the P–R interval). It should be no more than 0.2 s, which is 5 small squares; it is 7–8 small squares, or 0.32 s. (5) There is a prolonged P–R interval, therefore first-degree AV block.

Second-degree AV block: Mobitz type 2

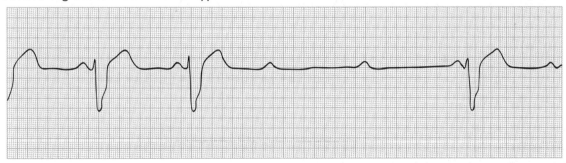

Figure 1.19 Second-degree AV block (Mobitz type 2)

Analysis. (1) There is a pause or gap. (2) The QRS complexes are irregular as some seem to be missing. (3) The P-waves are regular. (4) There are more P-waves than QRS complexes, but the P–R interval is constant. (5) There are two P-waves that are not conducted through to the ventricles (the two 'dropped beats'), therefore there is second-degree AV block.

Second-degree AV block: Mobitz type I

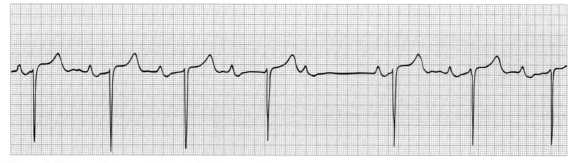

Figure 1.20 Second-degree AV block (Mobitz type I)

Analysis. (1) There appears to be a pause or gap. (2) The QRS complexes are irregular but narrow. (3) There are more P-waves than QRS, so there must be some kind of block. (4) Relationship between the P-waves and the QRS complexes is not constant. The P–R interval keeps changing. It gets wider and wider until a P-wave is not followed by a QRS. The P–R interval then goes back to normal and the pattern starts again. (5) Some conducted P-waves and some not conducted indicates second-degree AV block.

Third-degree AV block: complete heart block

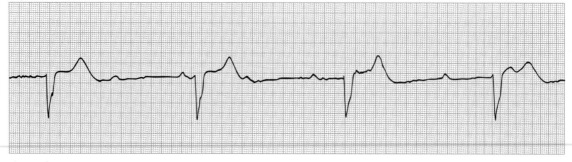

Figure 1.21 Third-degree AV block

Analysis. (1) The rate is slow at 40 beats/min. (2) The QRS complexes are regular but wide, therefore ventricular. (3) There are more P-waves than QRS complexes. The P-wave rate seems to be about 80/min. (4) There is no relationship between the P-waves and the QRS complexes. They are separate: the QRS rate is about 38/min. (5) Because there are more P-waves than QRS complexes there is some kind of block. The wide (slow) QRS complexes mean they are a ventricular 'escape' rhythm. The P and QRS are not related, so this must be third-degree (i.e. complete) AV block.

Managing cardiac arrhythmias

ACTIVITY   ?

Why is an abnormal heart rhythm bad for the cardiovascular system?

The two situations that are most concerning are when the cardiac rhythm is too slow and when it is too fast – bradycardia and tachycardia, respectively.

Bradycardia

When the rhythm is bradycardic, then one side of the equation *heart rate × stroke volume = cardiac output* is compromised. For example, if the heart rate is 35/min, then the stroke volume would have to compensate by increasing to about 140 mL to maintain a cardiac output of approximately 5 L. This level of compensation is unlikely, particularly in the seriously ill patient. The more likely scenario is that, if the heart rate drops substantially, then so will the cardiac output. If the heart rate falls to a level that is thought incapable of maintaining an adequate cardiac output, then attempts must be made to increase the rate. The approach to management of symptomatic bradycardia will be based on the underlying cause and the severity of the symptoms.

The most common rhythm associated with a symptomatic bradycardia is sinus bradycardia. This may be due to an increase in parasympathetic stimulation, such as in vomiting or while performing endotracheal suction. An important cause of sinus bradycardia is the effect of drugs that the patient may be taking, particularly beta-blockers or other antiarrhythmic drugs. Sinus bradycardia can also result from suppression of the SA node during myocardial ischaemia or infarction, and in the sick sinus syndrome.

A more severe and prognostically more sinister cause of symptomatic bradycardia is when there is a problem with conduction of the electrical activity of the heart between the atrium and the ventricle, usually referred to as 'heart block'. There are many forms and many causes. 'Heart block' can be used to describe slowing or blocking of the conduction in and around the SA node, the atrioventricular (AV) node, and the bundle branches. It is often AV block that is meant when clinicians refer to 'heart block', and this may be

the result of myocardial infarction or ischaemia, drug overdose (particularly beta blockers and digoxin), or as a complication following accidental or surgical trauma of the heart.

The basic problem in 'heart block' is that the conduction from the atrium to the ventricle through the AV node is either slowed or blocked altogether. Three stages or 'degrees' of AV block are described:

- first degree – where there is simply a delay in AV conduction (see Fig 1.18);
- second degree – where some impulses are conducted through the AV node and some are not (see Figs 1.19 and 1.20);
- third degree – where all the atrial impulses are blocked at the AV node and the slow ventricular escape rhythm takes over the ventricle (see Fig 1.21).

It will usually be second- or third-degree AV block that results in a bradycardia.

Management of bradycardia

Management will depend on the cause and the symptoms. Reversible causes must be addressed, such as sudden increases in vagal tone. In bradycardias that are symptomatic, atropine is the first-line therapy (up to 0.5 mg given intravenously). If the bradycardia is a result of AV block, it is quite probable that atropine will be ineffective. Second-line drug therapy is adrenaline 2–10 γg/min, or isoprenaline (Resuscitation Council UK 2005).

If the bradycardia is not a short-term acute problem, or if it is unresponsive to drugs, then artificial cardiac pacing will be indicated. Cardiac pacing most commonly involves inserting a pacing electrode in the form of an invasive catheter into the right ventricle via one of the large veins (usually the subclavian or internal jugular) and artificially stimulating the heart to initiate a contraction via a pulse generator.

Tachycardia

ACTIVITY   ?

If a heart rate of 70 beats per minute is good, then why is a heart rate of 170/min not better?

As explained earlier, the heart is dependent on an adequate preload to maintain stroke volume. The preload volume enters the left ventricle during diastole, and the diastolic period is inversely proportional to the heart rate. As the rate goes up the diastolic time decreases, so filling time and preload decreases. There is also an effect on myocardial oxygen supply and demand. As the coronary arteries fill during diastole, supply will fall; and as the number of contractions per minute increases, demand will go up. So, arrhythmias that are tachycardic result in:

- reduced filling time;
- reduced coronary blood flow;
- increased myocardial oxygen demands.

Management of tachycardia

As with bradycardia, the management of tachycardia will depend on the stability of the patient. Typically three scenarios could arise:

- the patient has a tachyarrhythmia but is stable with no adverse signs; or
- the patient has a tachyarrhythmia and is unstable with clinical features of low cardiac output – for example, low blood pressure or altered consciousness; or
- the patient has a tachycardia and no cardiac output.

The second situation is a medical emergency that requires immediate intervention with high-flow oxygen, intravenous access and specific antiarrhythmic treatment. The third situation is a cardiac arrest and therefore will require basic and advanced life support.

There are three options for treating a tachyarrhythmia: vagal manoeuvres, drugs, or cardioversion. In the stable patient a vagal manoeuvre such as carotid sinus massage may be tried, but this should be carried out only by appropriately trained staff as there is a risk of asystole and of cerebral embolism.

If the patient is stable, intravenous drugs will be used. There are many antiarrhythmic drugs available but a detailed discussion of them is outside the scope of this book. However, the choice of antiarrhythmic drug is important and depends on the correct diagnosis of the arrhythmia. The most important issue in choosing the right treatment is whether the tachyarrhythmia has a broad or a narrow QRS complex – these will be referred to as 'broad-complex tachycardia' (BCT) and narrow-complex tachycardia (NCT). As discussed earlier, this is based on the

assumption that BCTs are ventricular (see Fig. 1.16) and NCTs are supraventricular (see Fig. 1.14).

- For regular NCTs the current recommended treatment (Resuscitation Council UK 2005) is adenosine as a 6 mg rapid intravenous bolus followed by 12 mg if there is no response in 2 minutes. If there is still no response then expert opinion is sought and beta-blockers may be used.
- An irregular NCT is probably atrial fibrillation, which may be treated with a beta-blocker or amiodarone.
- For BCTs the initial treatment is with amiodarone 300 mg given intravenously over 20–60 minutes.

If the patient is haemodynamically unstable, then direct current (DC) cardioversion is the most appropriate option (Box 1.2). This is also the safest choice if there is any doubt about the correct diagnosis of the arrhythmia. In cardioversion, a DC shock is delivered to the patient's heart, the intention being to depolarize the myocardium, cancelling out the ectopic activity that is causing the arrhythmia. The first tissue to recover and to depolarize will recapture the rhythm, and this is usually the sinoatrial node, the heart's natural pacemaker.

Acute coronary syndrome

'Acute coronary syndrome' (ACS) is an umbrella term for a range of presentations of symptomatic coronary heart disease (CHD) that have in common unstable atherosclerotic plaque and myocardial ischaemia or infarction.

In the UK, despite a reduction in the past two decades, coronary heart disease remains the single most common cause of death in men and the second most common in women, aged under 65 years. There are estimated to be about 851 000 people in the UK between the ages of 35 and 75 who have had a heart attack. Chest pain accounts for about 700 000 A&E attendances per year and about a quarter of all acute medical admissions (British Heart Foundation 2010).

Pathophysiology

The processes leading to acute coronary syndrome are coronary atherosclerosis and plaque rupture.

Box 1.2 Procedure for DC cardioversion

- Following explanation to the patient, consent is obtained and a short-acting anaesthetic agent may be given. Sometimes intravenous diazepam may be used, particularly in a situation that is becoming rapidly unstable and requires immediate intervention.
- The patient should be adequately oxygenated before and during the procedure.
- The cardioverter–defibrillator is switched on and the monitoring leads attached, ensuring that a tall R wave is present on the screen. Some models will monitor through the defibrillator paddles; if so, make sure that the contact is good.
- Make sure that the defibrillator is set to 'synchronize'. This will ensure that the charge is delivered on the R wave of the ECG, so avoiding the vulnerable T wave.
- Ensure conducting pads are in place.
- Select the energy level. This will be determined by the rhythm and by the type of equipment being used.
- Place paddles firmly on the chest using 25 lb pressure. One paddle should be to the right of the sternum below the clavicle. The other is placed to the left of the nipple in the anterior axillary line.
- Press the charge button on the paddles. Check rhythm and ensure that everyone is clear of contact with the bed, equipment and patient.
- Press the 'shock' button and wait until the charge has been delivered. Note that with synchronized shocks there may be a short delay before the defibrillator delivers the shock as it waits for the next R wave.
- Assess the patient, including rhythm and cardiac output.

After several years of advancing disease resulting in a complicated atheromatous lesion in one or more coronary vessels, the atheromatous plaque ruptures. This leads to thrombosis in the coronary artery and to a spectrum of presentations that represent a continuum of increasing severity of myocardial damage, with irreversible injury beginning somewhere along this continuum (Wu 1998). Once the plaque has ruptured and clot has begun to form, the myocardium is at risk. The extent of the subsequent damage depends on a number of factors, but particularly the size and composition of the clot and whether it partially or completely occludes the vessel. The syndrome presents clinically as unstable angina and myocardial infarction (MI) – which is subdivided into a type with ST elevation on the ECG (STEMI) and a type without (NSTEMI).

No matter where the patient is on the spectrum of ACS, he or she is in a potentially life-threatening situation. Almost half of those experiencing an MI die within the first few hours of the event. Rapid access to medical help is essential, as is swift assessment and diagnosis so that appropriate interventions can take place.

Most episodes of ACS occur outside hospital, but it is important to recognize that MI is not an infrequent event in hospital and can occur in a number of situations. For example, perioperative MI is an important complication of surgery, particularly in elderly patients (Preibe 2005). It is therefore important for all staff working in acute areas to be able to recognize the signs and symptoms of ACS and to have some understanding of its management.

Presenting features, ECG and biochemical markers

The typical presentation of ACS is of sudden onset of severe, central chest pain. The pain is described as crushing or heavy, and has the classic feature of radiation to the left arm (or both), the lower jaw, neck and left shoulder. The pain will usually be continuous, last for longer than 15 minutes, and be unrelieved by rest or antianginal medication. The pain may be accompanied by extreme sweating, cold and pale skin, tachycardia, and fear.

While this typical presentation is well known and often cited as the symptoms of 'a heart attack', it must be recognized that many patients with ACS do not present in such an obvious and dramatic way, and some may not describe their initial symptoms as pain.

In a hospitalized patient, MI may be masked by other problems or interventions and so may be interpreted as non-specific deterioration, particularly in the elderly.

If ACS is suspected, a 12-lead ECG is performed and will be either normal or abnormal.

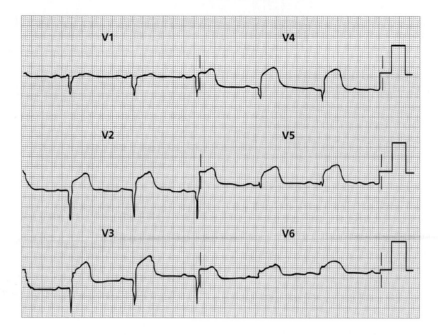

Figure 1.22 ST Elevation Myocardial Infarction

- If the ECG appears normal but there remains a high degree of suspicion for ACS, then the patient will continue to be monitored and further investigations performed in the form of blood tests for biochemical markers of myocardial damage.
- If the ECG is abnormal the patient may fall into one of two categories. One will confirm a diagnosis of STEMI, and one may suggest a diagnosis of NSTEMI. For STEMI, the presence of ST elevation of more than 1 mm in two adjacent leads (Fig. 1.22) or new left bundle branch block is required. For NSTEMI, the ECG is likely to show ST depression and/or T-wave inversion (Fig. 1.23).

This classification is important because it will determine the type of management – in particular whether the patient is referred for urgent reperfusion (Fig. 1.24).

The ECG diagnosis is assisted by biochemical markers of myocardial cell damage. Troponin I and T are cardiac-specific markers that detect even low levels of myocardial injury. Those with unstable angina, or MI without ST elevation with raised troponin, have a greater risk of serious cardiac events, and this information will trigger earlier aggressive management.

Troponin detection becomes reliable 3–4 hours after the event, so it should be taken both on presentation and 6–12 hours later. Any rise in troponin is important, but precise figures for 'normal' and 'abnormal' results vary between centres and continue to evolve as practice and research develops. As an example, a diagnosis of myocardial infarction may be made if the troponin concentration is above 0.03 ng/mL (Goodacre *et al.* 2009).

Management of ACS

The management of ACS is time critical. Many of the 140 000 people who die from a heart attack each year do so within the first hour of the onset of symptoms, and by 3 hours after the occlusion of the coronary artery most of the myocardium served by the affected artery will have died. The following discussion is based on current European guidelines (Bassand *et al.* 2007; Van de Werf *et al.* 2008).

Pain relief should be given immediately. Diamorphine is the drug of choice because, as well as being a potent analgesic, it has positive haemodynamic effects, particularly vasodilatation, which reduces myocardial oxygen demand. This should be given intravenously in sufficient amounts to achieve

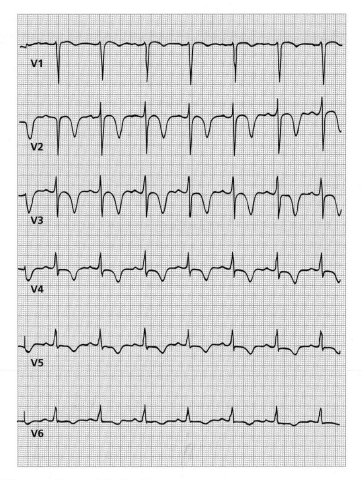

Figure 1.23 Non-ST Elevation Myocardial Infarction

pain relief; the dose will typically be between 2.5 and 10 mg but will depend on individual assessment.

The patient will be administered oxygen if there is any suspicion of hypoxia (SIGN 2007a), although there is no evidence for the routine administration of oxygen in ACS (Cabello *et al.* 2010); and 300 mg of aspirin is given to chew, unless clearly contraindicated. If there is ECG evidence of ischaemia/infarction or elevated cardiac troponin, clopidogrel 300 mg is also given. Both aspirin and clopidogrel are antiplatelet drugs.

In addition, patients with demonstrated ACS should be given low-molecular-weight (LMW) heparin or fondaparinux for anticoagulation.

Reassurance and early information giving are important during this stage. The often unasked question is 'Am I going to die?', so it is important for the patient to see that you acknowledge this fear and make him or her feel in safe hands. The American College of Cardiology have expressed this as presenting a 'warm and caring approach combined with professionalism and confidence' (ACC/AHA 1999). There can be long-term psychological problems caused by profound disturbing emotions experienced in the immediate aftermath of the MI (Whitehead 2005).

Continuous ECG monitoring is essential during the early stages to allow for the early detection of arrhythmia, as is careful observation for the signs of possible cardiac failure: rising heart rate, falling Sao_2, restlessness, dyspnoea, falling pulse pressure.

The critical intervention in the ACS patient is to re-establish an adequate blood flow to the myocardium. In the patient with ST-elevation MI this is

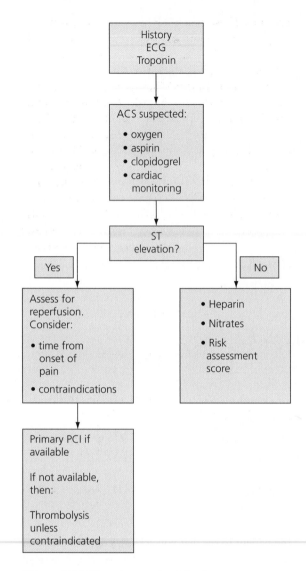

Figure 1.24 Management algorithm for acute coronary syndrome

balloon catheter into the coronary artery, inflating the balloon to open up the narrowed or blocked vessel, and then removing the balloon leaving a tubular framework called a stent to maintain patency. This procedure is carried out in a catheterization laboratory at specialist centres. To make this intervention available to the majority of the population there is an ongoing strategy in the UK to coordinate regional centres, district general hospitals, and the ambulance services to ensure that patients for whom this is a treatment option are rapidly assessed and transferred directly to an appropriate centre (MINAP 2009).

Thrombolysis

Not all patients will be suitable for PPCI because of either time delays or contraindications, so the second option of thrombolysis remains available.

Thrombolytic drugs work by activating the fibrinolytic system. The clot is broken down and the coronary vessel that is occluded has the potential to become patent once more, allowing reperfusion of the affected myocardium. As with all reperfusion strategies, the earlier this reperfusion can occur the more significant the results.

Current guidelines recommend fibrin-specific thrombolysis. The choice of agent for hospital-based administration is usually between one of the following:

- t-PA (alteplase);
- r-PA (reteplase);
- tenecteplase.

With all thrombolytics, bleeding represents a potential side-effect that should be monitored. Stroke is a small but important risk, with haemorrhagic stroke having a slightly higher incidence with t-PA (GUSTO 1993).

- *Absolute contraindications* are mainly those relating to increased potential for bleeding. They include: stroke; active internal bleeding; known bleeding disorder; suspected dissecting aneurysm; recent major surgery.
- *Relative contraindications* include: transient ischaemic attack (TIA) in the past 6 months; pregnancy; non-compressible punctures; traumatic resuscitation; refractory hypertension (systolic >180 mmHg); recent retinal laser treatment.

achieved by either thrombolytic drugs which break down the clot, or by an invasive procedure – a primary percutaneous coronary intervention (PPCI).

Primary percutaneous coronary intervention

PPCI is now the preferred option when patient and organizational circumstances allow. PPCI (also known as primary angioplasty) involves passing a

Additional therapies in the acute phase include beta-blockers, ACE inhibitors and statins, if not contraindicated.

> The key priority for patients with ACS is rapid assessment and decision-making so that they can benefit from the evidence-based interventions that are clearly set out in clinical guidelines.

Heart failure

One of the most common causes of admission to medical and elderly wards in acute hospitals is heart failure. It is estimated that heart failure accounts for at least 5 per cent of all elderly and medical admissions, and re-admission rates are high (Nichol *et al.* 2008). As heart failure is common in an ageing population it is likely that patients will be encountered in a variety of clinical settings where the current clinical problem is complicated by the presence of heart failure (e.g. the elderly surgical patient who has underlying heart failure).

'Heart failure' (HF) is the term used to describe the complex syndrome that results from the systemic and circulatory responses to the failing myocardium. This syndrome classically presents as fatigue, shortness of breath, orthopnoea, reduced exercise tolerance, and ankle swelling. These features are related to inadequate tissue perfusion and to the retention of fluid. The principal cause is left ventricular impairment, most commonly systolic dysfunction, secondary to coronary heart disease or hypertension. Heart failure is a long-term condition where a 'cure' is not possible. Here an overview of HF is given followed by a more focused discussion of acute HF.

Pathophysiology

One of the first points to establish is that chronic heart failure (CHF) is a multi-system disorder. The clinical manifestations of established heart failure occur as a result of a complex interaction between neuro-hormonal, immune, pulmonary and muscular responses. Here a simplified and limited account is given (Fig. 1.25).

As the forward pressure into the aorta begins to fall, the body responds by trying to preserve perfusion pressure. These changes in pressure are detected by baroreceptors in the carotid sinus and the aortic arch. The message that is given is that pressure within the system is falling.

The sympathetic nervous system is activated, the result being that there is an increase in circulating catecholamines, specifically noradrenaline. These changes produce a rise in heart rate and contractility, and in the degree of vasoconstriction, this through the stimulation of alpha- and beta-adrenergic receptors. The problem is that these responses, while creating an initial rise in perfusion pressure, have a negative effect on the myocardium in that they raise myocardial oxygen demands by the increase in heart rate and afterload, which increases myocardial workload.

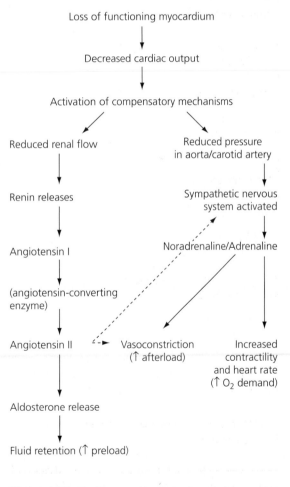

Figure 1.25 Compensatory mechanisms in heart failure

The kidneys detect the drop in pressure. The juxtaglomerular apparatus responds to falling renal artery perfusion pressure and to direct beta-2 stimulation and releases renin, which leads to the production of angiotensin II (see Chapter 3). Angiotensin II has a number of actions, but in particular:

- it is a powerful vasoconstrictor exerting direct effects on smooth muscle;
- it stimulates the production of aldosterone in the adrenal cortex, which leads to the reabsorption of sodium from the distal tubules, and therefore water retention.

In addition, antidiuretic hormone is secreted by the posterior pituitary in response to activity of atrial baroreceptors and the action of angiotensin II. The net haemodynamic result of the neurohormonal activity is:

- an increase in heart rate, due to the sympathetic stimulation;
- an increase in afterload, due to vasoconstriction;
- an increase in preload, due to the retention of sodium and water;
- an increase in contractility, due to the sympathetic stimulation.

This is the classic response to a threat to perfusion. The problem for the HF patient is that this initial compensatory response causes problems for the pump in both the short and long term.

- The increases in heart rate and contractility, although compensatory, significantly increase the myocardial oxygen demand and may lead to ischaemia, particularly if there is already ischaemic heart disease (IHD).
- The increase in afterload has a negative effect on the ventricular myocardium, which cannot overcome the increased resistance (Fig 1.26).
- The increase in preload, while beneficial in the normal heart, leads to pulmonary and systemic venous congestion in the failing heart.

The circulatory response is trying to maintain pressure within the system, but in doing so places increasingly intolerable demands on the already compromised heart. The response is designed to be a short-term regulatory strategy to maintain perfusion pressure, but chronic stimulation leads to molecular

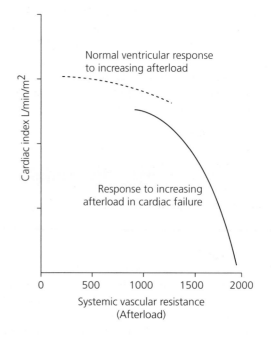

Figure 1.26 Effect of an increase in afterload on the ventricular myocardium

changes in the cardiac cells that result in severe left ventricular dysfunction.

Excessive volume retention overloads the pulmonary circulation, raising the hydrostatic pressure in the pulmonary vessels until it overcomes the osmotic pressure keeping fluid in the system, and pulmonary oedema results. A similar process in the systemic circulation results in systemic oedema.

Despite the attempts to drive cardiac output up through the activation of the sympathetic pathways, the failing heart cannot meet tissue oxygen demands, particularly when those demands increase through exercise.

As the condition progresses the patient may reach a point where cardiac function is so poor that adequate tissue oxygenation becomes impossible. This point may be referred to as *end-stage failure* and is similar to that seen in cardiogenic shock.

Management of CHF

Chronic heart failure may present slowly and insidiously with the classic symptoms of fatigue, reduced exercise tolerance and oedema. For the healthcare team this condition represents a significant challenge as the possibility of 'cure' is negligible. Half of the patients diagnosed with HF will die within four years, and of those with severe heart failure, up to half will die within one year (Hobbs *et al.* 2007). With this in mind, the aims of management are:

- to prolong survival;
- to increase exercise tolerance;
- to improve symptoms.

Management is based around pharmacological and non-pharmacological strategies.

Drugs for HF

The drug therapy used in heart failure is now well established and should be based on clinical guidelines (NICE 2010; SIGN 2007b; Opie 2008). The following drugs are used, but for a more complete account you should read the guidelines listed in the references or the *British National Formulary.*

Angiotensin-converting enzyme inhibitors

ACE inhibitors are now seen as the starting point for treatment of heart failure. This group of drugs act by blocking the conversion of angiotensin I into angiotensin II. This results in reduced vasoconstriction, and therefore afterload, and a decrease in sodium and water retention. The net therapeutic effects are of increased cardiac output and reduced volume overload, leading to improved quality of life and reduced mortality. All patients with heart failure due to left ventricular (LV) systolic dysfunction should be on the maximum dose that can be tolerated (e.g. lisinopril, starting at 2.5–5.0 mg daily, titrated up to 30–35 mg daily over several weeks).

An angiotensin II receptor antagonist may be an option for selected patients who cannot tolerate an ACE inhibitor (e.g. candesartan 4–16 mg daily).

Beta-blockers

Clinical trials have shown improvement in symptoms and survival with low-dose beta-blockers. These attenuate the sympathetic over-stimulation. Beta-blockers are initiated in patients with LV systolic dysfunction after ACE inhibitor and diuretic therapy (e.g. carvedilol 3.125 mg daily up to 25–50 mg daily).

Patients with HF should be taking both an ACE inhibitor and a beta blocker unless contraindicated.

Diuretics

Diuretics should be routinely used for the relief of symptoms of fluid congestion. The use of loop diuretics such as furosemide or bumetanide will increase the excretion of sodium and water, which will reduce both systemic and pulmonary oedema. They should be titrated up or down in response to symptoms and to evidence of fluid retention.

Aldosterone antagonists

Spironolactone improves symptoms and improves survival. A dose of 12.5–25 mg daily is used.

Digoxin

Digoxin has the dual effect of controlling the ventricular rate in atrial fibrillation (AF), which is common in cardiac failure, and increasing contractility. It is used in patients with HF and AF, and in those with severe HF despite the foregoing therapy.

Other measures

Sodium and water restriction

Sodium restriction and water limitation are important measures in heart failure. The degree of fluid restriction is assessed by the monitoring of fluid intake and output and of daily weight. A weight gain of 0.5 kg/ day is significant and is associated with volume retention. The patient will need to understand the reason for these restrictions if they are to comply with what may be an uncomfortable aspect of their care.

Exercise

Part of the approach to management is to reduce excessive demands for cardiac output that cannot be met. This usually means complete rest for the patient who has been hospitalized with HF. However the role of conditioning exercises has been increasingly recognized, and this can begin with gentle moves that maintain muscle tone but place little demands on the heart.

Oxygen

Supplemental oxygen will need to be administered if the arterial oxygen saturation is not adequate.

Psychological support and education

For many patients the prognostic reality is one of slow deterioration marked by steadily reducing exercise tolerance and increasingly distressing symptoms. This picture is made bleaker by the high incidence of sudden death. The level of support needed by both patient and family will be considerable. The nature of this support should probably be centred on an optimistic but realistic outlook and the motivation associated with the attainment of achievable goals. This is related to self-esteem and is likely to be most positively encouraged by an improvement in exercise tolerance that will contribute to the patient's independence. It must also be recognized that this is a terminal condition that the patient and family will need support to come to terms with.

The nursing role in managing heart failure is being increasingly recognized. The development of nurse-led HF services and monitoring have led to a reduction in readmission rates in the USA, and services in the UK are mostly based on the model developed in Glasgow (Stewart and Blue 2004).

Acute left ventricular failure

Presentation

Acute LV failure is a situation in which the left ventricle has failed suddenly and has become overwhelmed by the volume of fluid returning to it from the pulmonary circulation (hence this is also called 'acute cardiogenic pulmonary oedema'). This, by the mechanisms described earlier in the chapter, creates an acute rise in left ventricular diastolic pressure (preload), which is transmitted back through the pulmonary capillaries, giving rise to pulmonary oedema as the hydrostatic pressure in the vessels overcomes the osmotic pressure and fluid leaks out.

This leads to the all-too-familiar picture of acute left ventricular failure (LVF). The patient will be acutely and significantly breathless and distressed, tachycardic, possibly with systemic hypotension (although not always). There will be increased production of sputum that is classically 'frothy'. There may be cyanosis and confusion.

The diagnosis of acute LVF will be made on the basis of these signs, the presenting history, plus the objective evidence of pulmonary oedema that can be found on chest auscultation and examination of the chest X-ray and by the low oxygen saturation.

The underlying cause of acute LVF is usually an acute exacerbation of long-term heart failure and may be precipitated by both cardiac and non-cardiac causes. Cardiac triggers include ACS, tachyarrhythmia and valve disease. Non-cardiac triggers include chest infection, anaemia, fluid overload and non-compliance with medication.

Management of acute LVF

Management is aimed at improving the oxygen saturation by reducing the pulmonary capillary pressure. This is achieved by improving the myocardial oxygen supply/demand balance, reducing the amount of circulating fluid, and offloading the left ventricle. One must also consider the underlying cause. If tachyarrhythmia is the cause then the priority is to control it. The nursing role here will be central to the success of the therapeutic interventions.

The priorities are informed by the ESC guidelines (Dickson et al. 2008).

Patient positioning

The patient should sit upright if possible. This will have the effect of increasing the lung capacity, reducing the venous return and reducing the work of breathing. If the patient is profoundly hypotensive, however, this position should be avoided or at least modified.

Oxygen

Oxygen is administered via a high-percentage mask at a high flow rate of 8–10 L/min. If an adequate Sao_2 cannot be maintained, then recent clinical trials suggest the use of non-invasive ventilation as CPAP or BiPAP (Gray 2008; see Chapter 2).

Diuretic

The loop diuretic furosemide is usually the drug of choice and will be prescribed in doses from 40 to 80 mg IV. The effect of furosemide in this situation is a vasodilatory effect and a diuretic effect. The result is a reduction in the pulmonary capillary pressure and therefore pulmonary oedema.

Nitroglycerine

Unless the patient is profoundly hypotensive, a nitrate (nitroglycerine) will be prescribed, possibly sublingually, or by intravenous route at a dose of 0.25 γg/kg per minute, increasing every 5 minutes until there is a fall in blood pressure of 15 mmHg or if the systolic pressure falls to 90 mmHg. This will vasodilate, mainly on the venous side, and will reduce the volume of blood that is returning to the left ventricle, and therefore reduce left ventricular and pulmonary capillary pressures.

Diamorphine

The dose prescribed will be between 2.5 and 5 mg depending on the size of the patient, and should be administered intravenously. This will have a sedative effect that is beneficial in this situation where the fear and agitation of the patient increases the oxygen demand. Diamorphine also has a mild vasodilatory effect which contributes to the lowering of preload.

If the blood pressure fails to respond despite the compensatory mechanisms and above therapies, then the clinical picture becomes one of *cardiogenic shock* (discussed later).

It should be recognized that the above scenario represents a medical emergency and is life-threatening. For the patient this is all too apparent, and the distressing symptoms will create intense anxiety as the patient struggles to breathe. Complicated explanations are not appropriate at this time, but the patient will need simple assurances that you are doing something positive to relieve the distress. The mental state of the patient may change from anxiety and agitation to confusion and then to coma as the condition progresses.

Shock (circulatory failure)

The greatest threat in the seriously ill patient is the complete failure of the cardiovascular system to maintain effective pressure to meet tissue oxygen demands. When this failure begins to develop, a complex set of mechanisms are activated that attempt to compensate and to restore adequate perfusion. When these mechanisms fail then the term 'shock' is often used. Shock is a complex clinical syndrome that occurs as a result of acute circulatory failure and will often be the final pathway that leads to death from cardiovascular causes.

The shock syndrome can be described as 'a state in which there is a significant reduction in cardiac output, effective tissue perfusion and tissue oxygenation, resulting in multi-organ symptoms'. The unifying feature in all forms of shock is the critical reduction in the supply of oxygenated blood to the tissues.

Classification

To recall our earlier analogy, circulatory failure will arise because of a problem with either the pump, the pipes, or the volume. It will occur if:

- the pump cannot maintain adequate perfusion despite the constriction of the pipes;
- the volume is insufficient despite attempts to increase the pumping;
- the pipes are too dilated for the pump and the volume available to fill to an adequate pressure.

Shock is often classified on the basis of the causative pathophysiology, as follows:

- cardiogenic;
- hypovolaemic;
- distributive (septic, anaphylactic or neurogenic).

CASE STUDY 1.1

Patrick Hopkirk is a 67-year-old man who has been brought to A&E by ambulance following an episode of extreme breathlessness and collapse in a pub. On arrival he is distressed, very breathless and sweaty. He is finding it difficult to speak and is agitated and restless. No further history can be obtained from him. His wife says that he is 'under the doctor' for breathlessness and 'blood pressure' and is on 'water tablets'. She also reveals that he has been getting increasingly breathless over the past few weeks. The following are obtained: BP, 160/90 mmHg; heart rate, 115/min; respiratory rate >40/min; Spo_2, 88 per cent.

- What is the likely cause of this man's symptoms?
- What should be the initial management?

These are the shock scenarios most likely to be encountered when caring for the acutely ill hospital patient.

Cardiogenic shock usually results from severe impairment of cardiac muscle contractility. Specific causes include myocardial infarction, valve disease, cardiomyopathy, tamponade and myocardial dysfunction after cardiac surgery. In cardiogenic shock secondary to MI, 40 per cent or more of the myocardium is necrotic or injured and so does not contribute to contractility. By definition, therefore, cardiogenic shock usually implies the presence of extensive muscle damage. The prognosis for this shock state is extremely poor and the in-hospital mortality remains high.

In *hypovolaemic shock* there is a decrease in the intravascular volume of 15–25 per cent, with haemorrhage being the most common cause. Clinical scenarios associated with hypovolaemic shock include surgical blood loss, burns, peritonitis, trauma and excessive diuresis.

The *septic shock syndrome* is associated with the presence in the blood of micro-organisms or their toxins. This leads to a complex syndrome in which there is an extremely low systemic vascular resistance (a large hosepipe) leading to reduced preload and poor perfusion pressure, a decrease in myocardial contractility, and reduced cellular oxygen uptake.

The precise clinical picture of shock may vary. It is dependent on the cause of the disorder and on the stage of the shock. The following sections look at cardiogenic shock and hypovolaemia; sepsis is discussed in Chapter 5.

Cardiogenic shock

Pathophysiology

When there is a decrease in systemic blood pressure following, for example, extensive MI, the body initiates a series of compensatory mechanisms to maintain an adequate perfusion of the brain and the heart. This compensation is similar to that seen in heart failure (see Fig. 1.25). Baroreceptors detect the drop in pressure and, via the autonomic nervous system, stimulate the release of adrenaline and noradrenaline. These catecholamines act on the sympathetic receptors (principally beta-1 and alpha) to cause an increase in heart rate, contractility and vasoconstriction. The heart rate increases to assist in improving the cardiac output according to the equation *heart rate × stroke volume = cardiac output*. The increase in contractility attempts to augment the stroke volume.

The blood vessels to the skin, abdominal viscera, voluntary muscle and finally the kidneys constrict in an attempt to maintain the blood pressure and redirect blood flow to the more critical areas of the brain and heart. Both the venous and the arterial ends of the capillary bed constrict. The systemic vascular resistance (SVR) increases in response to this vasoconstriction.

Initially blood pressure is maintained and symptoms may be limited to tachycardia. In the absence of invasive haemodynamic monitoring this early stage may be missed.

As the condition progresses the vasoconstriction that has been maintaining the blood pressure creates key problems. The high SVR, because of the afterload effect, increases cardiac work and therefore myocardial oxygen demands. There is also an increase in the already elevated preload, which may ultimately lead to an increase in pulmonary artery pressures and pulmonary oedema.

In response to the reduced flow of blood to the kidneys in cardiogenic shock, the renin–angiotensin–aldosterone pathway is activated. The angiotensin causes further vasoconstriction and aldosterone release. Aldosterone causes sodium and water retention and potassium excretion. These changes further increase preload and afterload. The increase in afterload again increases myocardial oxygen demand and leads to a further decrease in contractility. The increase in preload contributes further to increased pulmonary artery pressures and pulmonary oedema, potentially reducing oxygen saturation (Sao_2).

As this situation progresses the systolic blood pressure falls and the diastolic blood pressure remains elevated secondary to the increased SVR. This can be seen clinically as a fall in pulse pressure (the difference between the systolic and diastolic pressures). Eventually, however, the falling cardiac output cannot maintain adequate arterial pressure despite the vasoconstriction, so arterial blood pressure will begin to fall. This sometimes happens precipitously.

Clinical picture in cardiogenic shock

If invasive monitoring is being used, then the following are typical measurements:

- cardiac index (CI) 1.6–2.2;
- systemic vascular resistance (SVR) 2000 dyne-s/cm^5;
- pulmonary capillary wedge pressure (PCWP) 25 mmHg;
- ejection fraction (EF) 30 per cent or less;
- mean arterial pressure (MAP) under 60 mmHg.

This typical intermediate or progressive stage is manifested clinically as the classic syndrome of shock. The skin becomes cool, moist and dusky, with the tip of the nose, the earlobes and the distal extremities becoming cyanotic, secondary to the intense vasoconstriction. The fall in cardiac output and vasoconstriction of the vessels to the kidneys cause decreased renal perfusion, which results in oliguria and eventually anuria. In spite of the compensatory mechanisms, the supply of oxygenated blood to the brain decreases resulting in such symptoms as dizziness, confusion, agitation and lethargy. This may progress to decreased levels of consciousness and coma.

The inadequate cellular perfusion causes cell anoxia and changes in cellular metabolism. Cellular anoxia results in a change to anaerobic metabolism; the cells are forced to metabolize glucose without oxygen. As a result, lactic acid accumulates within the cell, leading to lactic acidosis, or metabolic acidosis, with a decrease in serum pH.

In this stage of shock, no matter what the initiating factor, there is a downward spiral that is all but impossible to arrest. Severe lactic acidosis is potentiated by a decrease in carbon dioxide removal, due to a decrease in blood flow. The acidic environment stimulates vasodilatation of the arteriolar ends. The venous link from the capillary bed, however, remains constricted. Blood flows into the capillary bed but cannot return to the heart. Stasis and pooling of blood occurs in the capillary beds. Hypoxia, decreased serum pH and cellular acidosis contribute directly to cell membrane changes. Cellular, tissue and organ death are now imminent.

As shock progresses to this irreversible phase, multi-system failure results with the ensuing complications of further myocardial ischaemia and depression, and tubular necrosis in the kidneys. The multi-organ problems that occur as a result of the failing perfusion are summarized in Box 1.3.

Box 1.3 Multi-organ problems occurring as a result of failing perfusion

- **Brain**. There is decreased cerebral blood flow.
- **Myocardium**. The increasing mismatch of oxygen supply and demand leads to disorders of cell membrane and cell death.
- **Kidney**. Prolonged hypoperfusion leads to acute tubular necrosis and acute renal failure.
- **GI tract**. There may be mucosal ischaemia, ileus and full-thickness gangrene of the bowel with possible contamination with gut bacteria. There is also the possibility of GI bleeding.
- **Lungs**. Pulmonary oedema may occur.
- **Immune system**. Immune system depression will leave the patient at heightened risk of serious infection.
- **Skin**. Poor tissue perfusion and pooling within the interstitial space leave the skin vulnerable to breakdown.

Management of cardiogenic shock

The aims of management are:

- to improve and maintain perfusion of the vital organs;
- to improve the myocardial oxygen supply/demand ratio (possibly through revascularization);
- to recognize failure of treatment early, to allow a dignified and pain-free death.

Assessment and monitoring

Assessment and monitoring is an essential part of management. Decisions about therapeutic strategies will depend on the availability of accurate data on which to act. The patient will need the following:

- continuous ECG monitoring;
- hourly urine output monitoring;

- blood pressure monitoring;
- oxygen saturation monitoring via pulse oximetry;
- (if considered necessary) a pulmonary artery catheter to allow a more direct indication of LV function;
- pH and electrolyte assessment.

Therapeutic strategies

The therapeutic strategies employed will depend on the precise clinical picture and aetiology that presents. It must also be recognized that, if the cause of the shock is significant myocardial cell loss, then the mortality rate is very high. However, in established cardiogenic shock where the decision has been taken to pursue active treatment, some of the following specific treatments may be appropriate.

Arrhythmia

Any arrhythmia is corrected in order to optimize cardiac output.

Hypovolaemia

While the usual picture will be one of fluid *overload*, there are occasions when the patient is relatively hypovolaemic, in that the left-sided preload is not adequate (reflected by a low PCWP) and should therefore be corrected. This is particularly so in right ventricular infarction complicated by cardiogenic shock, where optimization of left-sided filling pressures is the immediate priority (Menon and Hockman 2002). It is important to recognize that in some cases of acute right ventricular failure increasing the volume load may not be sufficient and positive inotropic support will also be required.

Arterial hypoxaemia

Arterial hypoxaemia is treated by giving supplemental oxygen via a high-concentration mask. If this strategy fails to raise the pO_2 above 8 kPa, then the use of continuous positive airways pressure (CPAP) must be considered.

Metabolic acidosis

A metabolic acidosis may result from the impaired tissue perfusion. It may be treated with the judicious administration of sodium bicarbonate.

Electrolyte imbalance

Any electrolyte imbalance is corrected – particularly potassium, as a deranged potassium may predispose to cardiac arrhythmias.

Low cardiac output

An attempt is made to optimize cardiac output by the use of agents that will have a direct effect on preload, afterload and contractility. Contractility is increased by the administration of a positive inotropic agent. At present, dobutamine is the drug of choice in this context, although this may be supplemented by additional agents. Preload and afterload are reduced by the use of vasodilators such as nitrates. The usual scenario, however, is that the blood pressure is so low that nitrates are used only with caution to reduce the preload pressure on the left ventricle. Any vasodilator is unlikely to be used if the systolic blood pressure is less than 90 mmHg.

Profound failure of perfusion

Profound failure of perfusion, as evidenced by a MAP less than 60 mmHg, may prompt the use of a vasopressor agent such as noradrenaline. In practice this is likely to be seen only in a heart surgery patient as a final attempt to maintain perfusion. In the post-infarct patient, vasoconstrictors are usually avoided because of the disastrous effect a further increase in afterload may cause.

Low urine output

Renal support is provided initially by giving diuretics to increase the urine output.

Lowering oxygen demand

Tissue oxygen demands are kept to a minimum by ensuring the patient is resting completely. This may require the administration of small doses of diamorphine as the distress caused by the low cardiac output and the dyspnoea may result in considerable agitation. This must be supported by adequate explanations and reassurance. The presence of family members at this time may serve to reassure the patient.

Nutrition

Nutritional requirements via enteral routes at this time are limited to maintaining comfort. The poor tissue perfusion also affects the gut which may become ischaemic within the first 24 hours (Janssens *et al.* 2000).

Skin condition

The skin is particularly vulnerable in this situation and the potential for pressure sore development is high. Interventions to reduce this risk must be considered.

Emotional support

Consideration must be taken of the patient's family who are facing a situation that carries a very high mortality rate. Social and emotional support is essential if the needs of the relatives of the critically ill individual are to be met. These needs have been repeatedly identified as the need for hope, information, relief of anxiety and to feel useful, since the seminal study by Molter (1979).

Angioplasty

There is evidence for the benefit of early angioplasty in post-infarct cardiogenic shock. In centres where this is available it should be considered, particularly for patients under 75 years of age (Hockman 2001; Menon and Hockman 2002).

CASE STUDY 1.2

Mrs Brady is a 67-year-old woman who is on a medical ward following an anterior myocardial infarction 48 hours ago. This was her second heart attack. Overnight she has been getting increasingly breathless and agitated. Her blood pressure overnight has changed as follows (mmHg): 120/70; 110/70; 100/65; 90/65; 85/60. Her heart rate is 110/min. She is breathless and her skin is cold and sweaty. She has not passed urine overnight. The staff nurse coming on the early shift puts a pulse oximeter on which shows an SpO_2 of 89 per cent.

- What additional observations would be appropriate in this case?
- What is the likely initial management?

Inotropic drugs

One of the mainstays of drug therapy in the seriously ill is the use of positive inotropic drugs.

Inotropic substances are those that have an effect on myocardial contractility. Positive inotropes therefore are those agents that increase myocardial contractility.

The agents commonly referred to as inotropic drugs are also chronotropic (they affect the heart rate) and vasoactive (they have an effect on vascular smooth muscle cells). Their effect is therefore more complex than simply increasing the contractility of cardiac muscle cells.

The clinical effects of increases in contractility combined with a vasoactive action can be predicted to a point, but they must be considered in the context of a variety of factors, including:

- the agent or combination of agents used;
- the clinical scenario that is the indication for their use;
- the dose of the agent given;
- the haemodynamic status of the patient.

Inotropic agents are therefore not interchangeable and their use must be based on a good understanding of the underlying physiology and pharmacology and the evidence of patient-centred outcomes from clinical trials.

The majority of inotropic drugs are catecholamines and therefore dependent on their interaction with sympathetic adrenergic receptors. These receptors are alpha, beta-1, beta-2 and dopaminergic.

- Stimulation of the alpha receptors results in increased systemic and pulmonary vascular resistance.
- Beta-1 stimulation results in increased contractility, heart rate and conduction.
- Beta-2 stimulation results in mild vasodilation.
- Dopaminergic stimulation results in dilatation of the renal and mesenteric arteries.

Dopamine and the 'renal dose'

One review concluded that 'there is insufficient evidence to support the use of renal-dose dopamine in the intensive care unit' (Jones and Bellomo 2005). At doses of 2–3 γg/kg per minute dopamine may have a unique effect on dopaminergic receptors and dilate the renal arteries. However, there has been considerable discussion in the literature about the nature of this 'renal' effect, some suggesting that any case for the use of low-dose dopamine, either as a treatment for acute renal failure or as a prophylactic, is based more on opinion than on evidence (Bailey 2000). A randomized controlled trial showed no clinically significant protection from renal failure in at-risk patients with systemic inflammatory response syndrome (Bellomo *et al.* 2000). Similarly, no advantage of dopamine over adequate hydration was found in patients with mild to moderate renal failure undergoing coronary angiography (Gare *et al.* 2000).

At doses of 3–10 γg/kg per minute there is a strong beta-1 effect that increases myocardial contractility. There will also be an unpredictable rise in heart rate and myocardial oxygen demand.

At doses of 10–20 γg/kg per minute there are increasing inotropic effects but also strong alpha effects resulting in vasoconstriction.

Dobutamine

Dobutamine at doses of 2–20 γg/kg per minute has a potent beta-1 effect producing a predominantly inotropic response. There is some beta-2 effect that will produce mild vasodilation and may therefore lower left ventricular preload. The net result is of increased contractility without severe increases in myocardial oxygen consumption. Dobutamine continues to be recommended as the first-choice inotrope in cardiogenic shock, and in sepsis it has been recommended to be used if additional inotropic support is needed following fluid loading and correcting of SVR with pressor agents such as noradrenaline.

Adrenaline

Adrenaline is a potent beta-1 agonist that will increase contractility and heart rate significantly. At doses up to 2 γg/kg per minute there is also a beta-2 effect that causes a mild vasodilation. At higher doses the strong alpha effects will raise the SVR (afterload) and increase myocardial oxygen consumption. Adrenaline will tend to be used in situations where a rise in SVR combined with a rise in contractility is needed. The possibility of mesenteric ischaemia must be considered due to the pressor effects.

Noradrenaline

Noradrenaline is a powerful alpha agonist that also has some beta-1 effects. The predominant effect is to raise SVR which is positive in the appropriate circumstances, such as massive vasodilation, but the profound vasoconstriction can lead to renal or gut ischaemia . Dose is from 1 γg/kg per minute.

There appear to be differences between centres in the choice of inotropic agents used. There are certainly differences between settings, with different agents being used in general ICU, cardiac ICU and coronary care settings. Any lack of definitive consensus perhaps reflects the complexity of the agents themselves and of the conditions in which they are used.

When using an inotropic drug, consider the likely effects given the clinical context. For example, septic shock, cardiogenic shock and major trauma will produce quite different haemodynamic profiles and therefore require different approaches to circulatory support. In sepsis there is the need to raise the SVR with fluid and pressor agents as well as using an agent that has a positive inotropic effect to optimize MAP. In cardiogenic shock the aim is to increase MAP by using a positive inotropic agent and to endeavour to reduce SVR (and therefore afterload) by possibly using a vasodilator, although this latter may not be possible if adequate pressure cannot be achieved. In trauma patients, raising preload with fluids will have a better outcome than starting with a positive inotrope (Millar 1998). The choice of agents will be guided by the current best evidence for the particular scenario faced.

Hypovolaemia

One of the key aspects of maintaining a satisfactory perfusion pressure in the system is the regulation of adequate volume. Hypovolaemia requires restoration of fluids and the circulating plasma volume, but the choice of fluid and the amount given will depend on assessment of the clinical situation presented. This section will examine the clinical management of fluid resuscitation in the seriously ill patient. It is necessary to consider the normal distribution of fluid in order to better understand the approach to treatment. Further discussion can be found in Chapter 3.

Body fluid consists of water and its dissolved constituents. About 75 per cent of total body weight is body fluid, so there is about 40 L in a 70 kg person. This body water is distributed in the intravascular, interstitial and intracellular spaces which, in our example of a 70 kg person, will have about 5 L, 13 L and 23 L, respectively. Fluid is able to move between each of these spaces at certain points and under certain conditions. The intravascular space is separated from the interstitial space by the semipermeable membrane of the capillary walls. The interstitial space is separated from the intracellular space by the complex structure that is the cell membrane.

In the patient with acute circulatory failure secondary to, for example, haemorrhage, it is the volume in the intravascular space that is of immediate concern. Movement of fluid in and out of the intravascular space depends on the opposing forces of hydrostatic and osmotic pressure. The capillary membrane is permeable to water and small ions, for example sodium, but impermeable to large protein molecules found in the plasma. There is normally a hydrostatic pressure gradient between the capillaries and the interstitial space that pushes fluid out of the intravascular space. The osmotic pressure gradient pulls fluid back into the intravascular space, this being generated by the plasma proteins and other large molecules. When intravenous fluid is given it initially goes into the intravascular space. How much of the fluid stays in this space and how it is ultimately distributed among the three spaces depends partly on the nature of the fluid given.

There are basically two types of fluid that can be administered to the patient, crystalloid and colloid.

Crystalloids are electrolyte solutions that do not contain the oncotic particles that would restrict them to the intravascular space. Examples are 0.9% saline solution, Ringer's lactate and 5% dextrose. The distribution of crystalloids once infused is dependent mainly on the sodium concentration. As sodium is mainly extracellular (interstitial and intravascular), fluids with an isotonic concentration of sodium (e.g. 0.9% saline) will be confined to the interstitial and intravascular spaces, with three-quarters of the fluid

going to the interstitial space as this is much larger. The lower the sodium concentration, the more fluid will go to the intracellular space. For example, 5% dextrose contains no sodium and so is distributed proportionately over the three spaces; out of one litre infused, 520 mL will go to the intracellular space, 360 mL to the interstitial space and only 120 mL to the intravascular space. This makes it inappropriate for an acutely hypovolaemic situation where the goal is to increase the intravascular volume.

Colloids are fluids that contain particles that exert an oncotic pressure and are mainly confined to the intravascular space when given because the capillary membrane is not permeable to the large molecules. Colloids can be classified as those that have an oncotic pressure that is the same as plasma, such as blood and blood products and those with a higher osmotic pressure. While all colloids will pull fluid into the intravascular space, if the oncotic pressure of the colloid is higher than the natural oncotic pressure of plasma, then more fluid is pulled into the intravascular space. Such agents are called 'plasma expanders' as they are said to expand the plasma volume. Examples of plasma expanders are Haemaccel and hydroxyethyl starch (HES), the latter having the theoretical potential to expand the plasma volume by up to 170 per cent of the infused volume.

When deciding on fluid therapy the choice of fluid is dependent on the assessment of the fluid deficit in each space. In acute hypovolaemia, often secondary to haemorrhage, it is the volume in the intravascular space that is deficient. This can be estimated by the clinical picture that is presented. This is based on the degree of compensation undertaken by the pump and by the pipes, namely, the attempted increase in the output of the heart, and the degree of vasoconstriction. The guidelines in Table 1.2 are from the

Table 1.2 Clinical signs of fluid loss in intravascular spaces

Clinical sign	Blood loss < 15%	Blood loss 15–30%	Blood loss 30–40%	Blood loss > 40%
Systolic BP	Unchanged	Normal	Reduced	Very low
Diastolic BP	Unchanged	Raised	Reduced	Very low
Pulse pressure	Normal	Decreased	Decreased	Decreased
Heart rate	< 100/min	> 100/min	> 120/min	140/min
Mental state	Alert	Anxious	Anxious and confused	Confused or unconscious
Capillary refill	Normal	> 2 s	> 2 s	Undetectable

American College of Surgeons and provide an attempt to give an objective assessment. These guidelines are useful in that they require no invasive monitoring equipment and therefore can be used in any situation where there is a sphygmomanometer.

If invasive monitoring is available, then the CVP and/or the PCWP are used to titrate the volume replacement to the filling pressures of the heart.

The choice of fluid, then, will first be between a colloid, a crystalloid or blood, usually packed red blood cells (RBC). In the past there has been considerable debate about this choice with a 'colloids versus crystalloids' argument. Earlier thinking has been based on the belief that colloids are better because they will hold more fluid in the vascular space. More recently the evidence suggests that the previously held belief about the need for very large volumes of crystalloid as compared to colloids for fluid resuscitation is unfounded. Crystalloids are cheap and have few side-effects, whereas colloids are expensive and, in the case of blood products like albumin, can potentially lead to adverse reactions.

There is no strong evidence that any one colloid is better or safer than any other (Bunn *et al.* 2008). Also, there is no convincing evidence that colloids are more effective than crystalloids in fluid resuscitation in trauma, burns or surgery. As colloids are more expensive than crystalloids, a recent Cochrane review (Perel *et al.* 2007) concluded that there is no justification for their general use in acute fluid resuscitation, which suggests that crystalloids are the first choice in most situations.

Current guidelines for fluid management in the hypovolaemic patient are shown in Box 1.4.

Box 1.4 Guidelines for fluid management in the hypovolaemic patient (Powell-Tuck *et al.* 2008; Perel and Roberts 2007)

- Initial fluids should be a crystalloid such as Hartmans or Ringer's Lactate, alternatively 0.9% (normal) saline. Some guidelines allow for colloids as an alternative but suggest avoiding albumin, although evidence for harm resulting from albumin administration is limited (SAFE 2004).
- In trauma patients, fluid should be administered initially in a 250 mL bolus and the patient then reassessed.
- In haemorrhagic shock, blood is the preferred choice for fluid replacement but crystalloid should be given initially if there is delay.
- In surgical patients, if the diagnosis of hypovolaemia is in doubt then a 200 mL fluid challenge should be administered and the patients assessed before and after infusion.
- In patients who are dehydrated, 5% dextrose is used, as this will most successfully correct the intracellular deficit.

Conclusion

A good understanding of the cardiovascular system, including assessment and an overview of common cardiovascular problems, is an essential part of the knowledge base for any practitioner engaged in the care of acute patients with actual or potential serious illness. This chapter has combined the underlying physiology and pathophysiology with a discussion of general assessment and a focused discussion of specific cardiovascular problems and interventions. The key message from this chapter is to understand the factors that contribute to the maintenance of perfusion and to be able to relate this to assessment and management.

References

ACC/AHA (1999). *Guidelines for the Management of Patients with Acute Myocardial Infarction.* ACC/AHA

Bailey, J (2000) Dopamine: one size does not fit all, *Anesthesiology* **92**; 303.

Bassand *et al.* (Task Force for the Diagnosis and Treatment of Non ST segment ACS of the European Society of Cardiology, 2007). Guidelines for the diagnosis and treatment of non ST elevation acute coronary syndromes, *European Heart Journal* **28**; 1598–660.

Bellomo R, Chapman M, Finfer S *et al.* (2000). Low-dose dopamine in patients with early renal dysfunction: a placebo-controlled randomised trial, *Lancet* **356**; 2139–43.

Bern L, Brandt M, Mbelu N *et al.* (2007). Differences in blood pressure values obtained with automated and manual methods in medical inpatients, *Medsurg Nursing* **16**; 356–61.

British Heart Foundation (BHF, 2010). Heartstats. Available at www.heartstats.org/homepage.asp.

Bunn F, Trivedi D, Ashraf S (2008). Colloid solutions for fluid resuscitation, *Cochrane Database Syst Rev* (1):CD001319.

Cabello JB, Burls A, Emparanza JI, Bayliss S, Quinn T (2010). Oxygen therapy for acute myocardial infarction, *Cochrane Database Syst Rev* (6):CD007160.

Connors AF, Speroff T, Dawson NV *et al.* (1996) The effectiveness of right heart catheterization in the initial care of critically ill patients, *Journal of American Medical Association* **276**; 889–97.

Dickson *et al.* (2008). ESC guidelines for the diagnosis and treatment of acute and chronic heart failure, *European Heart Failure* **29**; 2388–442.

Gare M, Haviv Y, Rubinger D *et al.* (2000). The renal effects of low-dose dopamine in high-risk patients undergoing coronary angiography, *Journal of American College of Cardiology* **34**; 1682–8.

Goodacre S, Pett J, Arnold J *et al.* (2009). Clinical diagnosis of acute coronary syndrome in patients with a normal or nondiagnostic ECG, *European Medical Journal* **26**; 866–870.

Gray A, Goodacre S, Newby DE *et al.* (3CPO Triallists, 2008). Noninvasive ventilation in acute cardiogenic pulmonary edema, *New England Journal of Medicine* **359**; 142–51.

GUSTO (Global Utilisation of Streptokinase and Tissue plasminogen activator for Occluded coronary arteries, 1993). An international randomized trial comparing four strategies for acute myocardial infarction, *New England Journal of Medicine* **329**; 673–82.

Hakumaki M (1987). Seventy years of the Bainbridge reflex, *Acta Physiology Scandanavia* **130**(2); 77–85.

Hobbs FD, Roalfe AK, Davis RC *et al.* (2007) Prognosis of all-cause heart failure and borderline LVSD: 5 year mortality of the Echocardiographic Heart of England Screening Study (ECHOES), *European Heart Journal* **28**; 1128–34.

Hockman J *et al.* (2001). One-year survival following early revascularization for cardiogenic shock, *Journal of American Medical Association* **285**; 190–2.

Janssens U *et al.* (2000). Gastric tonometry in patients with cardiogenic shock and IABC, *Critical Care Medicine* **28**; 3449–54.

Jeavon P (2009). Blood pressure measurement, *Nursing Times*, February.

Jones D, Bellomo R (2005). Renal-dose dopamine: from hypothesis to paradigm to dogma to myth and finally superstition? *Journal of Intensive Care Medicine* **20**; 199–211.

Leach R, Treacher D (2002). The pulmonary physician in critical care: oxygen delivery and consumption in the critically ill, *Thorax* **57**; 170–7.

Lilly L (2003) *Pathophysiology of Heart Disease*. Baltimore: Lippincott, Williams & Wilkins.

Menon V, Hockman J (2002) Management of cardiogenic shock complicating acute myocardial infarction, *Heart* **88**; 531–7.

Millar P, Meredith JW, Chang MC (1998). Randomized, prospective comparison of increased preload versus inotropes in the resuscitation of trauma, *Journal of Trauma Injury, Infection and Critical Care* **44**; 107–13.

MINAP (Myocardial Ischaemia National Audit Project, 2009). *How the NHS Manages Heart Attacks*. London: National Institute for Clinical Outcomes Research.

Molter NC (1979). Needs of relatives of critically ill patients, *Heart & Lung* **8**; 332–9.

NICE (2010). *Chronic Heart Failure: National Clinical Guidelines for Diagnosis and Management in Primary and Secondary Care*. London: National Clinical Guidelines Centre.

Nichol E, Fitall B, Roughton M (2008). NHS heart failure survey: a survey of acute heart failure admissions in England, Wales and Northern Ireland, *Heart* **94**; 172–7.

Opie LH (2008) *Drugs for the Heart*, 7th edn. London: WB Saunders.

Perel P, Roberts I (2007). Colloids versus crystalloids for fluid resuscitation in critically ill patients, *Cochrane Database Syst Rev* (4):CD000567.

Powell-Tuck J, Gosling P, Dileep N, Lobo *et al.* (2008). *British Consensus Guidelines on Intravenous Fluid Therapy for Adult Surgical Patients* (GIFTASUP). London: BAPEN.

Preibe HJ (2005). Perioperative myocardial infarction: aetiology and prevention, *British Journal of Anaesthesia* **95**; 3–19.

Priebe HJ, Skarvan K (2000) *Cardiovascular Physiology*, 2nd edn. London: BMJ Books.

Resuscitation Council UK (2005). *Resuscitation Guidelines*. London: Resuscitation Council.

SAFE (2004). A comparison of albumin and saline for fluid resuscitation in the intensive care unit, *New England Journal of Medicine* **350**; 2247–56.

Santry (2010). Manual observation push to prevent deterioration, *Nursing Times*, June.

SIGN (2007a). *Acute Coronary Syndromes: A National Clinical Guideline*. Edinburgh: SIGN.

SIGN (2007b). *Management of Chronic Heart Failure: A National Clinical Guideline*. Edinburgh: SIGN.

Stewart S, Blue L (eds) (2004). *Improving Outcomes in Chronic Heart Failure*, 2nd edn. London: BMJ Books.

Stover J, Stocker R, Lenherr R *et al.* (2009). Noninvasive cardiac output and blood pressure monitoring cannot replace an invasive monitoring system in critically ill patients. *Anaesthesiology* **9**; 6.

Van de Werf *et al.* (Task Force for the Management of ST Elevation Acute Myocardial Infarction of the European Society of Cardiology, 2008). Management of acute myocardial infarction in patients presenting with persistent ST elevation, *European Heart Journal* **29**; 2909–45.

Wagner G (1994). *Marriott's Practical Electrocardiography*, 9th edn. Baltimore: Williams & Wilkins.

Whitehead D, Strike P, Perkins-Porras L, Steptoe A (2005). Frequency of distress and fear of dying during acute coronary syndromes and consequences for adaptation, *American Journal of Cardiology* **96**; 1512–16.

Williams B, Poulter NR, Brown MJ *et al.* (Fourth Working Party of the British Hypertension Society, 2004). Guidelines for management of hypertension: BHS IV, *Journal of Human Hypertension* **18**; 139–85.

Wu AHB (ed.) (1998). *Cardiac Markers*. New Jersey: Humana Press.

Tracey Moore and Catharine Thomas

LEARNING OUTCOMES

On completion of this chapter the reader will:

1 understand the importance of oxygen delivery for cell functioning

2 understand the role of respiratory mechanics on oxygen delivery and patient conditions that may compromise lung function

3 have an appreciation of the assessment and monitoring techniques that the nurse can use

   to aid the care of patients with a respiratory disorder

4 have an understanding of a number of specific respiratory disorders that impact upon oxygen delivery and the associated patient care and management.

Introduction

This chapter examines the purpose of the respiratory system, how this system may fail, and the nursing care and management of a patient with a failing respiratory system.

Patients needing acute care share the challenges of similar life-threatening situations. Whether the cause is cardiogenic shock, acute pulmonary embolus, septic shock or another condition, these patients have altered cellular metabolism from inadequate uptake, delivery or use of oxygen. Nurses caring for these patients need to understand the principles of oxygen delivery, methods of assessing a patient's oxygenation status, and interpretation of these results to be able to effectively intervene and attempt to correct tissue hypoxia.

Oxygenation of all body systems is essential to optimum functioning. Oxygen is needed to generate energy, which the cells use for metabolism. If oxygen is not available then cells may cease to function and ultimately die.

Oxygen contributes to energy generation by accepting electrons removed from hydrogen during the catabolism of substrates, especially fats and proteins. As the hydrogen is removed from the substrates (fats and proteins), electrons from the hydrogen are passed from one element to another through a series of chemical events in the Krebs (tri-carboxylic acid) cycle and cytochrome pathway (Fig. 2.1). As an electron is passed from one element to another, energy is generated. Some of this energy is captured by adenosine diphosphate (ADP), which is then converted to adenosine triphosphate (ATP). The conversion of ADP to ATP is termed *oxidative phosphorylation* because oxygen is needed for the process to continue. As the electron continues down the cytochrome pathway it is passed from one cytochrome to another cytochrome, and as it does so energy is produced which is again captured by ADP and converted into ATP. When the electron reaches the last cytochrome in the pathway it is accepted by oxygen to finally form water. This process is known as *aerobic metabolism* (i.e. metabolism using oxygen).

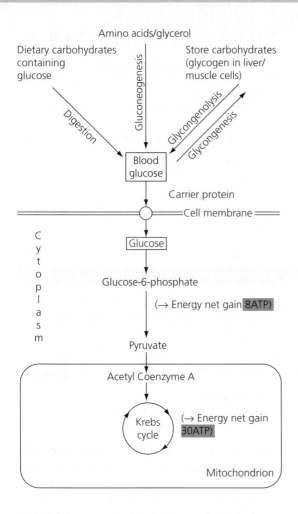

Figure 2.1 Glucose metabolism (cellular respiration)

If the amount of oxygen available for this process is inadequate, then electron transfer is inhibited and oxidative phosphorylation stops. At this point, anaerobic metabolism (i.e. metabolism without using oxygen) becomes the primary source for energy production. Anaerobic metabolism produces energy through the catabolism of carbohydrates and use of creatinine phosphate. However, both carbohydrates and creatinine phosphate are short-lived energy sources. While they may be invaluable as an energy source during a clinical emergency such as a cardiac arrest, they are unable to sustain cellular activities over time. This lack of energy will eventually result in a failure of all cellular functions, and then cell death.

Furthermore, as anaerobic metabolism increases so does the production of lactate. Systemic lactate accumulation is associated with decreased survival of patients because it reflects the lack of oxygen available for aerobic metabolism.

So, since it is clear that molecular oxygen must be continuously available to body tissues and cells in order to maintain aerobic metabolism, monitoring oxygenation in patients has to be a primary nursing concern. Many interventions are directed towards this goal in the acute care setting where accurate assessment and treatment of oxygenation disturbances may determine a patient's survival. Understanding the principles of oxygenation is crucial to the nurse's knowledge base.

The transport of oxygen and disposal of carbon dioxide to and from the organs and tissues of the body depends on effective pulmonary and cardiovascular functioning. This includes ventilation of the alveoli, diffusion of gases across the alveolar capillary membrane, perfusion of blood to the lungs, and gas transport to the tissues. These sequential steps to oxygenation can be expressed as:

- *oxygen uptake* – a means for extracting oxygen from the environment into the delivery system;
- *oxygen transportation* – a mechanism by which this uptake results in the delivery of oxygen to the cells;
- *oxygen utilization* – a metabolic need for molecular oxygen by the body cells.

For the sake of clarity the oxygenation process will be examined here using three stage headings.

- **Ventilation** is the movement of air from the atmosphere to the lungs' alveoli.
- **External respiration** is the diffusion of oxygen in the air from the alveoli, across the alveolar capillary membrane to the plasma, and its subsequent binding to the haemoglobin in the red blood cells.
- **Internal respiration** is the diffusion of oxygen from the arterial blood in the capillaries to the tissues and cells. Once inside the cells, oxygen is used to produce energy required for cell metabolism.

ACTIVITY   ?

Consider patients you have cared for whose condition compromised their ventilation (breathing). Make a list of the conditions.

The list you produced might look something like this:

- asthma
- chronic obstructive pulmonary disease (COPD)
- chest wall injury such as a flail chest segment or pneumothorax
- spinal cord injury
- Guillain–Barré syndrome
- head injury.

ACTIVITY   ?

Consider patients you have cared for whose condition compromised the diffusion of gases across the alveolar–capillary membrane. Make a list of the conditions.

The list you produced might look something like this:

- adult respiratory distress syndrome (ARDS)
- fluid aspiration
- pulmonary oedema
- atelectasis
- pulmonary embolus
- inhalation burns
- pneumonia.

ACTIVITY   ?

Consider patients you have cared for whose condition caused a drop in their serial haemoglobin count and in the ability of the blood to carry oxygen. Make a list of the conditions.

The list you produced might look something like this:

- haemorrhage
- haematological disorders, such as leukaemia
- inappropriate fluid replacement
- carbon monoxide poisoning
- haemoglobinopathies, such as sickle cell disease.

ACTIVITY   ?

Consider patients you have cared for whose condition compromised their cardiac output. Make a list of the conditions.

The list you produced might look something like this:

- hypovolaemia
- acute myocardial infarction
- cardiac tamponade
- dysrhythmias, such as atrial fibrillation and tachycardia
- septic shock.

ACTIVITY   ?

Consider patients you have cared for whose condition compromised the internal respiration process. Make a list of the conditions.

The list you produced might look something like this:

- hypovolaemia
- disseminated intravascular coagulation
- septic shock.

Ventilation consists of two phases: *inspiration* (the period when air is flowing into the lungs) and *expiration* (the period when gases are leaving the lungs). Alveolar ventilation is a mechanical process dependent on volume changes occurring in the thoracic cavity. When a change in volume occurs there is a corresponding change in pressure that in turn leads to a flow of gases to equalize the pressure. Boyle's law (an ideal gas law) provides an explanation for this relationship between volume and pressure: in a large volume, the gas molecules are far apart and pressure will be low, but as the volume decreases the molecules are compressed and the pressure rises. This forms the basis for inspiration and expiration.

Numerous gases that make up the Earth's atmosphere surround all of us. Each of these gases has its own *molecular weight*, and each gas is pulled down towards the centre of the Earth by gravity. *Atmospheric pressure* is the collective pressure exerted by all these gases. This pressure equals 760 mmHg at sea level (i.e. the downward force of all these gases will support a column of mercury 760 mm high). *Respiratory pressures are always described relative to atmospheric pressure.* For example, a negative pressure of minus 4 mmHg means that the pressure in that area of the lungs is 4 mmHg lower than atmospheric pressure (760 mmHg – 4 mmHg = 756 mmHg). *Remember that a respiratory pressure of zero is equal to atmospheric pressure.*

Mechanics of ventilation

To examine the principles of breathing (ventilation) the nurse must first understand the role of lung pressures in this process.

Ventilation is the process by which gases are exchanged between the atmosphere and lung alveoli. This flow of air occurs as a direct result of a *pressure gradient*. When the atmospheric pressure is greater than the pressure inside the lungs, then we breathe in (inspiration); when the pressure inside the lungs exceeds atmospheric pressure we breathe out (expiration).

Inspiration

The diaphragm is the major muscle of ventilation, but the accessory muscles of ventilation including the scalene, sternocleidomastoid, trapezius and pectoral muscles also provide a great reserve. As inspiration begins, the diaphragm and the external intercostal muscles contract. Contraction of the diaphragm causes it to be pulled down, increasing the volume of the thoracic cavity. Contraction of the external intercostal muscles elevates the anterior end of each rib causing the rib to be pulled upward and outward. This causes an increase in the anteroposterior diameter of the thorax. This overall expansion of the thoracic cavity causes the pressure inside the lungs to fall from 760 mmHg to 758 mmHg.

During normal breathing the pressure between the two pleural layers of the lung is always sub-atmospheric (756 mmHg). This is known as the *intrapleural pressure*. The overall increase in the volume of the thoracic cavity just before inspiration causes the intrapleural pressure to fall to 754 mmHg. This fall in pressure creates a partial vacuum that causes the lungs to be sucked outwards. Movement of the pleurae also aids expansion of the lung volume.

This overall increase in lung volume and consequent reduction of pressure within the thoracic cavity causes a pressure gradient to be set up between the

lungs and the atmosphere. Air then rushes from the atmosphere into the lungs in an attempt to make the pressure both inside and outside the lungs equal (Fig. 2.2).

Expiration

Because inspiration is initiated by muscle contraction it is referred to as an *active process*. Expiration, on the other hand, is largely a *passive process* determined more by the natural elasticity of the lungs than by muscle contraction.

As the inspiratory muscles relax, the diaphragm and external intercostal muscles resume their initial resting length, the rib cage descends and the lungs recoil. This results in a reduction in thoracic and lung volume with subsequent compression of the alveoli. This causes the intrapulmonary pressure to increase until it finally exceeds atmospheric pressure. Again this creates a pressure gradient between the lungs and the atmosphere which forces gases to flow out of the lungs. This causes a decrease in thoracic and lung volumes, and a normal resting phase resumes where atmospheric and lung pressures are equal (see Fig. 2.2).

Factors influencing ventilation

Several factors such as airway resistance, lung compliance and elasticity and alveolar surface tension may influence the passage of air between the lungs and the atmosphere, and therefore alter the efficiency of pulmonary ventilation.

Airway resistance

As already mentioned, the amount of gas moving in and out of the alveoli is determined by changes in pressure gradients between the alveoli and the atmosphere. Indeed, very small changes in pressure cause very large changes in the volume of gas flow. For example, a change in pressure of only 4 mmHg can bring about a gas flow of 500 mL into the alveoli. However, gas flow is influenced not only by changes in pressure gradients but also by airway resistance. The relationship is represented in the following equation:

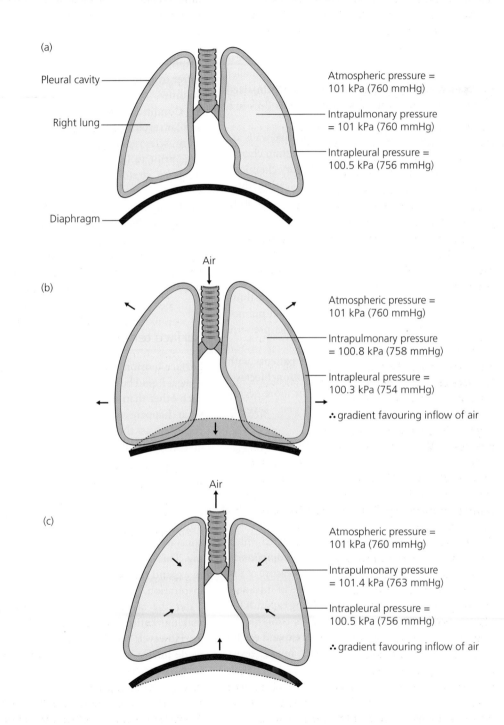

Figure 2.2 Pressure gradients during inspiration and expiration: (a) at end of normal expiration; (b) during inspiration; (c) during forced expiration

$$\text{gas flow} = \frac{\text{pressure gradient}}{\text{resistance}}$$

Airway resistance is determined by the diameters of the airway. In the larger air passages where the diameter of the airways is greatest, airway resistance is minimal and has little effect on gas flow. In the smaller air passages, for example in the medium-sized bronchi, airway resistance can influence air flow to a greater extent.

The smooth muscle cells of the bronchial walls are very sensitive to neural control and to certain chemicals. If we inhale irritant and inflammatory chemicals then our immune system responds by releasing *histamine*. Histamine release is part of the inflammatory response aimed at destroying the irritant. However, histamine also causes the smooth muscle cells of the bronchi to constrict, resulting in a narrowing of the airways. Narrowing of the airways increases resistance to air flow. This is the typical response of a person suffering an acute exacerbation of asthma where bronchial constriction is so great that pulmonary ventilation is inhibited despite the pressure gradients.

Mucus plugging of the airways in patients with bronchitis, pneumonia, asthma and bronchiectasis also increases airway resistance and in more severe cases pulmonary ventilation can be severely compromised.

Assessment and management of the patient with inefficient pulmonary ventilation will be examined in more detail later in this chapter.

Lung compliance and lung elasticity

Healthy lungs are very stretchy. The ease with which they can be expanded is defined as *lung compliance*. More specifically, lung compliance is a measure of the change in lung associated with a change in intrapulmonary pressure where the more the lung expands for a given rise in pressure the greater its compliance. High compliance means that the lungs expand easily, low compliance means that the lungs resist expansion.

However, lung compliance is determined not only by how stretchy the lungs are but also by the size of the thoracic wall, and any condition affecting either of these factors will affect lung compliance. For example, adult respiratory distress syndrome (ARDS), a form of respiratory failure that results from direct or indirect pulmonary injury, is characterized by stiff lungs. The lung tissue loses its ability to expand, resulting in decreased compliance. This in turn results in diminished pulmonary ventilation as a result of reduced tidal volumes. Similarly, patients with emphysema characterized by fibrosed lung tissue suffer from inelastic lungs and therefore lowered tidal volumes.

Conditions affecting the thoracic cage can cause similar results. For example, paralysis of the intercostal muscles reduces the outward movement of the rib cage prior to inspiration, reducing the space for the lungs to stretch into and therefore lowering tidal volumes.

Lung elasticity will also affect lung recoil during expiration. Reduced elasticity will make this process less effective, and the residual volume of air (i.e. the air left in the lungs following expiration) will be increased. However, elasticity and thoracic size are not the only determinants of lung compliance.

Surface tension

Surface tension is created when the liquid molecules at a gas liquid boundary are more strongly attracted to each other than they are to the gas molecules. This is what happens at the alveolar wall, which can be regarded as the gas liquid boundary. Imagine the alveoli as air-filled bubbles lined with water. The attractive force between the water molecules lining the alveoli causes them to squeeze in upon the air within the bubble. The attractive force is known as surface tension. The surface tension makes the water lining resemble highly stretched rubber. This rubber constantly tries to shorten and resist further stretching. This cohesion and tension makes it very difficult to expand the alveoli, and therefore the lungs during inspiration. Indeed, if the lining was made entirely of water the alveoli would collapse between breaths, making ventilation largely ineffective.

However, the liquid film lining the alveoli is not made purely of water but also contains a substance called surfactant. This is a lipoprotein produced by type II alveolar cells. It acts to reduce the surface tension by lessening the cohesive bond between the water molecules on the alveolar surface. This increases total lung compliance, enabling ventilation to be more effective, while also preventing total collapse of the alveoli on expiration.

Unfortunately, problems occur when insufficient amounts of surfactant are present. Adult respiratory distress syndrome is characterized by limited surfactant production. This causes surface tension to rise and as a result a number of alveoli collapse. This requires that the collapsed alveoli be completely reinflated on inspiration. This demands increasing amounts of energy, which in an already compromised patient can lead to exhaustion and worsening pulmonary insufficiency.

This principle can be explained by examining what happens when you blow up a balloon. When the balloon is new out of the packet and is completely deflated, the effort required to inflate the balloon is great. Once the balloon starts to inflate, filling it with more air becomes easier. When the balloon deflates again it never collapses as fully as when new and reinflating it is always easier.

External respiration

When inspiration is complete, oxygen diffuses from the alveoli into the blood for transportation around the body. Carbon dioxide is transferred from the blood into the alveoli for removal from the body during expiration. This 'external respiration' is optimized by several factors.

Fick's law, which describes diffusion through the tissues, states that the rate of transfer of a gas through a sheet of tissue is proportional to the tissue area and the difference in gas partial pressure between the two sides, and inversely proportional to the tissue thickness. The area of the blood–gas barrier in the lung is large, measuring between 50 and $100\,m^2$. Equally important is the thickness of the blood–gas barrier, more commonly referred to as the 'alveolar–capillary membrane', which is only $3\,nm$ thick in some parts. Together these form the ideal dimensions for diffusion.

The partial pressure of oxygen (Po_2) in a red blood cell entering a pulmonary capillary overlying an alveoli (deoxygenated blood) is $40\,mmHg$ and alveolar Po_2 is $100\,mmHg$. This creates a steep oxygen partial pressure gradient, which causes oxygen to diffuse from the alveolus into the red blood cell. The Po_2 in the red blood cell rises quickly until equilibrium is reached.

Carbon dioxide (CO_2) moves in the opposite direction, from the red blood cell into the alveolus, also as a result of a partial pressure gradient – since the Pco_2 of pulmonary deoxygenated blood is $45\,mmHg$ and that of the alveoli is only $40\,mmHg$. The carbon dioxide that diffuses into the alveolus is then eliminated during expiration.

For gas exchange to be most effective, ventilation (the amount of gas reaching the alveoli) and perfusion (the blood flow in the capillaries) must match closely. In alveoli where ventilation is inadequate the Pao_2 will be poor. In response to this, arterioles constrict and blood flow is directed to alveoli where oxygen uptake may be more effective. Alternatively, where alveolar ventilation is maximal pulmonary arterioles dilate, so increasing blood flow to the associated pulmonary capillaries. This *autoregulatory mechanism* exists to provide the most appropriate conditions for gas exchange.

When oxygen has diffused across the alveolar capillary membrane into the blood, it is carried in the red blood cells (bound to the haemoglobin) and dissolved in the plasma. Because oxygen is relatively insoluble in water, only 1.5 per cent is carried in the dissolved form, with 98.5 per cent being bound to haemoglobin.

Each molecule of haemoglobin can combine with four molecules of oxygen. The combination of haemoglobin and oxygen creates a substance called oxyhaemoglobin (HbO_2). When the first molecule of oxygen binds to the haemoglobin molecule, haemoglobin changes its shape. This change of shape makes it easier for the second oxygen molecule to attach itself to the haemoglobin molecule, which makes it even easier for the third to attach and easier still for the fourth.

When one, two or three sites are bound with oxygen the haemoglobin molecule is said to be *partially saturated*. Once all four sites are bound with oxygen the term changes to *fully saturated*.

In the same way that oxygen binding is enhanced as more sites become saturated with oxygen, so the removal of oxygen molecules at the tissues is made easier as more sites are unloaded with oxygen. The second oxygen molecule therefore is unloaded more easily than the first, and the third even more easily, and so on until all the oxygen has been unloaded.

Haemoglobin that has unloaded its oxygen molecule at tissue and cell level is referred to as *reduced* or deoxyhaemoglobin (HHb).

The next stage in external respiration, which will be examined in more detail in Chapter 1, involves the pumping of the oxygenated blood to the tissues (i.e. the cardiac output).

For delivery to be effective, the cardiac output – defined as the volume of blood ejected by either ventricle per minute – must be able to meet the current metabolic demands of the body. For example, if you are running for a bus then your metabolic demand will increase to give you more energy to run. Cells producing greater amounts of energy will need more oxygen. To increase the supply of oxygen to the cells your cardiac output increases. It is this ability of the body to alter cardiac output to meet metabolic demand that is central to the maintenance of tissue oxygenation.

In certain clinical conditions such as hypovolaemia, acute myocardial infarction and cardiac tamponade, this function is impaired and metabolic demand for oxygen can no longer be met. This results in *tissue hypoxia*.

Internal respiration

The final stage in the process of respiration involves the exchange of oxygen and carbon dioxide between the blood in the systemic capillaries and the tissue cells. The exchange results from diffusion driven by the partial pressure gradients of oxygen and carbon dioxide on each side of the exchange membranes.

As tissue cells use oxygen for metabolic activity they also produce equal amounts of carbon dioxide. This creates a situation where the Po_2 in the tissue cells is 40 mmHg due to the use of oxygen during metabolic function, and the Po_2 of the blood in the systemic capillaries is 104 mmHg. This results in the rapid diffusion of oxygen from the capillaries into the tissue cell that continues until equilibrium is reached.

At the same time, tissue cells are producing carbon dioxide as the end-product of cell metabolism. This results in a situation where the level of CO_2 in the tissue cells is greater than that in the blood, so CO_2 diffuses from the tissues into the blood until equilibrium is achieved.

Carbon dioxide is then expelled from the lungs during passive expiration. In a healthy individual the amount of CO_2 produced during cell metabolism and the amount expelled during expiration are equal. This state of equilibrium is known as *acid–base* balance.

Maintaining the acid–base balance

This part of the chapter examines the role of the respiratory system in acid–base balance.

Homeostasis

All functional proteins such as enzymes, haemoglobin and cytochromes are influenced by the hydrogen-ion concentration of their environment. The hydrogen-ion concentration is frequently expressed in terms of the pH of a solution, which is defined as a negative logarithm (to the base of 10) of the hydrogen-ion concentration:

$$pH = \log_{10} H^+$$

For example, a solution with a hydrogen-ion concentration of 1027 mol/L will have a pH of 7.0. A more acidic solution with a hydrogen-ion concentration of 1026 mol/L will have a pH of 6.0. Therefore, as the acidity increases the pH decreases and the change in pH from 7.0 to 6.0 represents a ten-fold increase in hydrogen-ion concentration.

Water is 'neutral' with a pH of 7.0. Solutions with a pH greater than 7.0 (i.e. solutions with a lower hydrogen-ion concentration) are called 'alkaline'.

*Extra*cellular fluid is slightly alkaline with a pH of 7.4. *Intra*cellular fluid tends to be slightly more acidic. At values outside of these limits, functional proteins reduce their ability to function and so biochemical reactions relying on their influence become less effective. In fact, a pH of less than 6.8 or greater than 7.8 is incompatible with life.

Therefore, *homeostasis* of pH is essential to survival. Indeed, for many seriously ill patients disturbance of this delicate balance can be life-threatening.

Regulation of blood pH

Despite the continual production of acid as a by-product or end-product of cell metabolism, the pH must be kept within normal limits. This balance is maintained through three systems:

* by chemical buffers in the blood;
* by the lungs;
* by the kidneys.

Chemical buffers are the immediate defence against acid base abnormalities, acting within seconds of the imbalance occurring. There are many systems in the body designed to buffer acids. These include:

- the bicarbonate and carbonic acid system;
- haemoglobins;
- plasma proteins;
- phosphates.

These buffers work by absorbing or releasing acid as required to maintain a normal pH. For example, if there is excess base or alkali in the blood the buffer system will release acid from buffering sites to mop up the excess alkali to a safe level. Alternatively, if there is excess acid in the blood then the buffer system will absorb the acid in an attempt to maintain pH homeostasis.

However, while they are an excellent short-term answer to acid–base imbalance, chemical buffers can maintain blood pH only for as long as they are available – so eventually other methods of restoring acid–base balance must be used. The lungs will attempt to resolve the imbalance within minutes of it occurring, followed by the kidneys hours or even days later. Therefore, effective functioning of both these systems is vital to the maintenance of acid–base balance.

Respiratory control of acid–base balance

As already mentioned, the respiratory system is responsible for eliminating carbon dioxide from the blood. Carbon dioxide, generated by cellular metabolism, enters the erythrocytes in the circulation and is converted to bicarbonate ions for transport in the plasma. This is shown by the following equation:

$$CO_2 + H_2O \rightleftharpoons H_2CO_3 \rightleftharpoons H^+ + HCO_3^-$$

The sign $\rightleftharpoons$ indicates a reversible equation. From the equation you will note that a reversible equation falls between dissolved CO_2 and H_2O on one side and H_2CO_3 (carbonic acid) on the other:

$$CO_2 + H_2O \rightleftharpoons H_2CO_3$$

A reversible equation also falls between H_2CO_3 and H^+ and HCO_3^-:

$$H_2CO_3 \rightleftharpoons H^+ + HCO_3^-$$

As a result of the reversible equation, an increase in any of these chemical substances will push the reaction in the opposite direction. For example, when CO_2 unloads in the lungs to be expelled during passive expiration, then the equation will shift to the left, and H^+ generated from H_2CO_3 will be reincorporated into H_2O. This means that hydrogen ions produced by carbon dioxide transport are not allowed to accumulate in the blood and therefore have little or no effect on the blood pH.

When a patient is unable to expel carbon dioxide, as a result of chronic obstructive pulmonary disease (COPD) for example, the high levels of retained CO_2 act as a stimulus on the medullary chemoreceptors in the brainstem. They respond by increasing both the respiration rate and depth of respiration in an attempt to try to 'blow off' the excess CO_2. In addition, a rising plasma hydrogen ion concentration resulting from any metabolic process, diabetes mellitus for example, will indirectly stimulate the respiratory centre, again causing breathing to become faster and deeper.

On the other hand, when the blood pH starts to rise (become more alkaline), then the respiratory centre will be depressed. As the respiration rate falls and breathing becomes shallower, then CO_2 will be allowed to accumulate. As CO_2 accumulates the reaction will be pushed to the right, causing hydrogen ion concentrations to rise once more. Again pH will be restored to within the normal range.

This method of maintaining an acid–base balance is an exceptional one and corrections to an abnormal balance are generally achieved within a minute or so. However, this method of control may be compromised by problems in the respiratory system. For example, any factor that causes a patient to hyperventilate – such as fear, anxiety or pain – will increase CO_2 elimination and the blood pH will rise. On the other hand, conditions such as chronic obstructive pulmonary disease, pneumonia or asthma will cause the patient to retain CO_2 and the blood pH will fall.

When the fall in blood pH is caused by an associated respiratory problem, then the person is deemed to have a *respiratory acidosis*. When the blood pH rises this is termed *respiratory alkalosis*.

The role of the kidneys in the maintenance of acid–base balance is examined more closely in Chapter 3. The next part of this chapter examines causes, signs and symptoms and treatment of patients with a metabolic or respiratory acidosis or alkalosis.

Assessing a patient with a respiratory disorder

Metabolic acidosis

This occurs when there is decreased bicarbonate, due either to increased loss or increased use in attempting to mop up or neutralize excess acid. Loss of bicarbonate may occur in patients with a fistula or severe diarrhoea.

Metabolic acidosis may also occur in patients with impaired kidney function. Ineffective urine excretion causes acid levels in the blood to rise as hydrogen ions formed during tissue metabolism accumulate. Diabetic ketoacidosis (an increased lactic acid production due to hypoxia, shock, heart failure or liver disease) may result in a metabolic acidosis due to the over-production of acid.

Patients suffering from metabolic acidosis may present with gasping respiration, lethargy, restlessness and disorientation, cardiac dysrhythmias, nausea and vomiting.

Treatment relies on being able to identify and reverse the metabolic acidosis. For example, if the cause is acute renal failure then dialysis may be indicated. Sodium bicarbonate may also be prescribed.

Metabolic alkalosis

This occurs where there is an increase in bicarbonate, as a result of acid loss or excess alkali.

- Causes of acid loss, resulting in an increase in the blood's pH, include diarrhoea and vomiting, prolonged, excessive nasogastric aspirations, gastrocolic fistula, and prolonged use of diuretics causing potassium ion (K^+) depletion (a low serum K^+ causes an increase in the excretion of H^+ ions instead of K^+ ions from the kidneys).
- Raised alkali levels may result from sodium bicarbonate administration and antacid abuse.

Patients suffering from a metabolic alkalosis may present with vomiting, restlessness, tremors, tingling of the extremities, tetany and convulsions.

Treatment is aimed at the primary cause. For example, where alkalosis is caused by over-ingestion of antacids then bicarbonate intake must be discontinued and acid fluids such as citrus fruit juices may be given. Where alkalosis is due to vomiting and diarrhoea then the cause must be treated, antiemetic and antidiarrhoeal drugs may be prescribed and appropriate fluid replacement treatment therapy maintained.

Respiratory acidosis

This is caused by carbon dioxide retention due to impaired ventilation resulting in an increase of carbonic acid in the blood. Impaired ventilation may result from conditions such as chronic obstructive pulmonary disease, emphysema and asthma which compromise gas exchange. Drug or alcohol overdose, trauma and neurological disorders such as Guillain–Barré syndrome and myasthenia gravis can also cause respiratory acidosis.

Respiratory acidosis may be characterized by a diminished mental state, drowsiness, muscle twitching, peripheral vasodilation and cardiac dysrhythmias.

Treatment is aimed at reversing the underlying cause of the acidosis. Typical examples are medication, correct patient positioning, chest physiotherapy and deep breathing. In more extreme cases it may be necessary to provide mechanical ventilatory support to help to 'blow off' the excess carbon dioxide.

Respiratory alkalosis

This occurs in patients who are hyperventilating, thus decreasing the level of carbon dioxide in the blood. Anxiety states, salicylate poisoning and pain are the most common causes of hyperventilation, but a neurological disorder such as a stroke, a tumour or breathing at a high altitude can also cause hyperventilation.

Symptoms of respiratory alkalosis may include impaired consciousness, seizures, increased muscle tone, tetany and hypokalaemia which may cause irregular heart rhythms.

Treatment is aimed at removing the underlying cause of the alkalosis. Typical examples are administering effective pain relief to reduce hyperventilation in a patient with pain, or asking an anxious patient who can breathe spontaneously to re-breathe his or her own carbon dioxide by breathing into a paper bag.

Arterial blood gas analysis

Arterial blood gas analysis ('ABGs') includes measurement of hydrogen-ion concentration (pH), partial pressure of carbon dioxide (Pco_2), partial pressure of oxygen (Po_2), bicarbonate (HCO_3) and base excess (BE). Normal ranges can be found in Table 2.1.

Table 2.1 Normal values of arterial blood gases

Measure	Value
pH	7.34–7.44
Pco_2	4.4–5.8 kPa
Po_2	10.0–13.3 kPa
HCO_3	20–24 mmol
BE (base excess)	−2.0 to +2.0

- Hydrogen-ion concentration or pH has already been defined.
- Pco_2 is an indicator of respiratory function and is a measure of acid secretion through respiration. A level of more than 6.0 kPa suggests too little ventilation resulting in the retention of CO_2. A level of less than 4.5 kPa indicates too much ventilation resulting in CO_2 dioxide being 'blown off'.
- Po_2 is not used in acid–base measurement but reflects the level of oxygenation in the blood.
- HCO_3 is an indicator of metabolic function. This is sometimes measured by means of the standard bicarbonate measurement (SBC). Here the plasma concentration is measured in relation to a normal Pco_2 of 5.3 kPa with fully saturated haemoglobin and at a temperature of 37.8°C.
- Base excess measures the degree of metabolic acidosis and alkalosis. It refers to the amount of acid or base/alkali that is needed to restore the pH to 7.4 at a normal Pco_2. Negative base excess, for example a BE of minus 5, is referred to as a 'base deficit' (acid surplus).

While pH does reflect the overall state of acidity or alkalinity of the blood, a normal pH alone does not necessarily indicate the absence of an acid–base disturbance. To have the whole picture, the pH, Pco_2 and HCO_3 must all be examined. If pH, Pco_2 and HCO_3 are *all* within the normal ranges then no acid–base disturbance exists. However, if any one of these values is abnormal then both the primary disturbance and the degree to which the patient is compensating for this acid–base disturbance must be determined.

Compensation

Compensation can be described as *total*, *partial* or *absent*. It relates to the degree to which one system, such as the respiratory or the renal system (metabolic system), is able to offset a change in the other and by so doing return the pH back to within normal limits.

When total compensation occurs the pH will fall within the normal range. However, theoretically total compensation is never complete because the pH will always fall closer to the side of normal that reflects the primary disturbance while still remaining between 7.34 and 7.44.

ACTIVITY ?

Determine the primary cause of the acid–base disturbance and the degree of compensation in the ABGs below:

- pH = 7.36 (normal, but close to the acidic side of the normal range);
- Pco_2 = 6.5 kPa (high, indicating respiratory acidosis);
- HCO_3 = 29 mmol (high, indicating metabolic alkalosis).

In this example the pH is normal but is closer to the acid end of the range (7.34–7.44), so if a disturbance is present it must be acidic in nature. The other parameters show that the level of CO_2 corresponds to a respiratory acidosis (i.e. the patient is retaining CO_2), while the level of HCO_3 is indicative of a metabolic alkalosis. The respiratory parameter is the one that matches the pH value (acidity) and is therefore described as the *primary disturbance*.

The metabolic alkalosis seen in this example occurs as the metabolic system attempts to compensate for the respiratory acidosis by retaining more HCO_3. Since the pH has been returned back to normal by the efforts of the metabolic system, this is defined as *total compensation*.

Remember that it may take the kidneys hours or even days to resolve an acid–base disturbance. As a consequence the attempted compensation by the metabolic system in this example would indicate that the respiratory disorder is chronic, not acute.

Partial compensation occurs when, despite compensatory efforts, the pH still remains outside the normal range.

ACTIVITY ?

Determine the primary cause of the acid–base disturbance and the degree of compensation in the ABGs below:

- pH = 7.30 (acidic);
- P_{CO_2} = 4.0 kPa (low, indicating respiratory alkalosis);
- HCO_3 = 17.3 mmol (low, indicating metabolic acidosis).

In this example the primary disturbance is a metabolic acidosis indicated by the low bicarbonate. The respiratory system has attempted to compensate for the imbalance of the metabolic system by 'blowing off' more CO_2, but this has not been completely successful because the pH value still lies outside the normal range, so the compensation is only partial.

A simple three-stage checklist helps with arterial blood gas interpretation, as follows:

1 Look at the pH. Is it normal, acidic or alkaline?
2 Determine the primary cause of the imbalance by checking the values of the other parameters. The parameter that matches the pH is usually the primary disturbance. For example, if the pH is acidic and the P_{CO_2} is elevated, then the primary cause of the imbalance will be the respiratory system.
3 Determine whether compensation has occurred. If it has, is it partial or complete?

While arterial blood gas analysis as described above provides valuable information relating to arterial oxygenation, it has drawbacks. The information is available only intermittently when the ABGs are taken. At times, in the acutely ill patient, this is not enough and other methods of monitoring the patient's oxygenation status are required.

Pulse oximetry

Pulse oximetry is a valuable, non-invasive monitoring technique that provides data rapidly. If used appropriately it enables the nurse to estimate the patient's arterial oxygen saturation and to follow trends of arterial oxygen saturation to help in assessing for hypoxia. It should not be applied to a patient unless the nurse is fully aware of both its uses and limitations.

It functions by positioning any pulsating vascular bed between a two-wavelength light source and a detector. The pulsating vascular bed, by expanding and relaxing, creates a change in the light path that modifies the amount of light detected. This produces the familiar waveform. The amplitude of the varying detected light depends on (a) the size of the arterial pulse change, (b) the wavelength of light used, and (c) the oxygen saturation of the arterial haemoglobin. The accuracy of pulse oximetry relies on several factors.

- The tissue must be reasonably transparent to the wave lengths of light being used. A finger, toe or ear lobe are the most common preferred sites. However, if the skin on the chosen area is thickened, for example on the fingers of a labourer, then the wavelengths of light may not be absorbed. In such instances a more suitable site must be selected.
- There must be pulsatile arterial blood within the tissues. If the patient is poorly perfused or hypotensive, for example, the reading may be inaccurate.
- Dark skin pigmentation, nail polish, nicotine-stained fingers and patient movement may all affect the accuracy of the reading.
- Arterial haemoglobin oxygen saturation levels of 85 per cent and above are accurate to within 1–2 per cent. However, as the saturation level falls below 85 per cent then the oximeter reading becomes less reliable.
- Delays can occur in the time it takes for the pulse oximeter to display any changes in arterial oxygen haemoglobin saturation. For example, if a patient has a drop in inspired oxygen concentration it may take up to 30 seconds for this fall in concentration to be detected by the pulse oximeter. In a seriously ill patient these 30 seconds could be vital.
- Flooding or extreme light directed at the pulse oximeter, direct sunlight for example, can cause a false reading.
- Using an incorrectly sized probe, such as a children's probe for an adult, will give an inaccurate reading.

- Abnormal haemoglobin will give a false reading. For example, a very small amount of carboxyhaemoglobin (COHb) will make the arterial haemoglobin oxygen saturation equal to 100 per cent. COHb is caused by inhaling even small amounts of carbon monoxide. Therefore the use of a pulse oximeter is not recommended in a patient who has been in or close to a fire, or has attempted suicide using car exhaust fumes, or is a heavy tobacco smoker.
- Other absorbants such as injected physiological dyes will cause inaccurate readings.
- Bounding veins and venules, as found in patients with tricuspid valve disease and hyperdynamic circulations, may cause inaccurate readings.

Guidelines for patient selection and knowledge of the limitations of pulse oximetry are central to the provision of safe nursing care and management. Pulse oximetry is an invaluable monitoring device when the data it provides are interpreted accurately and correctly, but a false reading can also cause a false sense of patient wellbeing and lead to poor nursing and medical management.

For example, one common misconception in clinical practice is that maintaining arterial haemoglobin oxygen saturation above 94 per cent is reassuring and can mean that the patient is clinically stable. However, an acceptable oxygen saturation does not necessarily imply adequate ventilation, tissue oxygenation, perfusion or oxygen transport.

So, in addition to monitoring devices nurses must also use their knowledge and skills to accurately assess a patient's clinical status. Objective measurements must be assessed in conjunction with other significant changes that may indicate ineffective ventilation and tissue hypoxia. These are summarized in Box 2.1.

Breath and chest sounds

Breath and chest sounds can be used as an additional indicator of abnormal or normal ventilation, and hence oxygenation status.

Auscultation

Auscultation (listening with the diaphragm of the stethoscope pressed firmly against the chest wall) is a

Box 2.1 Signs of ineffective ventilation and tissue oxygenation

- Absent or diminished breath sounds
- Decreased tidal volume and minute ventilation
- Change in respiration rate, depth and pattern
- Expiration time (In patients with any of the obstructive lung diseases, expiration time is 1.5 times the inspiration time.)
- Tachypnoea, defined as greater than 24 breaths/min
- Dyspnoea
- Air hunger
- Position of trachea (Is the trachea mid-line or is it deviated to one side or another? A pleural effusion or tension pneumothorax usually deviates the trachea away from the diseased side. Atelectasis pulls the trachea towards the diseased side.)
- Cough (Is it effective, or shallow and ineffective?)
- Cyanosis
- Low urine output
- Dysrhythmias
- Clammy, cold, sweaty skin
- Patient distress or anxiety
- Confusion
- Lethargy
- Drowsiness
- Coma

technique that allows the nurse to assess the intensity and loudness of the patient's breath sounds. Auscultation moves from side to side of the patient's chest and from top to bottom. The procedure needs to be performed on the anterior and posterior chest (Fig. 2.3).

First listen to the patient's breath sounds when he or she is quietly breathing. Then ask the patient to take a deep breath (but beware of hyperventilation). When a maximum deep breath is taken this will normally cause a four-fold increase in breath sounds. In patients with airway obstruction, chronic obstructive pulmonary disease or atelectasis, for example, the breath sounds will be diminished.

Restricting the movement of the diaphragm will cause diminished breath sounds in the area of restriction. This happens in obese patients and in pregnancy.

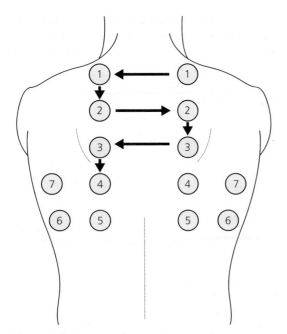

Figure 2.3 Locations for auscultation and percussion

Pleural thickening, pleural effusion, pneumothorax and obesity all insulate the breath sounds, making them less loud.

Normal breath sounds

Tracheal and bronchial breath sounds are most commonly heard over the trachea and mainstem bronchi. *Vesicular* breath sounds are heard throughout most of the lung and are the sounds the nurse is most likely to hear.

Abnormal breath sounds

Abnormal breath sounds are described as normal breath sounds that are heard in lung areas other than those in which they originate. When lung tissue loses its air (e.g. where alveoli fill with fluid, as in consolidation) it transmits high-pitched sounds more effectively. As a result bronchial breath sounds replace normal vesicular breath sounds in the airless areas. Therefore if a patient has lobar pneumonia, for example, bronchial breath sounds will be heard over the involved area rather than the normal vesicular breath sounds.

Added breath sounds

Added (also called adventitious) breath sounds can be:

- rales/crackles (fine or coarse, short interrupted crackling or bubbling sounds heard during inspiration);
- rhonchi (loud gurgling continuous noises in the larger airways, usually more prominent on expiration);
- wheezing (whistling noises);
- expiratory grunt.

Chest percussion

To percuss the chest you need to send vibrations through the chest wall. To do this, hyperextend the middle finger of your left hand and press its distal interphalangeal joint to the surface of the chest area. The middle finger of the right hand (called the hammer finger) now strikes the distal interphalangeal joint of the middle finger of the left hand using a quick, sharp, but relaxed wrist action. Both the anterior and lateral chest should be percussed, moving from side to side and comparing each as one moves along (see Fig. 2.3).

- In a healthy person the chest will give a hollow percussion note.
- If there is air in the chest (e.g. in a patient with a pneumothorax) the percussion note will be hyper-resonant (a drum-like sound).
- A dull or flat sound will occur when an area with no air is percussed. Atelectasis, pneumonia, a pleural effusion, thickened pleura or a mass lesion will all cause a percussion note to be dull or flat.

Chest palpation

Palpation is used to identify any areas of tenderness or deformity. With pleurisy, for example, tenderness will be felt over the inflamed pleura.

Palpation assesses the expansion and symmetry of the chest. This is performed by placing your hands on the patient's back, thumbs together at the midline, and asking the person to breathe deeply. Note the distance between your thumbs as they move apart during inspiration. A one-sided decrease in chest expansion may occur with diseases such as lobar pneumonia and pleural effusion.

Summary

We have established how important it is for a nurse to understand the physiological mechanisms fundamental to the delivery of oxygen to the tissues. We have also examined how the nurse can use this knowledge to assess the patient's clinical status and to interpret both objective and subjective measurements that may indicate a change in the patient's condition.

When performing a respiratory assessment the nurse must remember that a patient with an underlying *neurological disorder* with characteristic muscle weakness may not necessarily exhibit the usual signs of respiratory distress associated with an increase in the work of breathing. In such a patient the nurse must be able to observe for other indicators of ineffective ventilation.

Oxygen administration

This section examines the various methods available for administering oxygen therapy to a patient.

ACTIVITY ?

List as many methods as possible that are used for administering oxygen therapy to patients.

Principles

Oxygen is widely available and commonly prescribed by medical and paramedical staff. When administered correctly it may be life-saving, but oxygen is often given without careful evaluation of its potential benefits and side-effects. As with any drug, there are clear indications for treatment with oxygen and the method of delivery. Inappropriate dosage and failure to monitor treatment can have serious consequences, so vigilant monitoring to detect and correct adverse effects swiftly is essential.

When prescribing oxygen, the risk of carbon dioxide retention is regarded as secondary to the danger of severe hypoxaemia, which is life-threatening.

Following release of the British Thoracic Society's guidelines for oxygen use in adult patients, oxygen is required to be prescribed by *target saturation ranges*. These target ranges are based on the patient's actual clinical condition. For example, a patient with COPD may require a target saturation of between 88 and 92 per cent, whereas a patient with no lung disease may require a target saturation of 94–98 per cent. These

ranges satisfy their normal oxygen requirements in stable episodes of health. The target oxygen saturation enables therapy to be titrated for escalation and weaning by nurses, physiotherapists and medical staff appropriate to the patient's status. The BTS guidelines aim to reduce the risks surrounding oxygen therapy while prompting appropriate escalation and weaning of therapy in a timely manner.

Oxygen can be delivered in a variety of ways. Whichever method is chosen, it is essential that this is the most appropriate device. The oxygen delivery device should deliver a consistent concentration of oxygen and, as far as is possible, be comfortable for the patient. Oxygen delivery systems can be divided into low-flow systems and high-flow systems.

Low-flow systems

Low-flow systems include nasal cannulae and the medium-concentration (simple) face mask.

Nasal cannulae deliver 100 per cent oxygen at a flow rate that is commonly 1–4 litres per minute. Normal inspiratory flow rates vary from 25 to 30 L/min, which far exceeds the flow given by the nasal cannulae, so the patient also takes in room air to meet inspiratory demand. This means that the typical oxygen concentration available from the nasal cannulae is diluted down to between 24 and 40 per cent (although, because of variations in respiratory rate and depth, this is not accurately measureable).

Inspiratory flow rates will often increase during respiratory distress, sometimes exceeding 60 L/min, so that inspiratory flow demands of the patient will not then be met. Therefore, even if a patient is saturating satisfactorily, the nasal cannula is not the interface of choice. A Venturi mask should be used instead (described later) as this will deliver both the flow and oxygen required for the patient. Mouth breathing predominately takes over at flow rates exceeding 35 L/min, which is when patients have a need for a face mask or nasal high-flow interface, which are discussed later.

Nasal irritation and dehydration develop quickly when using dry oxygen. This increases airway resistance and places further physiological stress on the patient already under respiratory compromise. Therefore it is important that, even with nasal cannulae, the patient be assessed for nasal irritation and the oxygen interface changed if required.

A medium-concentration (simple) face mask works in a similar way to nasal cannulae. The mask delivers variable amounts of oxygen based on the flow rate that is set and the patient's respiratory rate and depth. Owing to this imprecision, the mask is usually used in theatres or postoperatively for short-term use. Its use with a patient who requires a specific oxygen concentration is not recommended. If the mask is set at a flow rate below 4 L/min there is a risk of rebreathing carbon dioxide. In an emergency situation these masks should not be used as they have no reservoir facility to give extra oxygen supply on demand from the breathless patient, and the percentage of oxygen delivered is less than that available by using a non-rebreathing mask. All things considered, these masks are not the interface of choice for ward care.

High-flow systems

The term 'high flow' in respiratory medicine is used to describe the provision of gas flow equal to, or greater than, that required by the individual throughout the respiratory cycle at various minute volumes. Systems that deliver high-flow oxygen include the Venturi mask, the high-concentration reservoir (non-rebreathing) mask and nasal high flow (NHF).

Venturi mask

Venturi systems provide an accurate form of gas delivery via set oxygen concentrations ranging from 24 to 60 per cent. They can if required be humidified via cold or warm nebulizers.

The mask works on the principle of the Bernoulli effect. Oxygen passes through a narrow orifice, producing a high-velocity stream that draws a constant proportion of room air in through the base of the Venturi valve. This air entrainment depends on the jet velocity (determined by the size of the orifice and the oxygen flow rate) and the size of the valve ports. This ensures that an exact percentage of oxygen is delivered to the patient.

The practitioner must ensure that the minimum correct LPM (litres per minute) is set for the desired percentage. If the patient is short of breath but saturating well, the practitioner can increase the LPM by 50 per cent up to 15 L/min, which increases the

flow the patient receives without affecting the oxygen percentage delivered. If the LPM is set below the minimum required amount stated on the mask for the set O_2 percentage, then the patient will not be receiving the desired amount of oxygen or the necessary LPM to relieve the acute shortage of breath.

At lower oxygen concentrations, the total flow rate received by the patient exceeds inspiratory demand. However, as the oxygen concentration increases up to 60 per cent, total flow rate reduces to around 30 L/min as less room air is entrained into the mask through the Venturi orifice, which is often inadequate at meeting the patient's inspiratory flow demands. Thus, the demands of a patient requiring higher levels of support are often not met and the patient can cascade into respiratory fatigue. It is advisable then to consider more intense respiratory support interfaces if a patient is deteriorating and showing progressively higher oxygen requirements. Such support may be gained via continuous positive airway pressure (CPAP) or non-invasive ventilation (NIV).

Reservoir mask

The high-concentration reservoir (non-rebreathing) mask is recognized by most institutions as the 'front-line' device to support the acutely deteriorating patient. It should be used in acute situations only and should be set at a flow rate of 15 L/min.

When a patient requires the non-rebreathing bag then a diagnosis and reason for the deterioration must be made. Prompt referral to a doctor, senior nurse, respiratory physiotherapist, outreach team, anaesthetist or cardiac arrest team should be made.

This mask is designed to deliver an oxygen concentration of between 60 and 90 per cent, depending on the patient's respiratory rate and depth. It is advisable not to reduce the flow below 15 L/min, despite manufacturers' claims that it can be used at between 10 and 15 L/min. This is because the patients who require this level of respiratory interface are unstable and should be given the maximum potential support the mask is designed to give, until otherwise stated by an appropriate clinician. The flow meter should never be set below 10 L/min as this reduces the ability for expired carbon dioxide to be flushed out from the mask into the atmosphere, resulting in the patient rebreathing it. Rebreathing carbon dioxide may push the patient into a narcosed state.

Before using this system it is prudent to ensure that all the valves on the mask are working and that the reservoir bag inflates and empties properly.

When the patient is ready to wean, the Venturi system is usually used to continue supporting the patient with a flow even if low concentrations of oxygen are required.

Nasal high-flow delivery

Nasal high flow (NHF) provides humidified oxygen therapy via the nasal passages using large-bore cannulae (unlike simple nasal cannulae that provide low-flow dry gas at 1–4 L/min).

Nasal high flow works by reducing the alveolar dead-space, which is achieved by setting the flow above the patient's own respiratory demands (30 L/min is the minimum recommended high-flow setting). The high flow of incoming gas flushes the anatomical dead-space with positive-pressure flow, resulting in support for the respiratory work. The high flow creates a positive-pressure nasopharyngeal reservoir of gas, allowing for immediate delivery of gas upon diaphragmatic contraction, bypassing the normal physiological dead-space. This 'storage' of positive pressure in the dead-space effectively reduces the anatomical dead-space, which subsequently improves fractions of alveolar gases (both carbon dioxide and oxygen). Furthermore, owing to the dead-space washout, NHF provides increased oxygen delivery compared with mask therapies, thereby reducing inspired oxygen requirements (Fig. 2.4).

Nasal high flow may require the patient who is experiencing increased respiratory demands to create less negative pressure within the thorax to stimulate adequate alveolar ventilation, resulting in decreases in energy expenditure and increasing the time to fatigue. This may prevent the patient from deteriorating into type I or type II respiratory failure.

To reduce the work of breathing for patients, NHF should be set greater than the patient's respiratory demands (30 L/min minimum setting). The flow generated will minimize the normal resistance associated with the nasopharynx. This reduction in resistance will reduce the resistive work of breathing experienced in both resting and exercising individuals.

Humidification

Inspired gases that are cold and dry (such as bottled medical gases) may cause bronchoconstriction, which counteracts the beneficial effect of NHF (dead-space washout and overcoming nasal inspiratory resistance). Therefore, NHF systems are humidified to the physiological environment of 44 mg/L at 37°C to prevent deleterious changes to the lungs. Ideally all oxygen therapy should be humidified to optimal humidity, but it is a costly option.

There is a significant energy cost associated with gas conditioning, so any high-flow support that exceeds the patient's normal ability to heat and humidity may compromise the patient's energy

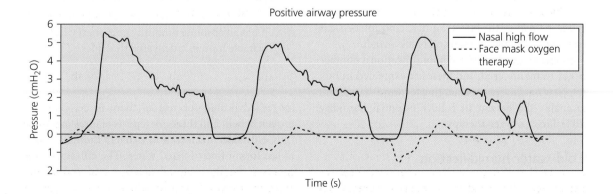

Figure 2.4 Pressure diagram for non-invasive ventilation (NIV)

resources and adversely affect his or her rehabilitation tolerance.

Heated humidification

The use of heated humidification is intended to maintain or restore the natural balance of the airway. In the normal airway, heat and moisture is added on inspiration, and this is recovered to some extent on expiration. However, the nasopharynx (the only part of the airway specifically designed for humidification purposes) can easily be overwhelmed by any increase in flow, drop in temperature or lower level of humidity for even relatively short periods. Patients remove their face masks, complaining of drying in the nose, and for this reason oxygen therapy protocols recommend that nasal cannulae should not be used for flows above 4 L/min. Patient compliance to treatment is, of course, a real benefit and is not unrelated to clinical outcome.

In all respiratory patients with compromised airways, maintenance of the mucocillary transport system is imperative as this will maximize the patient's ability to remove inspired pathogens and so reduce the risk of infection. Any patient with copious and tenacious secretions will benefit from heated humidification.

Infection risk is reduced also by the use of water vapour. Water vapour molecules have a size of 0.0001 microns, whereas cold-water nebulized systems produce droplets sized between 1 and 40 microns. Viruses and bacteria range in size from 0.017 to 10 microns, so a water droplet can transport these pathogens but water vapour cannot.

Another reason why heated humidification is beneficial is that it will optimize the lungs' capacity for gaseous exchange, as the airway resistance is not increased due to the effects of dry, cold inhaled gas and secretions will not pool and block alveoli.

When discussing heated humidification a number of key terms are used, and these are explained in Box 2.2. New modalities are emerging for ward based care to enable the patient to receive essential humidity (EH) during oxygen therapy.

Cold-water humidification

Humidification therapy in the ward environment is commonly delivered via cold-water nebulization or 'bubble-through' systems. However, the latter are no

Box 2.2 Terms used to describe humidity

- Absolute humidity (AH) is the total amount of water vapour in a given volume of gas in which it is contained. AH is measured as a mass divided by volume of gas (mg/L). When the water in a litre of gas is condensed out and measured in milligrams, ideally this would be 44 mg.
- Relative humidity (RH) is the actual humidity expressed as a percentage of what the gas could hold at the same temperature. For example, if a litre of gas could hold up to 44 mg of water vapour, but it actually contains only 11 mg of water vapour, then it is said to have a relative humidity of 25 per cent (11/44).
- Maximum capacity is the actual amount of humidity a gas can hold at a specific temperature and is stated in mg/L. A warm gas can hold more water vapour than a cold gas, which is why heated humidification compared with humidification alone is important.
- Optimal humidity is what the body expects in the lungs at 37°C. If the absolute humidity is 44 mg/L, this is expressed as '37/44'. This is critical for tracheostomy patients and those having nasal high-flow therapy.
- Essential humidity (EH) is the condition of the gas as it normally leaves the nasopharynx. If the nose is overwhelmed by any increase in flow, reduction in temperature or humidity, then the essential humidity is not achieved. EH is the condition of gas that needs to be supplied to the patient to prevent adverse effects. EH is considered to commence at 31°C at 100 per cent relative humidity, which means it has an absolute humidity of 32 mg/L. This is suitable for mask-delivered therapies.

longer advocated for use as there is no clinically proven benefit and there are reports of infection risks.

Cold-water nebulization delivers humidification in the form of aerosolized water. The efficacy of the gas carrying the water droplets is reduced as the temperature will vary from 12°C to 22°C, resulting in an absolute humidity of only 0.3–20 mg/L and a relative humidity of only 2–50 per cent (see Box 2.2).

An AH of at least 31 mg/L is required to avoid mucosal drying in the healthy adult, and we can expect this to be higher in the hospitalized patient.

Portable heated units can be applied to cold-water nebulization systems. However, the temperature is not measureable, the units are noisy, and much of the effectiveness is lost through heat dissipation and condensation.

Continuous positive airway pressure

Continuous positive airway pressure (CPAP) is a method of delivering oxygen therapy to a patient who has type I respiratory failure and who cannot be stabilized or reversed adequately with standard oxygen therapy alone. CPAP has in the past been a treatment delivered in high-care areas, but an increasing number of acutely unwell patients are seen now on wards, so more supportive means of delivering oxygen therapy need to be considered for ward-based provision. The future will see CPAP and other non-invasive ventilation methods being applied outside the high-care setting, which will allow more timely intervention for ward patients when required. Box 2.3 shows common indications, cautions and benefits of CPAP.

CPAP is a method of enhancing a patient's oxygenation by recruiting and utilizing more alveoli for gas exchange (external respiration). In its most basic form CPAP delivers a positive pressure of oxygen to the patient and prevents full exhalation, resulting in a predetermined volume of air being kept in the lungs. By preventing full expiration more alveoli can be used in the process of gas exchange, which increases the surface area for oxygen diffusion.

The amount of gas that is prevented from being exhaled is measured in centimetres of water pressure (cmH_2O). Typical settings for CPAP therapy range from 5 to 15 cmH_2O.

When a person exhales there is a certain amount of gas left in the lungs, known as the *functional residual capacity* (FRC). Continuous positive airway pressure simply enhances the FRC, which reduces with age, disease and poor positioning (supine or slumped). On increasing the FRC, inspiratory effort will be reduced. The idea of CPAP is to set the pressure to overcome the surface tension and resistance in the lungs by splinting open the conducting

Box 2.3 Common indications, cautions and benefits of continuous positive airway pressure (CPAP)

Indications
- Type 1 respiratory failure: $Pao_2 < 8\,kPa$
- Obstructive sleep apnoea (OSA): acts as a pneumatic splint to the airways
- Pulmonary oedema

Benefits
- Recruits and maintains the airways in an open state, throughout the respiratory cycle. It must be remembered that any true atelectasis will require higher pressures than that used in CPAP to recruit lung tissue. In such cases the physiotherapist can be called to recruit established atelectasis
- Improves alveolar gas exchange
- Allows more time for diffusion
- Allows the decrease in FiO_2 and subsequent risk of O_2 toxicity by using more surface area for gas exchange
- Decreases the intrapulmonary shunt, improving ventilation/perfusion matching
- Decreases the resistance to airflow, making it easier for the patient to inspire, so decreasing the work of breathing
- Maintains alveolar expansion in lungs with reduced surfactant production
- Redistributes extra-alveolar lung water
- Aids in unloading the myocardium in heart failure

Contraindications
- Undrained pneumothorax
- Subcutaneous emphysema: needs investigating

Cautions
- Bullae
- Bronchopleural fistula
- Recent oesophageal/bronchial surgery
- Large tumour in proximal airways
- Facial trauma
- Hypovolaemia

airways and alveoli so that the patient's inspiratory effort is used to produce a tidal volume and not wasted on overcoming resistance. This is particularly relevant when the patient has an elevated respiratory rate and the inspiratory time is significantly reduced, as the whole of inspiration can be used for alveolar ventilation.

If you examine a patient having CPAP you should be able to see an improved tidal volume almost immediately, if the pressure is set appropriately. It follows that, as the person is breathing on a more compliant part of the pressure volume curve, the work of breathing will be reduced. However, CPAP can be set too high for the patient, against which the patient must exhale. If there is too much positive pressure in the lungs the patient may recruit expiratory respiratory accessory muscles, which can quickly cascade the patient into excessive increases in work of breathing, respiratory fatigue, and type II respiratory failure. To prevent this it is important that the patient be assessed for expiratory effort and the CPAP adjusted accordingly to balance both inspiratory and expiratory requirements. Full observation monitoring and ABGs are required.

The tidal volume of the patient is entirely dependent on his or her own respiratory efforts. Despite CPAP therapy the patient may continue to deteriorate and fatigue into type II failure, requiring non-invasive ventilation.

Non-invasive ventilation

Non-invasive ventilation (NIV) is a treatment modality recommended by the British Thoracic Society (BTS) and the National Institute for Clinical Excellence (NICE) for the treatment of COPD patients in type II respiratory failure. However, increasingly NIV is also being used for a growing variety of clinical conditions that result in type II respiratory failure, including asthma, congestive heart failure, and weaning from invasive ventilation. NIV is used to help reverse type II failure, where the patient is unable to produce effective alveolar ventilation independently.

NIV provides ventilation support via the upper airway by using facial interfaces such as the full face mask, nasal mask, nasal pillows or a helmet. In acute type II failure, a full face mask is often used as the first-line therapy because there is a tendency for the patient to mouth breathe when demanding inspiratory flows of above 35 L/min.

NIV is essentially CPAP (described earlier) with pressure support. However, commonly the CPAP setting in NIV machines is often referred to as *expiratory positive airway pressure* (EPAP).

The pressure-support aspect of NIV aims to augment the tidal volume to improve alveolar ventilation and thus exhale carbon dioxide. It involves presetting the inspiratory positive airway pressure (IPAP), and then the patient triggers the pressure-support function in the ventilator by making a small inspiratory effort. This tells the machine to deliver gas under positive pressure until the preset IPAP is met. The machine then stops giving inspiratory support and the patient is able to expire. The *pressure difference* between the EPAP and IPAP is the pressure support; the larger the gap the greater the tidal volume. The clinician can increase or decrease the IPAP to achieve the tidal volume required by the patient to both rest the respiratory muscles and expel the carbon dioxide.

Box 2.4 shows common indications, cautions and benefits of NIV.

Care and treatment of patients with specific respiratory disorders

In the introduction to this chapter the three stages specific to oxygen delivery were considered: (a) ventilation (breathing), (b) external respiration, and (c) internal respiration. In what follows, each stage will be considered and clinical conditions identified that will compromise that stage. We will examine in turn the pathophysiology, assessment and nursing management of patients suffering from COPD, pneumonia and atelectasis.

Supporting a patient with chronic COPD

Chronic obstructive pulmonary disease is a leading cause of morbidity and mortality worldwide, especially in those aged over 40 years. There are probably 210 million sufferers worldwide, one million of them residing in the UK.

While it is generally accepted that tobacco smoking is a major risk factor, an estimated 24–45 per cent of patients with COPD have never smoked. Emerging evidence now suggests that other risk

Box 2.4 Common indications, cautions and benefits of non-invasive ventilation (NIV)

Indications in acute respiratory failure (type II failure)

- Acute exacerbation of COPD with respiratory acidosis (pH 7.25–7.35, $P_{CO_2} > 6.0$, H^+ > 45 mN) that persist despite maximal medical treatment and appropriate controlled oxygen therapy. Patients with pH < 7.25 or H^+ > 56 mN respond less well and should be managed in a HDU or ICU
- Hypercapnic respiratory failure due to chest wall deformity (scoliosis, thoracoplasty) or neuromuscular disease

Indications in acute respiratory failure (type I failure)

- Low arterial–alveolar (A–a) oxygen pressure gradient. Patients with severe, life-threatening hypoxaemia are more appropriately managed by tracheal intubation
- Cardiogenic pulmonary oedema unresponsive to CPA
- Weaning from tracheal intubation

Absolute contraindications

- Impaired consciousness with inability to protect the airway
- Life-threatening hypoxaemia
- Fixed obstruction of the upper airway
- Facial burns or severe trauma

Relative contraindications

- Recent upper gastrointestinal surgery
- Copious respiratory secretions
- Severe co-morbidity: is it appropriate, are the other conditions treatable?
- Confusion/agitation
- Bowel obstruction
- Pneumothorax: intercostals drain should be inserted
- Vomiting: uncontrolled/unpredictable
- Extensive fibrosed bullae

factors are important, such as smoke from biomass fuel, occupational exposure to dusts and gases, a history of pulmonary tuberculosis, chronic asthma, respiratory-tract infections during childhood, outdoor air pollution, and poor socioeconomic status.

What is COPD?

The definition of COPD has changed over the years, but there is now agreement that it is a lung disease characterized by chronic obstruction of lung airflow that interferes with normal breathing, is usually progressive, is not fully reversible, and does not change markedly over several months.

The more familiar terms 'chronic bronchitis', 'bronchiectasis' and 'emphysema' are no longer used officially, but are now included under the heading of COPD.

Care of a patient with COPD demands management from a range of individuals with various professional backgrounds. Optimizing the care of a patient with compromised lung airflow requires a range of functions that define the necessary multidisciplinary team activity. For the purposes of this discussion, multidisciplinary team activities include diagnosis and assessment, management of care, and palliative care of the patient.

Diagnosis and assessment of COPD

There is no single test to diagnose COPD, so the diagnosis relies on taking a history, physical examination and spirometry. COPD should be considered in those over 35 years of age with a risk factor (usually smoking), breathlessness on exertion, chronic cough, and sputum production – often with worsening of symptoms in the winter months (NICE 2004). Further factors need to be considered when confirming the diagnosis: weight loss, waking at night, ankle oedema, effort intolerance, and occupational risk.

The diagnosis is confirmed by a simple spirometry test. This measures how deeply a person can breathe in and how fast air can move into and out of the lungs. Spirometry should be considered in any patient who has symptoms of cough, sputum production or dyspnoea (difficult or laboured breathing), and/or a history of exposure to risk factors for the disease. Where spirometry is unavailable, the diagnosis of COPD should be made using all available tools. Clinical symptoms and signs, such as abnormal shortness of breath and increased forced expiratory time, can be used to help with the diagnosis. A low peak flow is consistent with COPD, but may not be specific to COPD because it can be caused by other lung diseases and by poor performance during testing. Chronic cough and sputum production often precede the development of airflow limitation, although not all individuals with cough and sputum production go on to develop COPD (WHO 2010).

NICE (2004) recommends the use of the Medical Research Council (MRC) dyspnoea scale as an aid to diagnosis. This scale grades the degree of breathlessness present in the patient measured by the level of exertion needed to generate it. A score of 1 equates with 'not troubled by breathlessness except on strenuous exercise', and a score of 5 equates with 'too breathless to leave the house, or breathless when dressing or undressing' (Box. 2.5).

Box 2.5 Medical Research Council scale for grading breathlessness (dyspnoea)

1 Not troubled by breathlessness except on strenuous exercise
2 Short of breath when hurrying or walking up a slight incline
3 Walks slower than contemporaries on the level because of breathlessness, or has to stop for breath when walking at own pace
4 Stops for breath after about 100 m or after a few minutes on the level
5 Too breathless to leave the house, or breathless when dressing or undressing

---

Medication for chronic COPD

Inhaled bronchodilator therapy

Short-acting bronchodilators are the initial empirical treatment for breathlessness and exercise limitation. If symptoms persist following this, treatment is increased to include either long-acting bronchodilators or combined therapy (a short-acting beta agonist and a short-acting anticholinergic).

Theophylline

Theophylline is used only after an unsuccessful trial with inhaled bronchodilator therapy, or in patients unable to tolerate inhaled therapy. Theophylline therapy requires plasma levels and interactions to be monitored.

Corticosteriods

- *Inhaled corticosteriods* should be reserved for patients with a forced expiratory volume (FEV) less than or equal to 50 per cent of predicted who are having two or more exacerbations of COPD in a 12-month period.
- *Oral corticosteriods* are not ususally recommended for patients with chronic COPD. People with advanced disease may require a maintenance prescription following an exacerbation.

Combination therapy for chronic COPD

Combination therapy is used in patients who remain symptomatic following single therapy. Effective combination therapies include the delivery of oxygen in various modalities.

Oxygen therapy

Long-term oxygen therapy

Long-term oxygen therapy (LTOT) is indicated in patients with:

- $Pao_2 < 7.3$ kPa when stable;
- $Pao_2 > 7.8$ and < 8 kPa when stable and also having one of the following conditions: secondary polycythaemia, nocturnal hypoxaemia measured by $Sao_2 < 90$ per cent for more than 30 per cent of the time, peripheral oedema or pulmonary hypertension;
- severe airflow obstruction measured by FEV < 30 per cent of predicted;
- oxygen saturations less than or equal to 92 per cent on air breathing.

Assessment of patients having LTOT requires analysis of ABGs taken on two occasions 3 weeks apart.

For LTOT to be of benefit, patients must breathe supplemental oxygen for a minimum of 15 hours daily. Greater benefit is seen in those who breathe supplemental oxygen for 20 hours a day.

Short-burst oxygen therapy

This should be considered only when a patient has periods of severe breathlessness that cannot be corrected by any other treatments.

Non-invasive ventilation

NIV should be considered for patients with chronic hypercapnic ventilatory failure (i.e. those with chronically high levels of retained CO_2) who have required ventilatory support during disease exacerbation, or those who are on LTOT who are hypercapnic or acidotic.

Other management considerations

Pulmonary rehabilitation

This involves a multidisciplinary programme of care for patients with COPD (usually $\geq$ MRC grade 3). The programme includes physical training, disease education, nutritional advice and psychological support.

Vaccination and antiviral therapy

This includes the pneumococcal vaccine and annual influenza vaccine.

Lung surgery

Bullectomy can be considered for those with a single large bullae (diagnosed by CT scan) and a FEV < 50 per cent of predicted. Lung volume reduction can be considered for those with FEV > 20 per cent of predicted, $Paco_2$ < 7.3 kPa, and emphysema in an upper lobe.

Other treatment possibilities

- Alpha-1 antitrypsin replacement therapy
- Mucolyptic therapy
- Physiotherapy
- Self management advice.

Note that there is insufficient evidence to recommend treatment with prophylactic antibiotics for those with stable COPD.

Palliative care in COPD

In patients with end-stage COPD, unresponsive to other treatments, opioids should be used as appropriate to palliate breathlessness. The person should be supported with pharmacotherapy to manage depression and anxiety, and oxygen therapy. The patient, his or her family and carers will need access to a full range of services to support them during this end-stage of the disease. These will be provided by a multidisciplinary palliative care team and may include admission to a hospice.

CASE STUDY 2.1

Jack is aged 80 years and is known to have COPD. He is admitted to the Medical Admissions Unit with increasing shortness of breath. You are the nurse allocated to Jack. You note that he is very distressed and agitated with an increased work of breathing. He is pursed-lip breathing and using his accessory muscles. His breathing is noisy and he finds it difficult to speak in full sentences. Jack is also coughing and states that he has been producing copious amounts of thick green sputum.

- What observations and assessment would you undertake immediately?

Managing acute exacerbations of COPD

What is an acute exacerbation?

An exacerbation can be simply described as a worsening of symptoms with a change in the patient's baseline dyspnoea, cough and/or sputum. These changes are beyond the normal day-to-day variations, are acute in onset and may require a change in medication. In addition, NICE (2004) describe symptoms of increased sputum production and changes in sputum colour. Other signs and symptoms may include upper airway symptoms, wheeze, chest tightness, increased dyspnoea with exercise (more than baseline for that patient), fluid retention and increased fatigue. As respiratory distress becomes more marked the patient may exhibit acute confusion, new-onset cyanosis and tachypnoea.

Several micro-organisms are responsible for exacerbations, the most common being *Streptococcus pneumoniae* and *Haemophilus influenzae*. *Staphylococcus aureus* may be the responsible causative micro-organism during the influenza season, and *Pseudomonas aeruginosa* can also cause exacerbations. Known viral causes include rhinoviruses, influenza, parainfluenza, coronavirus, adenovirus and respiratory syncytial virus.

Exacerbations of COPD can be triggered also by common pollutants, especially nitrogen dioxide, sulphur dioxide, particulates and ozone.

Assessment of exacerbations of COPD

Observation

Along with the symptoms noted earlier, the patient may also demonstrate:

- pursed-lip breathing;
- use of accessory muscles (sternomastoid and abdominal) to aid breathing when at rest;
- new-onset peripheral oedema;
- marked reduction in activities of daily living.

In deliberate pursed-lip breathing the person inhales through the nose over several seconds with the mouth closed, and then exhales slowly over 4–6 seconds through pursed lips held in a whistling position. This slows down the respiration rate. That reduces the resistive pressure drop across the airways, thus decreasing airway narrowing during expiration and helping to reduce dyspnoea. The technique is useful during or following any activity that makes the patient tachypnoeic or dyspnoeic.

Auscultation

Relatively high-pitched wheezes throughout the chest may be heard on auscultation. This is consistent with narrowing of the airways. However, as airflow is very limited in patients with COPD the chest may be quiet, making auscultation more difficult (Bickley and Szilagyi 2009).

Percussion

Generalized hyper-resonance – where the percussion note has a very loud intensity, lower pitch and relatively long duration – is typically heard in the over-inflated lungs evident in COPD as a result of 'air trapping'.

Palpation

An increase in anterior/posterior diameter of the chest giving a barrel shaped appearance to the chest may be present. This affects ventilation in the patient as the thorax is unable to expand and recoil enough to create sufficient pressure gradients between the chest and atmosphere to aid the movement of gas in and out of the chest.

Vital signs

A low blood pressure, tachycardia, tachypnoea and arterial haemoglobin oxygen saturation (pulse oximetry) less than 90 per cent usually indicate of the need for hospital admission (NICE 2004).

ACTIVITY   **?**

In case study 2.1, observations of Jack identify fatigue, pursed-lip breathing and the use of accessory muscles. Auscultation reveals high-pitched wheezes throughout the chest. Generalized hyper-resonance on percussion and palpation reveals limited movement and an increased anterior/posterior chest diameter. Observation of vital signs notes tachycardia, tachypnoea, low blood pressure and an SpO_2 of 87 per cent. What further investigations would you suggest, if any? Should Jack be hospitalized?

Investigations for exacerbations of COPD

Chest X-ray

A chest X-ray is not recommended routinely for those presenting with an exacerbation of COPD, but it should be considered in the recovery stage for patients who are not making sufficient progress (SIGN 2005).

Arterial blood gas analysis

ABGs assess PaO_2, $PaCO_2$ and acid–base status. Repeat regularly if necessary. Generally a PaO_2 under 7.3 kPa or a $PaCO_2$ above 7.0 kPa with accompanying acute or acute-on-chronic respiratory acidosis suggests acute respiratory failure and is an indication for hospital admission (Wouters 2004).

Electrocardiogram

An ECG is recommended to rule out co-morbidities (NICE 2004).

Sputum culture

The evidence on sputum analysis is controversial, but it does seem to have a role in patients exhibiting an exacerbation of COPD. The main indication for sputum analysis is its purulence. Green sputum is a fairly reliable sign of a significant bacterial infection needing antibiotic treatment, whereas those with an exacerbation but no sputum purulence seem to improve without antibiotic treatment.

Blood analysis

- Consider blood cultures if the patient is pyrexial.

- Bloods: full blood count (FBC), white cell count (WCC), C-reactive protein (CRP), urea and electrolytes (U&E), liver function test (LFT), bone, glucose.

Management of exacerbations of COPD

Pharmacological

- Bronchodilator therapy: high-dose short-acting bronchodilators (NICE 2004; Wouters 2004; SIGN 2005).
- Antibiotics: recommended for any exacerbation causing increased dyspnoea, increased sputum volume and sputum purulence (NICE 2004; SIGN 2005; Quon *et al.* 2008).
- Oral corticosteroids: evidence suggests a reduction in hospital stay for patients prescribed prednisolone 30 mg daily for 7–10 days, but there is no advantage to prolonged corticosteroid treatment (Aaron *et al.* 2003; NICE 2004; Wouters 2004).

Oxygen therapy

- Oxygen should be given to maintain Sao_2 above 90 per cent. NICE guidelines state that oxygen should be prescribed for patients who are breathless during an exacerbation even in the absence of oximetry or arterial blood gas analysis (NICE 2004). However, within an acute environment pulse oximetry and arterial blood gas analysis are essential. ABG should be maintained at Pao_2 above 6.6 kPa without a fall in pH below 7.26, or at above 7.5 kPa if pH is within the normal range (Wouters 2004).
- Respiratory stimulants such as doxapram may be prescribed, but reports demonstrate only minor short-term improvement in blood gas partial pressures (Wouters 2004). In addition NICE (2004) recommend their use only when non-invasive ventilation is unavailable.
- Non-invasive positive-pressure ventilation (NPPV) as an adjunct to other treatment has shown favourable outcomes, including reduction in mortality, reduced risk of endotracheal intubation, shortened hospital stay (by more than three days) and reduced risk of treatment failure (Lightfowler *et al.* 2003; NICE 2004; Wouters 2004).
- Endotracheal intubation and mechanical ventilation in intensive care is appropriate for patients where NPPV is contraindicated or for those where NPPV is not successful.
- Physiotherapy using positive expiratory pressure masks should be considered for selected patients, to help with clearing sputum.

Supporting a patient with pneumonia

For ease of reference, conditions that may compromise external respiration can be divided into:
- those affecting the diffusion of gases at the alveolar capillary membrane;
- those affecting haemoglobin concentration and the ability of the blood to carry oxygen;
- those affecting cardiac output.

We now consider one of those conditions in detail.

What is pneumonia?

Pneumonia is a significant clinical and public health problem. It affects up to 11 in 1000 adults each year in the UK, especially during autumn and winter months. Pneumonia can affect a person of any age, but in some groups it is more common and can be more serious. Examples are:

- babies, young children and elderly people;
- people who smoke;
- people with other health conditions, such as a lung condition or a lowered immune system.

People in these groups are also more likely to need treatment in hospital.

Primary influenza pneumonia occurs most commonly in adults and may progress rapidly to acute lung injury requiring mechanical ventilation. Secondary bacterial infection is more common in children. *Staphylococcus aureus*, including methicillin-resistant strains, is an important cause of secondary bacterial pneumonia and carries a high mortality rate.

Defining and predicting pneumonia is difficult but important, and assessment of severity of pneumonia is key to the appropriate management of the disease. Consequently, several new predictive models and more sophisticated approaches to describing pneumonia have been proposed to be used in conjunction with clinical judgement. They include the Pneumonia Severity Index (PSI) to gauge patient

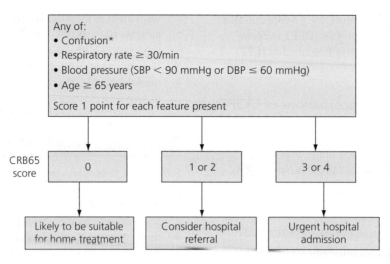

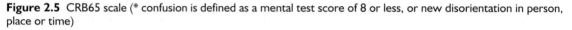

Figure 2.5 CRB65 scale (* confusion is defined as a mental test score of 8 or less, or new disorientation in person, place or time)

risk and necessary treatment, and the CRB65 (BTS 2009; Fig. 2.5).

Both those systems perform well, but the CRB65 has gained popularity because it is easy to remember and to compute, being based on four parameters: confusion, respiratory rate, blood pressure and age. If the patient scores 2 on the CRB65, hospital referral and admission should be considered. For those scoring 3 or more, urgent hospital admission is needed as their risk of death is high (BTS 2009). For a patient scoring 4 or 5, specific consideration for transfer to high-dependency care or intensive care should be made. In addition, patients with an oxygen saturation of less than 92 per cent also require urgent hospital admission.

The development of pneumonia depends on a pathogen reaching the alveoli and the host defences being overwhelmed by the virulence or size of the pathogen. Endogenous sources for the pneumonia-causing pathogen are nasal carriers, sinusitis, oropharynx, gastric or tracheal colonization, and haematogenous spread (Alcon *et al.* 2005). Infection causes inflammation of the alveoli and bronchioles, which in extreme cases causes hypoxaemia.

Symptoms can include raised temperature, hypoxaemia, tachycardia, tachypnoea, and flu-like symptoms. Most people with pneumonia will have an acute cough, purulent sputum, shortness of breath and chest tightness (BHF 2010). Occasionally patients may complain of a sharp pain in the side which

increases with inspiration; this is consistent with inflammation of the pleura (pleurisy).

Investigations for pneumonia

- Vital signs: temperature, blood pressure, respiratory rate, mental status and Spo_2 at least twice a day, but more frequently in those with severe pneumonia or prescribed oxygen therapy (BTS 2009).
- Chest X-ray: recommended to confirm the diagnosis, and where possible prior to antibiotic treatment (BTS 2009).
- Oxygen saturations and arterial blood gas analysis.
- Further blood sampling investigations, including urea and electrolytes (U&E), full blood count (FBC), C-reactive protein (CRP), and blood cultures (SIGN 2005; BTS 2009). CRP is the best test to distinguish between pneumonia and non-pneumonic lower respiratory tract infection.
- Sputum culture.

Treatment of pneumonia

- Antibiotic therapy is essential for patients with pneumonia (SIGN 2005; BHF 2010) and should be administered within 4 hours of confirmation of the diagnosis.
- Oxygen therapy is indicated, including

monitoring of oxygen saturations and inspired oxygen concentration to maintain Pao_2 above 8 kPa and Spo_2 at 94–98 per cent (BTS 2009).

- Intravenous fluid therapy is needed for patients where dehydration is evident.
- Nutritional support is needed especially where illness is prolonged.

CASE STUDY 2.2

Mary arrives at the walk-in centre and you are allocated as her nurse. She is aged 68 years, has an increased work of breathing and a respiration rate of 30 breaths/min. Her heart rate is 90 beats/min and her blood pressure is 150/60 mmHg. You use pulse oximetry to determine a saturation of 90 per cent.

- Calculate Mary's CRB65 score
- Describe your subsequent plan of care for her.

Supporting a patient with atelectasis

What is atelectasis?

The term 'atelectasis' originates from the Greek words *ateles* and *ektasis*, which translates to 'incomplete expansion'. Clinicians usually refer to atelectasis as diminished lung volume, which for the acute clinician is often highlighted secondary to increasing demands for oxygen therapy.

The incidence of atelectasis is not well known. Postoperative and lobar atelectasis are the most common types seen in the acute setting, with no predilection for race or sex.

The pathologies that causes atelectasis are multiple in origin. They can be divided into obstructive and non-obstructive categories (Table 2.2).

Atelectasis presents with a wide range of symptoms which depend on the cause, speed of onset, percentage of involved lung tissue and the presence or absence of infection. In slowly developing atelectasis, such as right middle lobe syndrome, there may be minimal or no symptoms. The most common types that exhibit in the acute wards are typically acute and require progressive intervention.

The treatment of atelectasis depends on the underlying aetiology so it is important to try to ascertain the cause. A chest X-ray is the crucial investigation that can guide the diagnosis as well as identifying the area of lung concerned.

Clinical assessment of atelectasis

The nurse must assess the airways to ensure that ventilation from the atmosphere to the alveoli can occur. This is the first stage in oxygen therapy.

Respiration rate

If there is a significant area of atelectasis, the nurse will note either a progressive or a sudden elevation in respiratory rate (RR) in an attempt to compensate for the hypoxia. Occasionally hypoxic vasoconstriction can fully compensate for the area of atelectasis, so the RR may be within normal range.

Auscultation and percussion

Both are extremely useful assessment tools to identify the extent and location of the pulmonary problem. Atelectasis commonly causes absent, diminished or bronchial breath sounds over the affected area, and if the collapse were due to secretions one may hear some added noises of crackles or sputum-induced wheeze. It is important to listen to the patient breathing at tidal breaths, deep breaths and after a cough to identify how reversible the condition is. For example, if the breath sounds improve on the deep breath and cough then the interventions required will be far less complex than if no change is heard at all. Percussion over the area auscultated can help confirm collapse, a dull percussion note indicating airlessness.

Palpation

Palpation of the thorax should reveal some changes in normal excursion over the area of collapse. The expansion may be diminished, or the inspiratory expansion delayed. There may be some accessory muscle involvement to overcome the lack of available expansion. If the patient is starting to fatigue, inspiratory recession may be noted with or without partial paradoxical movement.

Central cyanosis

In acute atelectasis the patient may demonstrate signs of central cyanosis from reduced ventilation, shortness of breath and difficulty speaking full sentences

Table 2.2 Pathologies causing atelectasis, divided into obstructive and non-obstructive categories

Category	Cause	Examples
Obstructive	Reabsorption of alveoli gas when communication between alveoli and tracheal is obstructed	Foreign body, mucus, tumour Obstruction of a lobar bronchus is likely to produce lobar atelectasis Obstruction of a segmental bronchus is likely to produce segmental atelectasis
Non-obstructive		
Relaxation or passive atelectasis	Elimination of contact between pleura, leading to decreased volume Generally the uniform elasticity of a normal lung will preserve lung shape	Pleural effusion, pneumothorax or large emphysematous bulla Pleural effusions are more likely to collapse the lower and middle lobes, whereas the upper lobe may be more affected by a pneumothorax
Adhesive atelectasis	Surfactant deficiency	ARDS results in decreased production leading to inactivation of surfactant production, leading to alveolar instability and collapse Other causes include smoke inhalation, prolonged shallow breathing, cardiac bypass surgery
Compression atelectasis	Space-occupying lesion of the thorax	The lesion will force air out of the alveoli The mechanism is similar to relaxation atelectasis Common conditions include loculated collections of pleural fluid, or chest wall, pleural or intraparenchymal masses
Cicatrization atelectasis	Diminution of volume as a consequence of severe parenchyma scarring	Conditions causing this include granulomatous disease, necrotizing pneumonia, chronic tuberculosis and idiopathic pulmonary fibrosis
Replacement atelectasis	All alveoli within a lobe are filled by tumour, resulting in volume loss	Can occur with bronchioalveolar cell carcinoma

because of the low saturations, and possibly airway obstruction if the hypoxia has resulted in a reduced consciousness level.

Fatigue

If there are signs of fatigue it is extremely urgent to consider more supportive methods of oxygen therapy, to reduce the risk of the patient developing type II failure, although this is extremely rare as a consequence of atelectasis.

Heart rate and temperature

Atelectasis that causes hypoxia will inevitably cause an elevated heart rate (HR) in an attempt to deliver more oxygen to the body. If the condition has been deteriorating over a few days the patient may be

hypotensive through insensible loss and lack of fluid intake, which could also cause a compensatory elevation in HR. If the nurse finds that the capillary refill time is not prolonged (returns in under one second) the tachycardia and hypotension may be the result of sepsis. This would be further confirmed by an increased temperature.

Abdominal distension

The nurse may identify an acute abdominal distension that may be the cause of atelectasis, in which case a surgical review should be prioritized. If the patient is found to have neuromuscular thoracic weakness, the nurse should consider using CPAP or NIV to help reverse and prevent atelectasis. The physiotherapy team will be able to advise on specific adjuncts of use.

Investigations for atelectasis

- Chest X-ray is the crucial investigation to diagnose the cause and extent of the atelectasis and help choose between treatment options. The nurse should request a portable CXR and ensure a doctor and physiotherapist review it.
- Oxygen saturations and ABGs will help in assessing the extent of the oxygenation problem.
- The patient should be cannulated and a full blood count (FBC) and urea and electrolytes (U&E) taken. If infection or sepsis is suspected, lactate, liver function test (LFT), C-reactive protein (CRP) and a clotting profile should also be taken. If sepsis is highly likely the nurse should also take blood for culturing.

Management of atelectasis

Interventions should be responsive to the clinical presentation. Airway manoeuvres and the use of adjuncts may be required,.

Intravenous fluids

Bolus and maintenance IV fluids should be initiated to restore circulation.

Patient positioning

Consider sitting the patient in a supported upright position, or preferably position the person in a 30- to 45-degree elevated three-quarters side-lying position with the atelectasis in the uppermost lung. This can help with ventilation and relax the patient.

Oxygen therapy

Oxygen therapy via a non-rebreathing mask is required until a full assessment has been made and stabilization has been achieved. Modalities potentially required to meet with pathophysiological response subsequent to extensive atelectasis may involve high-flow, CPAP or NIV. The nurse must be aware early on of the limitations of normal mask therapy and closely monitor for deterioration.

Some argue that high-concentration oxygen therapy can exacerbate the atelectasis by the displacement and washout of nitrogen. This is certainly a consideration, but until the full assessment has been made no assumptions of cause and therefore oxygen intervention should be made. The priority is to maximize saturations to prevent hypoxic damage.

Bronchodilator therapy

Bronchodilators decrease muscle tone in both the large and small airways and may increase ventilation, thus improving oxygenation.

Humidification, nasopharygeal suction and respiratory physiotherapy

The nurse should consider setting up humidification or saline nebulizers to help the mucocillary escalator to clear retained secretions. Consider whether the patient is unable to clear upper airway secretions. Respiratory physiotherapy is very effective at reversing collapse and sputum retention, so it is imperative to involve a physiotherapist urgently.

Medication

An antipyretic can be given if required. If an infection from atelectasis is confirmed, then an appropriate antibiotic should be commenced. If sepsis is suspected or confirmed, the sepsis bundle should be initiated immediately after cultures have been taken.

Pain is common with atelectasis. The degree of pain needs assessment and appropriate analgesia given. This is important because adequate pain control may enable the patient to take deeper breaths, to cough and to mobilize, which should be encouraged in an attempt to reverse the atelectasis.

Conclusion

Maintaining optimum oxygenation in acutely ill patients must be a primary nursing concern. This chapter provides the information needed to understand the physiological principles underpinning oxygen delivery, methods of assessing a patient's oxygenation status, and the skills needed to interpret the results. By using this information effectively the nurse will be able to intervene more appropriately and attempt to correct tissue hypoxia.

Nurses caring for acutely ill patients need to have the knowledge and skills that equip them to manage life or death situations. Appropriate nursing care can dramatically improve a patient's oxygenation and improve his or her outlook for recovery.

References

Aaron SD, Vandemheen KL, Herbert P *et al* (2003). Outpatient Oral Prednisone after Emergency Treatment of Chronic Obstructive Pulmonary Disease, *New England Journal of Medicine* **348**: 2618–25.

Alcon A, Fabregas N *et al* (2005). Pathophysiology of Pneumonia, *Clinics in Chest Medicine* **26**(1): 39–46.

Bickley LS, Szilagyi PG (2009). *Bates' Guide to Physical Examination*, 10th edn. London: Lippincott, Williams & Wilkins.

Bott J, Keilty SE, Brown A, Ward EM (1992). Nasal intermittent positive pressure ventilation, *Physiotherapy* **78** (2); 93–96.

BHF (British Heart Foundation, 2010). Available at www.bhf.org.uk/.

BTS (British Thoracic Society, 2009). *Guidelines for the Management of Community Acquired Pneumonia in Adults*. British Thoracic Society Report 1(3), London.

Global Initiative for Chronic Lung Disease (2008). *Global Strategy for Diagnosis, Management, and Prevention of COPD*. Available at www.goldcopd.org (accessed May 2010).

Higgins C (1996). Principles and practice of blood gas measurement, *Nursing Times* **92**(46); 45–7.

Huber G (1979). *Arterial Blood Gas and Acid–Base Physiology*. New York: Upjohn.

Lightfowler JV, Wedzicha JA, Elliott MW, Ram FS (2003). Non-invasive positive pressure ventilation to treat respiratory failure resulting from exacerbations of COPD. Cochrane systematic review and meta-analysis, *British Medical Journal* **326**; 185.

Marieb EN (1992). *Human Anatomy and Physiology*, 3rd edn, chs 3 and 23. California: Benjamin/Cummings.

NICE (National Institute for Clinical Excellence, 2004). *Chronic Obstructive Pulmonary Disease in Adults in Primary and Secondary Care*. Clinical guideline.

Parke R, McGuiness S, Eccleston M *et al.* (2009). Nasal high-flow therapy delivers low-level positive airway pressure, *British Journal of Anaesthesia* **103**; 886–90.

Place B (1997). Using airway pressure, *Nursing Times* **93**; (37), 42–4.

Quon BS, Gan WQ, Sin DD (2008). Contemporary management of acute exacerbations of COPD: a systematic review and meta-analysis, *Chest* **133**, 756–66.

SIGN (Scottish Intercollegiate Guidelines Network, 2005). *Exacerbations of COPD*. Available at www.sign.ac.uk (accessed May 2010).

Souhami RL, Moxham J (1990). *Textbook of Medicine*, ch. 14. London: Churchill Livingstone.

Tortora GJ, Anagnostakas NP (1990). *Principles of Anatomy and Physiology*, 6th edn, ch. 23. London: Harper & Row.

Walsh M (1997). *Watson's Clinical Nursing and Related Sciences*, 5th edn. London: Ballière Tindall.

West JB (1995). *Pulmonary Pathophysiology: the Essentials*, 5th edn. London: Williams & Wilkins.

World Health Organization (WHO) (2010). *Chronic Respiratory Diseases*. Geneva: WHO Press.

Wouters EFM (2004). Management of severe COPD, *Lancet* **364**; 883–95.

LEARNING OUTCOMES

On completion of this chapter the reader will:

1   understand the role of the kidneys in maintaining homeostasis

2   have an appreciation of the pre-renal, renal and post-renal causes of acute renal failure

3   have an understanding of the altered physiology of renal failure

4   be able to describe the management of a patient with acute renal failure

5   have an overview of the care of a patient with chronic renal failure.

Introduction

Renal failure, either acute or chronic, is a common problem. It presents a challenge in assessment and in the planning and implementation of care.

• Acute renal failure (ARF) has been shown to affect 1–25 per cent of patients in critical care, and mortality is 15–20 per cent (Kellum *et al.* 2008).

• Chronic renal failure (CRF) has an increasing incidence and is often associated with age-specific conditions and the increased survival rates in such conditions as diabetes.

The perception that renal dysfunction can be treated only by 'high-tech' interventions carried out by specialist personnel is being questioned. Rapid, conservative interventions have proved effective in the treatment of mild to moderate renal failure, while techniques such as haemofiltration have enabled critical care areas to instigate effective mechanical renal replacement therapy without recourse to renal units.

The number of patients with existing CRF and receiving long-term renal replacement therapy who present in acute nursing areas is increasing. This is due to the higher survival rates of CRF patients and the increasing age of initial presentation and treatment. Such patients often have other pathologies requiring interventions from other specialties and the subsequent need for high-dependency care.

The aim of this chapter is to outline the range of potential presentations of renal dysfunction, describe the conservative approach to the care of people in renal failure, identify the potential mechanical renal replacement therapies available that enable care to be initiated as soon as possible – to improve the ARF patients' survival rate and minimize the complications to longstanding CRF patients (Box 3.1).

ACTIVITY   ?

List the main functions of the kidneys.

Box 3.1 Three principles in care of a patient in acute renal failure (ARF)

- To treat the cause or causes
- To protect the patient from the consequences of the renal dysfunction in terms of the effects that ARF will have on other body systems, and ultimately the potential death of the patient from such problems as hyperkalaemia and cardiac overload
- To control homeostasis functions in the presence of very different demands as the ARF progresses through the stages to recovery

Basic anatomy and physiology

The kidneys provide a stable internal environment in the face of wide fluctuations in the intake of protein and its metabolism, the intake of water and electrolytes, and the body's production of hydrogen. In addition the kidneys have a major role in maintaining the body's *homeostatic status* in terms of calcium and phosphate, red blood cell production and the active control of blood pressure.

The means by which the kidneys achieve these functions lie in their highly vascular structure, their ability to control the movement of fluids through the semi-permeable membranes of their nephrons, and the way in which concentrations of substances stimulate the production of hormones produced directly by the kidneys or from other sites acting on them.

The kidneys are in the upper, posterior portion of the abdominal cavity on each side of the spinal column. Leaving them are the two ureters that extend down to the bladder. Entering the pelvis of each kidney is the blood supply of the renal arteries, which are branches of the aorta. The renal vein drains into the vena cava. Blood flow is approximately 20–25 per cent of the cardiac output, accounting for between 1000 and 1200 mL per minute in an adult.

The kidney structure is divided into two distinct areas (Fig. 3.1). The *medulla* consists mainly of the collecting ducts draining into the pelvis of the kidney. The outer layer, the *cortex*, contains the 'working units' of the kidney – the *nephrons*.

The nephrons are blind-ended tubes where they form the junction between the capillaries and the Bowman's capsule (Fig. 3.2). The capillary, as it enters the capsule, forms a fine meshwork, the *glomerulus*, through which filtration takes place. Blood pressure

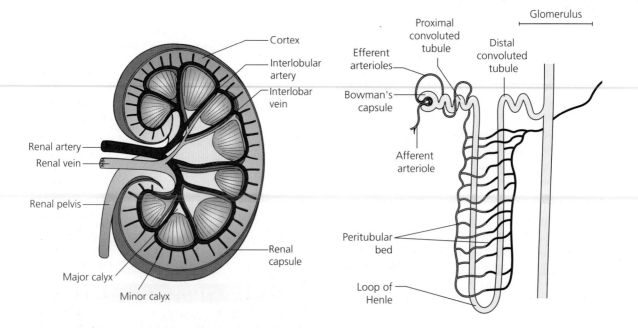

Figure 3.1 Structure of a human kidney

Figure 3.2 Structure of a human nephron

gives rise to the principal filtration force that drives plasma water, containing all substances smaller than plasma protein, through the capillary wall into the Bowman's capsule. The blood vessel then leaves the capsule and forms a capillary bed surrounding the nephron.

The three major processes in the production of urine are:

- filtration
- reabsorption
- secretion.

Filtration occurs across the glomerulus, reabsorption generally across the proximal and distal convoluted tubules, and secretion along the entire length of the nephron.

Reabsorption occurs as a result of the difference in osmotic pressure between the blood as it leaves the glomerulus and the much weaker filtrate within the tubule. Having lost approximately one-fifth of its volume, principally plasma water, the blood has increased its osmotic pressure from a normal value of 25 mmHg to 30 mmHg. The highly permeable walls of the proximal tubule allow the passive transport of water back into the circulation. In addition, active transport of sodium, glucose and amino acids ensures that 99 per cent of essential substances are also reabsorbed, so that the volume of the filtrate is reduced by approximately 26 per cent by the time it reaches the Loop of Henle.

Within the Loop of Henle the filtrate's concentration is altered by the 'countercurrent mechanism', which allows the movement of sodium and chlorine ions from the filtrate to the interstitial space and on into the circulation. In this way, body water is conserved.

The distal convoluted tubule is where the 'fine tuning' of homeostasis takes place under the influence of antidiuretic hormone and aldosterone. The movement of water back into the circulation from the filtrate is accompanied by an exchange of sodium and potassium into the filtrate as part of the systemic regulation of these electrolytes.

Within the collecting duct the final movement of water occurs in response to the osmotic gradients created in the Loop of Henle. At this point the filtrate is finally urine – water, salts, acids and nitrogenous wastes.

Functions of the kidneys

The main functions of the kidney are summarized in Box 3.2.

Box 3.2 Main functions of the kidneys

- Excretion of nitrogenous wastes: urea and creatinine
- Homeostatic control of water
- Homeostatic control of electrolytes
- Control of blood pressure
- Acid–base balance
- Erythropoiesis
- Vitamin D conversion to its activated form
- Calcium and phosphate homeostasis
- Excretion of drugs and toxins

Excretion of waste, drugs and toxins

The kidneys excrete nitrogenous wastes, urea, creatinine, 'middle-sized molecules' of unknown origin and larger molecules typified by B2 microglobulin, hippuric acid and parathormone. Drugs and toxins will also be excreted according to their size, protein binding and water solubility.

Fluid and electrolyte homeostasis

Fluid and electrolyte homeostasis, especially of sodium and potassium, occurs through the kidneys' response to antidiuretic hormone and aldosterone (Fig. 3.3). Increases in serum osmolarity, caused by fluid loss or increase in sodium concentration (also glucose), stimulate osmoreceptors in the hypothalamus. These in turn stimulate the ADH-secreting cells of the posterior pituitary gland. ADH is released into the circulation and travels to the tubule where it alters the permeability of the wall, resulting in a movement of water from the filtrate in the distal convoluted tubule and collecting duct back into the circulation. As a consequence of this, sodium is lost to the filtrate while potassium is reabsorbed with the water.

The action of aldosterone in the control of fluid homeostasis is closely tied to the control of *blood pressure* by the kidneys. Any fall in blood pressure threatens the filtration pressure of the kidney.

Therefore the juxtaglomerular cells, found in the capillary immediately leaving the glomerulus which is sensitive to pressure, secretes an enzyme (renin) directly into the blood. Renin then acts on a plasma protein to form angiotensin, which has two effects.

- The first effect is to produce vasoconstriction.
- The second effect is to stimulate the production

of aldosterone from the cortex of the adrenal gland.

Aldosterone then acts on the distal convoluted tubule, stimulating the reabsorption of water and increasing circulatory volume. As a consequence of this movement, potassium is lost to the filtrate while sodium is reabsorbed with the water. As both ADH

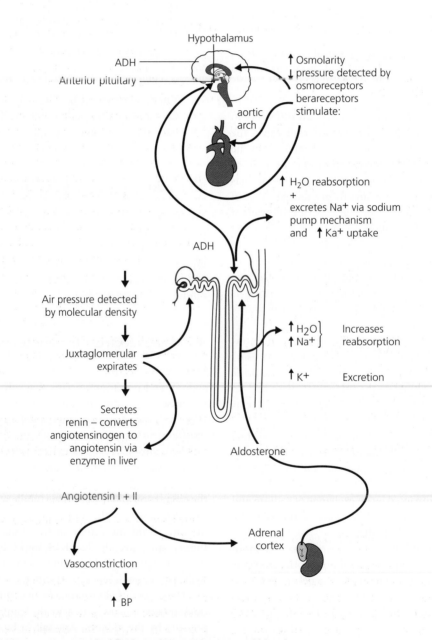

Figure 3.3 Homeostatic control of fluids, sodium, potassium and blood pressure

and aldosterone tend to work in conjunction with each other, not only is circulatory volume maintained but the balance between sodium and potassium concentrations is maintained despite the movement of such large volumes of water.

Acid–base balance

The metabolic processes of the body result in the production of high concentrations of hydrogen ions. These not only have to be excreted in order to maintain a blood pH of 7.4, they also need to be transported safely through the body to where they can be excreted. The kidney therefore serves two functions: the actual excretion of the hydrogen, as well as the production and maintenance of the means of such transport.

The wall of the nephron is the site at which hydrogen is transported into the filtrate by the process of secretion. The carbonic acid, a product of cellular metabolism, is split to form a 'free' hydrogen ion, which is passed into the filtrate, leaving behind bicarbonate, which is reabsorbed into the circulation.

This process is accentuated when there is an excess of hydrogen to be excreted through the production of ammonium. The nephron cells combine hydrogen with amino acids to form ammonia. This is passed into the filtrate where it picks up yet more hydrogen, forming ammonium. The overall effect is to acidify the urine, usually to a pH of 6.

The buffering system of the body relies on the availability of bicarbonate created by the kidneys, but also on the availability of the other principle buffers, plasma proteins and red cells. By conserving plasma proteins at the filtration level as well as providing the stimulus to the production of red cells, the kidneys have not only a primary role but also a secondary role in acid–base balance.

Erythropoiesis

Erythropoietin is a hormone responsible for stimulating the production of red blood cells in the bone marrow. Ninety per cent is produced by the juxtaglomerular cells in the kidneys, the remaining 10 per cent being produced by the liver. Sensors in the kidneys are stimulated by a fall in oxygen saturation

and increased amounts of erythropoietin are produced. This stimulates the bone marrow to convert stem cells into red cells. A peak in production will be achieved after about five days and continue as long as the hypoxia remains. Once hypoxia is corrected the production of erythropoietin returns to normal.

Control of calcium and phosphate homeostasis and vitamin D activation

Calcium has many functions in the body – not just for the development of bone but also in the regulation of the excitability of nerve fibres, contractions of the heart, blood clotting, and maintenance of normal membrane permeability. The body must have sources of calcium readily available not only from the diet but also from the internal 'stores' of the bones. Regulation of these sources is controlled by the kidneys.

Vitamin D, in its activated form, enables calcium to be absorbed across the gut wall. When the calcium has been absorbed it is stored within bone so that a consistent amount is available to the circulation in the face of an intermittent dietary supply. The relationship between calcium and phosphate in the serum regulates the rate at which the calcium is either liberated from bone or reabsorbed into bone through the action of the parathyroid hormone. Excess of either calcium or phosphate are excreted by the kidneys in response to the presence or absence of this hormone in a complex negative-feedback system. In a healthy body, serum calcium levels are maintained and the skeletal structure is remodelled continuously.

Acute renal failure: causes and classification

ACTIVITY ?

What would you expect to be the signs of renal failure?

In 2003, a survey in England and Wales of the management of acute renal failure (ARF) in the critically ill indicated that a change had occurred over the previous 10 years in the transfer rates of patients in ARF to specialist renal centres (Wright *et al.* 2004).

Patients, rather than being transferred, were more likely to be managed locally in acute and high-dependency units. There was also a trend for treatment to be managed not by nephrologists and renal nurses but by general medical staff, anaesthetists and acute and critical care nurses. This reflects the trend towards the use of continuous venovenous haemofiltration within high-dependency areas as a means of controlling a patient's fluid and electrolyte balance.

This change increases the demands on nurses undertaking the care of these patients. The key to effective planning and implementation of such care is an understanding of the causes and the effects of ARF.

Causes of acute renal failure

The classic approach to identifying the causes of ARF is to consider whether it is due to factors affecting the whole body (pre-renal causes), factors affecting the kidneys themselves (renal causes), or factors that produce problems in the renal tracts (post-renal causes). These factors are summarized in Boxes 3.3 to 3.5.

Definition and stages of acute renal failure

Acute renal failure – or 'acute kidney injury' (AKI) as it now tends to be called – is generally seen as a sudden or rapid decline in the renal filtration function. However, there has been difficulty in establishing an agreed definition in terms of its extent and severity.

In 2004, a conference of the Acute Dialysis Quality Initiative (ADQI) group developed a consensus definition and classification system that has gained extensive support. In order to assess the patient with

---

Box 3.3 Pre-renal cause of acute renal failure

- Severe reduction of renal perfusion due to hypovolaemia from loss of blood or plasma, therefore haemorrhage from trauma or surgery or burns
- Severe reduction of renal perfusion due to impaired cardiac function, following congestive cardiac failure, myocardial infarction, arrhythmias, pulmonary embolism, pericardial tamponade or cardiogenic shock
- Loss of glomerular perfusion pressure due to severe vasodilatation, which may be secondary to septicaemia, use of vasodilatory drugs or ACE inhibitors
- Vasoconstrictive effects of non-steroidal anti-inflammatory drugs(NSAIDs) used for analgesia, resulting in constriction of the afferent arteriole and therefore hypoperfusion of the glomerulus
- Fluid and electrolyte depletion due to extracellular fluid loss or dehydration, therefore bowel obstruction, severe vomiting and diarrhoea, gastric infections, fluid losses and volume shifts in pancreatitis and peritonitis (for example)

Box 3.4 Renal causes of acute renal failure

- Acute-on-chronic presentation of a pre-existing renal condition, often undiagnosed (e.g. glomerulonephritis, pyelonephritis, diabetic nephropathy, hypertensive nephrosclerosis)
- Inflammatory causes (e.g. the effects of infective agents such as *Streptococcus*, or vasculitic causes such as an acute presentation of polyarteritis nodosa, or systemic lupus erythematosus)
- Acute tubular necrosis due to prolonged pre-renal causes (see Box 3.3), including hypoperfusion, hypotension and hypovolaemia
- Effects of nephrotoxic substances such as myoglobulinurea and haemoglobinuria from crush injury and fractures
- Nephrotoxic damage from drugs such as antibiotics (particularly penicillin derivatives), paracetamol and radiographic contrast medium
- Toxic poisons from bacteriological sources such as *Clostridium welchii*, and substances such as organic solvents, ethylene glycol and mercuric chloride

Box 3.5 Post-renal causes of acute renal failure

- Mechanical or functional obstruction to the upper or lower renal tract (e.g. ureteric stricture, calculus, blood clot, retroperitoneal fibrosis, tumour compressing the ureters, benign prostatic hypertrophy, urethral strictures, or even obstruction of urinary catheters)
- Obstruction of the upper renal tract caused by intrarenal blockages brought about by such things as myeloma protein or uric acid crystals
- Damage to the nerve supply to the bladder and ureter through spinal cord damage or disease preventing adequate micturition and promoting retention

Box 3.6 The RIFLE classification

- *Risk.* Glomerular filtration rate (GFR) decreased by >25 per cent and creatinine increased to 1.5 times baseline. Urine output <0.5 mL/kg an hour for 6 h. In this situation the injury is still potentially reversible, so intervention strategies designed to prevent renal deterioration will help preserve renal function.
- *Injury.* GFR down by 50 per cent and creatinine increased to 2 times baseline. Urine output <0.5 mL/kg an hour for 12 h. At this stage a determination of whether the renal dysfunction is pre-renal in nature or intrarenal can help in preventing the development of tubular ischaemia and so acute tubular necrosis (ATN). Restoration of circulating volume, aggressive treatment of sepsis and removing neprotoxic agents could all play a part in the restoration of function.
- *Failure.* GFR down by 75 per cent and creatinine increased to 3 times baseline. Urine output <0.3 mL/kg an hour for 24 h, or anuria. At this stage the initiation of renal replacement therapy is necessary to correct the life-threatening symptoms associated with the cardiac effects of fluid overload, hyperkalaemia or metabolic acidosis, and the correction of other electrolyte imbalances.
- *Loss.* Persistent complete loss of renal function for more than 4 weeks. This criterion takes account of those patients who have pre-existing, underlying but undiagnosed renal dysfunction, as well as those whose renal damage is such that they become dialysis dependent even after the acute episode. As renal deterioration is also age-related, this group of patients could potentially increase in the future.
- *End-stage kidney disease.* Kidney disease for more than 3 months. This criterion is a logical extension of the 'Loss' phase in which permanent renal replacement is required.

acutely diminished renal function, a system of evaluation has been developed with the acronym RIFLE (Bellomo *et al.* 2004; see Box 3.6). RIFLE defines three grades of increasing severity of acute kidney disease: *risk*, *injury* and *failure* (the 'RIF' of the system). Two further aspects relate to the outcome variables: *loss* and *end-stage* kidney disease (the 'L' and 'E' of the system).

The classification includes separate criteria for creatinine and urine output. Changes in serum creatinine or changes in urine output, or both, can fulfil the criteria of AKI.

Urine and creatinine production

Urinary output can be a confusing sign in a patient with an acute kidney injury or acute renal failure. It can range from anuria to polyuria. However, certain changes to the urinary volume do suggest specific types of acute failure.

- Anuria with a daily output below 100 mL could represent lower urinary tract obstruction or even renal artery obstruction.
- Oliguria with a daily output below 300 mL suggests a pre-renal cause.
- Nonoliguria with a daily output above 400 mL could indicate acute interstitial nephritis, acute glomerulonephritis, or nephrotoxic and ischaemic acute tubular necrosis.

Further examination of the urine and blood can provide evidence of the potential site of injury. Pre-renal failure, characterized by hypoperfusion, will result in a change in the urea/creatinine ratio, from the normal 10:1 to greater than 20:1. This is due to the increased reabsorption of urea from slowly moving filtrate in the renal tubule.

Urine has a high osmolarity and specific gravity, while the urine sodium concentration is low and there are few, if any, sediments. This reflects the intact structure of the tubules which are attempting to respond to changes in the stimuli controlling their function.

Renal causes will be associated with oliguria or anuria with a normal urea/creatinine ratio – both, however, being raised. Urine osmolarity and specific gravity are low, indicating the failure of the tubules to concentrate the urine, while urinary sediment will show the presence of renal epithelial cells, casts and protein.

Post-renal causes will be typified by a normal urea/creatinine ratio (both being raised) and, as with pre-renal failure, urine osmolarity and specific gravity that are high. However, as time passes the urine will become less concentrated and the sodium content will rise. The oliguria may well fluctuate with polyuria with an output over 6 L a day, depending on the location and type of obstruction. Haematuria is a common feature in prostatic obstruction.

The progression of acute renal failure, from the disruption of urine formation to the recovery of function, is classically divided into:

- the oliguric/anuric phase;
- the diuretic phase;
- the concentration or post-diuretic phase.

Following the oliguric stage, after a period ranging from hours to weeks, the diuretic phase is marked by an increase of filtration. The tubules' ability to reabsorb remains compromised, however, so large volumes of dilute 'urine', which is more pure filtrate, is passed. It is during this phase that the principles of care appropriate to the oliguric stage are reversed in terms of fluid and electrolyte control and blood pressure regulation.

Finally the concentration or post-diuretic recovery phase is reached in which tubules recover the ability to reabsorb and to respond appropriately to hormone stimulation. This stage can last for anything up to a year before total control is re-established. During this phase there is usually sufficient normal function to ensure health.

Major effects of acute renal failure

To appreciate the assessment, investigation and management of patients with ARF, an understanding of the pathophysiology and of the three main causes of mortality and morbidity is essential. These are the cardiovascular impact, the effects of fluid disruption and the effects of acidosis.

Cardiovascular impact of ARF

The impact of ARF on the cardiovascular system is due largely to the effects of electrolyte derangement on excitation and contraction of the heart, and of the loss of glomerular filtration pressure, as a result of either hypovolaemia or congestive cardiac failure.

In the case of hypovolaemia (e.g. through dehydration or blood loss) or the vasodilatory effect of sepsis, the impact on the failing kidney will be the same as for the loss of circulatory pressure due to decreased cardiac output (see Chapter 1). Ultimately circulatory failure is the cause of death. In this situation the vasoconstrictive compensatory measures being brought about by the failing cardiac output result in further and rapid deterioration of cardiac efficiency. Peripheral shutdown occurs with cyanosis and hypotension. Any residual renal function fails and the patient's metabolism changes from aerobic to anaerobic, creating an exacerbation of the acidotic state brought about by renal failure. Cell membrane destruction and cell death herald multiple organ failure.

The effects of renal failure on the excitation and contraction of the heart are also life-threatening. Movement of nerve impulses along nerve fibres, as well as the contraction of heart muscle fibres, is the result of the movement of sodium and potassium from the intracellular to the extracellular spaces of heart and nerve cells. The rate of movement is determined by the availability of calcium. Therefore any disruptions of the levels of sodium and potassium have the potential to cause cardiac arrhythmias.

Of these, hyperkalaemia is the most dangerous. As the extracellular potassium concentrations increase, the cardiac cells depolarize to the extent that they cannot repolarize. Cells in this state are non-excitable, meaning that no further contractile activity occurs. Mild hyperkalaemia will result in 'tingling' sensations, muscle weakness or even frank paralysis, but it is frequently asymptomatic until cardiac toxicity occurs. Cardiac arrest may eventually result due to ventricular asystole or fibrillation.

In addition to these effects there will be a disturbance of the acid–base balance, and the excess of hydrogen ions results in metabolic acidosis (see Chapter 2). Further cardiac compromise will occur in acidosis through the effect of excess H^+ depressing myocardial contractility and via the action of ammonium formation, which is a normal part of the hydrogen cycle and the means by which excess hydrogen is excreted in the renal tubules. When there is renal dysfunction, ammonium formation still occurs but now it is liberated into the body to create inflammatory processes within the gut, pleura and, in this case, the pericardium. Pericardial rubs and effusions can result leading to pericardial tamponade. Finally, the disruption of the calcium metabolism that occurs in renal failure may contribute to the overall myocardial dysfunction in acute renal failure.

Effects of fluid disruption

In considering the fluid balance of the patient, attention must be given not only to volume but also to location and its availability for removal.

Initially the problem with fluid balance could well be one of classic oedema affecting the tissues, but progressing to left ventricular heart failure with pulmonary oedema. Alternatively the problem could be hypovolaemia due to dehydration, or volume loss due to haemorrhage or dehydration. This will present with hypotension, which soon becomes a problem of fluid overload in the face of increased fluid intake in the presence of oliguria. This, in turn, will result in generalized tissue oedema as the kidneys fail to regulate and excrete excess fluid, leading to raised central venous pressure (CVP). Pulmonary oedema will result in dyspnoea and the associated cardiac failure will exacerbate the situation.

In terms of 'location', consideration must be given to the ability of the fluid to move between the intracellular and tissue compartments and the circulatory system. The distribution of fluid between the three compartments of the body – the circulatory compartment, the interstitial compartment and the intracellular compartment – will be determined by a variety of forces that, in health, determine the correct hydration of all three. These forces include capillary

hydrostatic pressure, interstitial oncotic pressure, plasma oncotic pressure and interstitial fluid hydrostatic pressure – known collectively as Starling forces (Fig. 3.4). In addition, the lymphatic drainage and vascular compliance regulates the speed with which fluid moves through the tissues.

At the arteriolar end of capillaries, high pressure drives fluid through the semi-permeable walls into the tissues. However, as blood flows through the capillaries there is a pressure drop and so a reduction in filtration. The increased plasma oncotic pressure, generated by the concentration of plasma proteins increasing as fluid is lost from the circulation, brings about an osmotic gradient pulling fluid back into the arterioles.

If more fluid is absorbed than filtered, the overall blood volume increases. This is called 'passive refilling' since the process does not require energy and is a natural response to fluid depletion of the vascular compartment. The rate of refilling depends on the pressure in the capillary and interstitial space, the permeability of the capillary membrane and the oncotic forces established as protein concentrations are increased. Adequate plasma protein (albumin) is absolutely crucial for retention of fluid in the vascular compartment and the avoidance of oedema.

One of the key functions of cellular activity is the maintenance of osmotic equilibrium on each side of the cell membrane. If the concentration of an osmotically active solute is decreased in the extracellular space, a disequilibrium is established across the cell membrane. Water is then absorbed from the extracellular space into the cell to restore the equilibrium. The levels of these solutes in both the cellular and interstitial spaces 'lend' their relative strength to the fluid until equilibrium is restored.

The *lymphatic system* allows drainage of the interstitial spaces and the return of protein and fluid to the circulation which has 'leaked' into the tissues from the capillaries. An intrinsic pumping mechanism and series of one-way valves directs the lymph fluid back into the vascular space. The rate of lymph flow is determined largely by the pressure in the interstitial space. Normally the lymphatic system returns up to 4 L of fluid a day back to the blood, but in oedema this can be increased 20-fold.

In ARF the problems of fluid distribution and availability for removal concerns disruption of the hydrostatic forces, hypertension associated with overload or hypotension with its associated venous

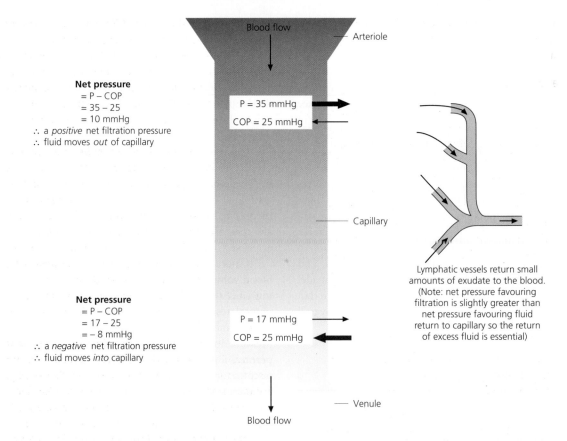

Net pressure
= P − COP
= 35 − 25
= 10 mmHg
∴ a *positive* net filtration pressure
∴ fluid moves *out* of capillary

Blood flow

Arteriole

P = 35 mmHg

COP = 25 mmHg

Capillary

Lymphatic vessels return small
amounts of exudate to the blood.
(Note: net pressure favouring
filtration is slightly greater than
net pressure favouring fluid
return to capillary so the return
of excess fluid is essential)

Net pressure
= P − COP
= 17 − 25
= − 8 mmHg
∴ a *negative* net filtration pressure
∴ fluid moves *into* capillary

P = 17 mmHg

COP = 25 mmHg

Venule

Blood flow

Figure 3.4 Fluid exchange between plasma and interstitial fluid across the capillary wall. The net movement of fluid into or out of the capillary will depend largely on the difference between the pressure favouring outward movement (the hydrostatic or blood pressure in the capillary, P) and that favouring inward movement (the osmotic pressure caused by plasma proteins, called the colloid osmotic pressure, COP)

'pooling' in the tissues. In addition there is a problem with the loss of serum protein (normal level 60–80 g/L) through catabolism, and therefore the loss of the osmotic 'pull' back to the circulation where the fluid would be available to any functioning tubules. This reduced osmotic gradient means that fluid forced from the circulatory system to the tissues by the hydraulic pressure of the heart remains trapped in the tissues, the result being intractable tissue oedema.

Hypoproteinaemia, associated with a fall in serum albumin to below 35 g/L, presents the problem of tissue oedema that is unresponsive to diuretics or mechanical methods of removal. It can occur as a result of specific renal disease causing proteinuria, such as nephrotic syndrome, or as a result of the effects of secondary causes of ARF resulting in gross protein loss, such as malnutrition or burns.

The classic presentation of problems associated with protein loss in renal dysfunction in the presence of non-oliguric output is that of the *nephrotic syndrome*. This is characterized by proteinuria with loss greater than 3.5 g per 24 hours resulting in hypoproteinaemia. The severe oedema resulting from loss of osmotic pressure is exacerbated by the loss of circulatory volume either to the tissues or from the osmotic diuresis that occurs resulting in polyuria. The corresponding hypotension stimulates the release of antidiuretic hormone and the subsequent reabsorption of water via tubules that are still functioning. At the same time the glomerulus will have responded to the fall in pressure by increasing the production of renin, resulting in increased production of angiotensin and aldosterone and a subsequent increase of sodium uptake and retention.

To summarize, the problems arising from fluid overload include the disruption of the regulatory functions that exacerbate the fluid overload problem, causing additional complications to patients' treatment.

Cardiac efficiency

The influence of cardiac efficiency on the control of fluid is related to the hormonal influence of aldosterone, the renin–angiotensin cycle, and their influence on blood pressure through changes in peripheral resistance and blood viscosity.

In normal renal function the features of volume control (in addition to those regulated by extracellular osmolarity as discussed above) are changes in circulatory volume and circulatory pressure.

Where there is a decrease in either sodium intake or blood pressure, the juxtaglomerular apparatus responds by releasing the enzyme renin, which leads, via angiotensin I, to angiotensin II.

Angiotensin II has two principal effects to bring about changes to the circulatory volume and pressure:

- active vasoconstriction of blood vessels, thus affecting peripheral resistance;
- stimulation for the release of aldosterone.

The point of the vasoconstriction is to reduce the loss of fluid in the filtrate by 'closing down' the afferent arterioles in order to reduce the filtration rate. In addition there is a systemic rise in blood pressure.

The aldosterone enhances sodium reabsorption in the tubules, which brings about a corresponding reabsorption of water, thus reducing plasma osmolarity and increasing circulatory volume. The effects of aldosterone tend to be slow and prolonged, lasting several hours, while the action of angiotensin in the stimulation of vasoconstriction produces an immediate effect on the blood pressure. In addition to these actions, aldosterone also produces an excretory effect on potassium.

Cardiovascular status

Fluid absorption, distribution and removal are, to a large extent, dependent on the adequacy of the cardiovascular status. If there is hypertension, as a consequence of either fluid overload itself or of overproduction of renin, then the capillary hydrostatic pressure is greater than the potential for the reversal of its effect by plasma oncotic pressure. In addition, the oedema and malnutrition reduce the ability of the tissues to generate an adequate fluid hydrostatic pressure to assist the return of fluid to the circulatory compartment. There is a further problem created by the failure of the disordered kidney to adequately control sodium. When there is hypernatraemia, the sodium will 'lend' its osmotic influence to the area in which it is contained (in this case the tissues), further reducing the efficiency of interstitial fluid oncotic pressure.

As the fluid overload increases, the cardiac efficiency reduces until blood pressure falls as a consequence of cardiac failure. Where there is residual renal function this fall in blood pressure is recognized and interpreted – incorrectly – as a need for an increase in water and salt. Renin is produced by the juxtaglomerular apparatus leading to a reabsorption of water and salt by the functioning nephrons. The consequence of this is a rapid deterioration in cardiac efficiency as the overload and hypernatraemia become worse, and so a vicious cycle continues to accelerate the damage.

In the case of renin/angiotensin-dependent hypertension – where the gradual destruction of the renal capillaries as a result of vascular disease (e.g. diabetic nephropathy) is the precipitating disorder – the principal effect will be a severe (accelerated) hypertension. Once again, the macula densa interprets the hypovolaemic situation to the glomerulus as a dehydration, giving rise to the increased production of renin. The resulting hyperaldosteronism, vasoconstriction, hypernatraemia and eventual fluid overload produces further damage to an already compromised kidney, hastening the ultimate destruction of viable renal tissue (Thomas *et al.* 2004).

Effects of acidosis

Metabolic acidosis is a feature of both acute and chronic renal dysfunction. The former produces life-threatening morbidities. The latter produces an underlying abnormal blood biochemistry that contributes to, and accelerates, other morbidities associated with renal failure, including anaemia, renal bone disease and hyperkalaemia. The mechanism of acid–base balance discussed earlier in the chapter will be challenged in acute renal failure in three ways.

- Metabolic acidosis induced by renal failure will increase muscle breakdown and therefore increase basal metabolic rate, thus increasing the production of H^+. In this way the acidosis will

Box 3.7 Effects of acidosis (Donald 2003)

Neurological

- Tinnitus, blurred vision, vertigo, lethargy, stupor, confusion, grand mal fitting, coma

Cardiovascular

- Decreased cardiac output due to reduced myocardial contractility, hypotension, congestive cardiac failure, bradycardia, reduced tissue perfusion
- Increased liberation of potassium from the cells combined with reduced potassium excretion leading to cardiac arrhythmias, ventricular fibrillation
- Irritation from increased ammonium production leading to pericardial effusions and tamponade

Pulmonary

- Increased stimulation of central and peripheral chemoreceptors that control respiration, leading to increased alveolar ventilation
- Kussmaul respirations, 'air hunger', intense respiratory effort, hyperventilation, respiratory failure
- Uniferous breath (acetone on breath), dry and coated tongue and oral mucosa
- Irritation from increased ammonium production, leading to pleural effusions

Gastrointestinal

- Gastric irritation, indigestion, anorexia, weight loss, increased metabolic rate, gastric ulceration and bleeding, diarrhoea, abdominal pain

Musculoskeletal

- Increased muscle breakdown with consequential increase in urea production, increased negative nitrogen balance, malnutrition
- Increased and accelerated renal bone disease due to increased stimulus to the parathyroid glands and production of parathyroid hormone
- Increased parathyroid cell production, leading to parathyroidism
- Increased stimulus to osteoclast activity and bone demineralization.

'feed' itself: the worse the acidosis the more rapidly the acidosis will progress. In addition, the renal damage to the tubules will reduce the ability of the kidneys to excrete fixed acids, those from the metabolism of dietary protein, and so the concentration of 'free' hydrogen in the blood increases.

- The production and maintenance of the buffers is compromised by, for example, bicarbonate production failing.
- The production of ammonia is disordered, leading to ammonium formation in the blood. This will create irritation of the gastric system, pleura and pericardium.

Consequences of acidosis (Box 3.7)

- In chronic renal failure, metabolic acidosis can result in a variety of changes in neurological, cardiovascular, pulmonary, gastrointestinal and musculoskeletal functions.
- In acute renal failure, the consequences of acidosis can rapidly prove fatal from disruption of the potassium control resulting in hyperkalaemia and cardiac arrhythmias.

Further systemic effects of ARF

Respiratory problems

Respiratory function is compromised in ARF due to fluid overload, pulmonary oedema and congestive cardiac failure, resulting in (initially) hyperventilation, then progressively to respiratory distress and eventually collapse. Tissue hypoxia, confusion and dyspnoea are all potential symptoms.

Hiccough is a particularly distressing symptom for the patient in ARF. The cause is unknown, but it is thought to be associated with a vasovagal stimulation. It can continue for days at a time and is extremely debilitating.

Central nervous system problems

Central nervous system disturbances are due to excess of metabolites, electrolytes and acidosis. The manifestation of CNS disturbance in ARF are sometimes ascribed to uraemia. The specific manifestations are confusion due to the high serum urea and creatinine, an increase in pH, and hypocalcaemia and hyperphosphataemia from the disturbance to the ability of the body to control calcium and phosphate homeostasis. Hyperkalaemia can result also in coarse muscle twitching and cardiac manifestations of ventricular arrhythmias or even fibrillation. Hypertension associated with fluid overload or an uncontrolled renin–angiotensin cycle can exacerbate the muscular twitching and cognitive disturbance, while the hypernatraemia can cause fluid to be drawn away from the brain into the vascular system by an increased osmotic gradient resulting in minute brain haemorrhages and convulsions.

Generalized neuromuscular weakness, lethargy and fatigue are symptoms of the overall toxic state of the patient, often accompanied by a reduced tissue saturation of oxygen from such things as blood loss, septicaemia, respiratory failure, or a loss of erythropoietin production causing a drastically lowered red cell count.

Digestive and nutritional problems

Gastrointestinal effects of ulceration, nausea, vomiting, loss of taste and anorexia are due to a combination of factors, primarily the initial insult that results in ARF, but then the effects of the failure. Here the ammonia of hydrogen metabolism fails to be excreted by the kidney and so it is accumulated in the body where it attacks the gastrointestinal tract. The acetone on the patient's breath (also a symptom of acidosis) reduces taste, while pulmonary oedema leaves the patient severely restricted when it comes to eating.

What makes these effects so dangerous in a patient in ARF is the effect on metabolism. The patient becomes hypercatabolic as he or she utilizes muscle mass as a source of energy, the body's requirement having accelerated due to the initial insult and now also as a result of the effects of ARF. This, in turn, accentuates the 'toxic background' of uraemia, driving up the levels of urea, creatinine and the hydrogen concentration, which in turn worsens the hypercatabolism.

Skin problems

The skin is compromised not only by the presence of oedema, especially over bony prominences, but also by the effects of acute disease processes resulting in ARF, and acidosis. Acute presentations of vascular disorders such as systemic lupus erythematosus (SLE) can result in purpuric rashes, while maculopapular rashes suggest either drug allergy or interstitial nephritis. Such rashes provide ample opportunity for skin breakdown, especially where there is severe itching and scratching. The reduced oxygenation of the tissues, which are waterlogged, and with a background of toxins is a perfect recipe for opportunistic infection and breakdown.

The effect of ARF on the immune response, with reduced macrophage activity, makes the treatment of such infections difficult, especially as antibiotics are nephrotoxic and could further compromise renal function.

Patient assessment and investigations in ARF

Attention must be paid to the cause of the renal insult and the needs generated by that cause. So, for example, a victim of trauma may well have haemorragic shock, have been subject to nephrotoxic drugs in the surgical stabilization of the injuries, received large doses of antibiotics and non-steroidal anti-inflammatory drugs postoperatively, and as a consequence developed acute renal failure. In addition to the care required with the original injuries, assessment of the effects of the ARF will generate very different requirements that must be taken into consideration if the patient is not to succumb to either permanent renal damage or death (Fry 2006).

Investigation results will take into account the RIFLE classification of changes to urinary output via the GFR and creatinine increases (see Box 3.6). However, other changes in both urine quality and content, as well as blood biochemical changes and other investigation findings, will help in the formulation of not only the diagnosis but also the specific clinical challenges that will require immediate attention.

Urine

- Urine is examined for changes to its specific gravity. A value above 1.020 could indicate pre-renal failure. A value between 1.010 and 1.020 could indicate intra-renal failure.
- A positive protein on reagent strips of 3+ or 4+ is indicative of intrinsic glomerular disease.

- Blood in the urine suggests a glomerular aetiology or lower urinary tract obstruction.
- White cells and casts point to interstitial nephritis, tubular necrosis or drug-induced nephropathy.

Blood chemistry

- Serum potassium (normal range 3.5–5 mmol/L) may well be raised owing to the failure of the kidneys to excrete the potassium load. There will also be a shift of intracellular potassium to the extracellular space caused by the acidosis associated with ARF, hypoxia, infection and an increased metabolism resulting in a catabolic state. Potentially lethal hyperkalaemia can result in increased myocardial excitability and arrhythmias, ventricular tachycardia and eventual ventricular fibrillation where the potassium is greater than 7 mmol/L.
- Serum sodium (normal range 135–147 mmol/L) can actually fall in ARF owing to the diluting effects of fluid overload and water retention. However, this may mask a total increase in total sodium within the body. The effects of such an increase will produce problems associated with the over-stimulation of antidiuretic hormone (ADH) and the stimulation of thirst and the active reabsorption of water from the tubules even in the presence of existing oedema.
- Serum creatinine (normal <120 ymol/L), and urea (normal <7 mmol/L) are recorded.
- Metabolic acidosis will be indicated by a fall in blood pH below 7.35 and a plasma bicarbonate below 22 mmol/L. This is due to failure to excrete hydrogen ions via the kidneys and a failure of the kidneys to conserve sodium bicarbonate.

These tests will give an indication of the presence of the renal dysfunction, but the speed of their elevation can indicate an immediate need to intervene clinically as in the case of hyperkalaemia and acidosis.

Haematology

- Haematology values will include haemoglobin (normal >12 g/dL) which will be decreased in cases of haemorrhagic causes of ARF or could indicate an acute-on-chronic aetiology.
- Elevated eosinophils (normal 2–4 per cent) could indicate acute interstitial nephritis.

- Leucocytosis, with a white cell count above $25–30 \times 10^9$/L (normal $3.5–9.5 \times 10^9$/L) is indicative of infective nephritis.
- Thrombocytopenia, with a fall in normal platelets below the norm of 150 000 to 450 000/mm^2, suggests inflammatory disease, while the presence of red cell fragments indicates other microangiopathies.

Circulation

Investigations into changes in the cardiovascular and circulatory volume status will include pulse rate and blood pressure recording, lying and standing. Examination of the jugular venous pulse, clarity of the lung fields, skin turgor and evidence of tissue oedema will be taken into account when establishing the presence of hyper- or hypovolaemia, as discussed earlier.

Imaging

An abdominal X-ray, along with ultrasound examination of the urinary tract, can help establish the nature of the renal failure. Small kidneys are usually associated with chronic failure possibly presenting as an acute-on-chronic condition. Normal sized or enlarged kidneys are indicative of acute failure, especially where there is no evidence of anaemia or other signs of chronic renal failure such as fatigue, pruritus, gastric ulceration and so on.

Electrocardiogram

An ECG will be recorded where there is any evidence of cardiac damage, either as a cause of the renal dysfunction (such as myocardial infarction) or where there is evidence of hyperkalaemia. The initial effects of hyperkalaemia on the ECG will be high and peaked T waves with a widening of the QRS complex.

Conservative management of acute renal failure

The first approach to care is to identify the specific cause or causes of the renal disruption and provide the specific therapies related to them. The second consideration is to protect the patient from the effects and consequences of the acute renal failure, enhancing any residual renal function or replacing it mechanically in order to, potentially, shorten the oliguric phase and to maintain the homeostatic functions, avoiding the lethal consequences of ARF.

Cardiovascular interventions will be aimed at either the correction of a hypotensive hypovolaemic state or the removal of excess fluid and the correction of the hypertensive state. These will be discussed in the section dealing with fluid disruption.

Other aspects of cardiac care in ARF centre on stabilization of the cardio-electrical control of the myocardium. Hyperkalaemia can be approached in four ways (Box 3.8).

Other cardiovascular impacts can result from disruption of coagulation or irritation of the gastrointestinal tract leading to bleeding.

Fluid management

What is required?

Fluid interventions will be based on correction of either the renal hypoperfusion resulting from hypovolaemia or the hypotensive effect of a reduced cardiac output as a result of fluid overload.

A careful estimation of fluid intake and output from all sources as far as is possible will be the first step in the establishment of fluid balance. Triangulation of this information, which is notoriously inaccurate, with the patient's daily weight and weight gain over short time scales will increase its accuracy. As 1 kg weight gain equates to about 1 L fluid gain, it is easy to identify fluid overload trends.

The association of fluid and blood pressure is a further measurement that can give greater accuracy to the assessment, but this must be supported by assessment of the location of the fluid. In order to achieve this, examination of serum total protein and serum albumin, as well as the normalized catabolic rate, will be of use to identify loss of fluid to the tissues in hypoproteinaemia and therefore the unavailability of the fluid to removal via mechanical or pharmacological means. Ultimately the hydration status will be accurately established through the measurement of the patient's central venous pressure.

Conservative therapy to address problems associated with the patient's hydration status will depend on whether there is evidence of dehydration, in which case a fluid intake sufficient to maintain a central venous pressure (CVP) between 5 and 8 cmH$_2$O will be required. The nature of the replacement fluid must be considered in relation to the evidence of the patient's serum protein, and human protein plasma fraction may well be in order, as well as the use of sodium chloride in relation to the patient's serum sodium.

Oral fluid intake has traditionally been based around the concept of a 500 mL loss through routes such as respiration and sweat, requiring replacement, with the rest of the fluid allowance being made up of the volume of the previous 24 hours' output. This approach, while providing a starting point, should

Box 3.8 Four approaches to hyperkalaemia (Fry and Farrington 2006)

- *Stabilize the myocardium.* The use of calcium gluconate or calcium chloride given as a slow infusion antagonizes the effects of potassium, so reducing the incidence of arrhythmias.
- *Reduce the potassium in the serum.* Since much of the potassium in ARF states is from the intracellular compartment, inducing it to return inside the cells will reduce the serum potassium level. Dextrose 50% and soluble insulin given as an infusion over 10–20 minutes will have this effect. This will buy only a few hours of time, so the cause of the migration of the potassium from the cells must be corrected during this respite. Careful monitoring of the serum glucose over the following 6 hours is also necessary.
- *Remove the potassium.* The kidney is not the only exit route for excess potassium in the body. The use of ion-exchange resins given either orally or rectally can induce the loss of potassium via the gut. Calcium resonium will exchange potassium for calcium or sodium across the gut wall and bind it to the stool. This is considered an approach suited to mild to moderate hyperkalaemia as it takes 2–3 hours to act, but is also useful in the maintenance of serum potassium once a reduction has been achieved.
- *Dialysis.* The final approach is to control the potassium, along with all the other electrolytes, via mechanical means.

not be ritualistically adhered to. Rather, fluid modification to meet the individual patient's needs, responsive to the physiological changes occurring throughout the genesis of ARF, is required. The problem with the formula '500 mL plus the volume of the previous 24 h' is that it makes no concession to fluid overload or dehydration but can simply maintain a fluid overload state or dehydrated state.

Enhancement of whatever renal function remains is of prime importance, not only in relation to fluid balance, but also the maintenance of other homeostatic functions. Correcting circulatory imbalances in order to minimize the effects of hypertension or hypotension will assist in maintaining glomerular filtration rate, while the use of loop diuretics, particularly furosemide or bumetanide, will enhance fluid removal. Potassium-sparing diuretics should be avoided. The thiazide groups are relatively ineffective once the glomerular filtration rate falls below 25 mL/h and may accumulate, causing side-effects (Thomas 2004).

In the case of poor renal perfusion due to cardiovascular causes, such as through left ventricular failure, hypovolaemia or cardiac ischaemia, agents such as noradrenaline and vasopressin may increase cardiac efficiency and also preserve renal function. There is no evidence that the use of dopamine is beneficial in such a situation (Lameire *et al.* 2003).

Tissue oedema is a particularly distressing feature of ARF, presenting problems in pressure area care and immobilization (McMillan 2007). Consideration must be made of where gravity puts tissue oedema. In a prone patient it can be found along the legs, sacrum, back and shoulders, and even in the scalp. More mobile patients will more likely present with the classic 'swollen legs'. To adequately address this problem, attention must be paid not only to volume but also the location of the fluid. As has been said, low serum protein levels will allow fluid loss to the tissues, which will prove difficult to remove, so the patient's nutritional status must be addressed.

Nutritional requirements

The problems of poor nutritional status in the acutely ill have been well-documented (e.g. Caimi *et al.* 2005), as have the consequences of such poor nutritional intake. Muscle loss and decreased body mass have been implicated in the development of depressed respiratory function, cardiac function and mobility. Subsequent impaired immune functioning associated with decreased nutritional intake has also been seen to contribute to chest infection, cardiac failure and increased risk of thrombosis and pressure sores. Apathy, depression and fatigue form the returning link of the cycle by further depressing nutritional intake.

In patients with ARF the problem is accentuated by their hypercatabolic state brought about by the initial physiological insult and the systemic effects of the renal dysfunction, such as cardiac failure, overload etc. (Krenitsky 2004). The problem of protein restriction used to reduce the workload on the renal system simply accelerates the hypercatabolic state. There is no benefit in protein restriction in catabolic ARF (Renal Association 2008); sufficient protein, nitrogen and carbohydrate sources must be maintained to compensate for catabolic loss.

Enteral feeding is the method of choice as it preserves the gastrointestinal barrier and so protects against bacterial infections. However, *total parenteral nutrition* (TPN) may be the only available route in the unconscious or ventilated patient. If so, then great care must be taken to take account of electrolyte content and to avoid overload, the potential for suppression of the immune response already suppressed by the ARF, and the danger of septicaemia.

Efficient prevention and treatment of malnutrition will make a major contribution to the patient's survival. It not only avoids the potential complications of catabolism, but also helps in the control of fluid balance by maintaining serum protein levels, and so allows for the oncotic shift of fluid between the cellular, intracellular and circulatory compartments of the body. In this way tissue oedema can be corrected through the enhancement of renal function or by mechanical replacement therapy, while in the hypoproteinaemic patient the fluid is not available for removal, trapped in the intercellular compartments.

Control of infection

Infection is a leading cause of death in patients with ARF (Sweeney *et al.* 2003). Common presentations are pneumonia, urinary tract infection (UTI) and wound sepsis, the progression of which are enhanced by the patient's immunosuppressed condition. Good nursing practice in the institution of central or peripheral venous lines and bladder catheters is essential.

Any evidence of infection should be treated with a narrow-spectrum antibiotic, care being taken as to the nephrotoxicity of such drugs and the appropriately modified dosage used. Broad-spectrum antibiotics, especially tetracycline, should be avoided owing to their severe nephrotoxicity.

Bladder catheters in the oliguric or anuric patient are contraindicated. They serve only as an irritant and potential source of a UTI. Frequent cultures of sputum, wound swabs and urine are required, and any early signs of infection (rise in temperature, fever etc.) should be acted on with speed. Early removal of lines (central venous pressure lines, venous cannulae, enteral feeding etc.) is recommended, as is early mobilization of the patient to alleviate the problems associated with bed rest and immobility.

Renal replacement therapy

Ultimately, the survival of a patient in acute renal failure may not be possible using conservative measures, even though the initial physiological insult may have been dealt with. The hypercatabolism, fluid overload, hyperkalaemia and acidosis can prove too great a stress on the body systems, resulting in multiple organ failure. Then, mechanical renal replacement therapy will be the treatment of choice to take over the main functions of excretion of nitrogenous waste, drugs and toxins, control of fluid balance, control of electrolyte balance and the correction of acidosis.

Mechanical renal replacement therapy is indicated where the extent of the symptoms of ARF have produced uncontrolled fluid overload, catabolic production of high urea and creatinine, severe acidosis and hyperkalaemia requiring such interventions as dextrose and insulin to prevent cardiac arrhythmias. In addition, in the face of malnutrition and oliguria, 'space' needs to be created to allow for adequate feeding, either orally with liquid supplements or intravenously via TPN (Vincente et al. 2008).

In the acute situation, renal replacement therapy serves as a rapid life-saving intervention. However, its use is generally restricted to areas where there is the necessary equipment and the expertise to use it is readily available, so it requires the infrastructure of an intensive-therapy unit, high-dependency unit or renal unit.

Types of replacement therapy

The available renal replacement therapies can be divided into the continuous and the intermittent, plus those used in combination. The indications for their use will depend on the specific demands created by the stability or instability of the patient's physiology (Box 3.9).

- The continuous systems are typified by *continuous venovenous haemofiltration* (CVVH) or *continuous venovenous haemodiafiltration* (CVVHDF).
- The intermittent systems are based on 'traditional' haemodialysis or the more recent haemodiafiltration. Intermittent therapies can be combined – with, for example, CVVH being interspaced with haemodialysis for a limited period daily or on alternate days.

All therapies rely on the formation of a vascular circuit from the patient's circulation, via a blood pump, through either an artificial kidney or filter and back to the patient. The porous membrane of this filter allows the passage of plasma water, electrolytes and waste products from the patient's blood to the other side and then removal. Depending on the system in use, a variety of forces are used to maximize the efficiency of such removal.

Continuous venovenous haemofiltration

In CVVH, the force of convection is the principle by which large amounts of solute (waste products, excess electrolytes etc.) are 'dragged' across the semi-permeable membrane of the filter from the circulation with the plasma water. The limiting factor is the volume of plasma water available in the circulation and the efficiency of its replacement from the tissues in response to this removal before a hypovolaemic situation is created.

CVVH will remove plasma water very efficiently through highly permeable membranes at a rate of up to 1–1.5 L an hour. When the patient's fluid overload has been corrected, the circulatory volume must be maintained via the delivery of a physiological electrolyte substitution fluid. This will also have the effect of

Box 3.9 Advantages and disadvantages of specific renal replacement therapies

Intermittent haemodialysis

- Rapid but 'aggressive' fluid removal. Can generate 'space' in the vascular compartment to be 'filled' in the periods between dialysis with nutritional support, such as total parenteral nutrition (TPN) or IV drugs.
- Efficient removal of waste products, but this effect will be compromised by hypercatabolic states creating a steep rise in uraemic toxins between dialysis sessions.
- Effective removal of excess electrolyte, thus correcting hyperkalaemia and hypernatraemia and aiding the correction of acidosis via the donation of bicarbonate to the patient from the dialysis fluid. Again, the effectiveness is limited by other physiological considerations during the intradialitic period, such as the movement of potassium from the cells to the serum under the influence of metabolic acidosis.

Continuous venovenous haemofiltration (CVVH)

- Controlled fluid balance that allows for continuous nutritional support, IV drug administration etc. Far more gentle in terms of fluid shifts within the body, and therefore greater control of blood pressure.
- Continuous removal of waste products which mimics glomerular filtration owing to the convective solute removal, therefore greater control of the 'uraemic' status.
- Continuous correction and maintenance of electrolyte balance, especially of potassium, sodium and hydrogen.
- The continuous need for anticoagulation during this therapy is a major consideration for patients with disrupted clotting patterns, recent surgery, bleeding problems, etc.

Continuous venovenous haemodiafiltration (CVVHDF)

- Offers either intermittent or continuous delivery of therapy combining the advantages of CVVH and haemodialysis. It has the additional benefit of allowing periods off therapy for patients requiring mobilization, or transfer from a high-dependency area to general care.

providing the volume for further fluid removal and so the continuation of the convective force generating the 'solvent drag'.

Careful calibration of the fluid removal with the fluid replacement means that haemodynamic stability is maintained despite the high filtrate production.

Haemodialysis

In haemodialysis the three forces of diffusion, ultrafiltration and osmosis are responsible for the removal of plasma water, waste products and excess electrolytes in a more 'controlled' way.

Diffusion of solutes from a higher concentration to a lower concentration allows the movement of excess electrolytes from the blood to a dialysate fluid, which flows on the opposite side of the semi-permeable membrane. As essential electrolytes are present at the 'correct' levels in the dialysate fluid, excess in the blood is lost but only down to this correct level. In addition, essential electrolytes, especially bicarbonate, will pass from the dialysate fluid to the blood to correct the sub-optimal level due to renal acidosis. As there is no 'waste product' present in the dialysate, urea, creatinine, middle molecules, B2 microglobulin and so on will be continuously lost to the dialysate.

Ultrafiltration is created by the drive of plasma water across the semi-permeable membrane through pressure generated in the artificial kidney by the blood pump. This positive pressure in the blood compartment of the artificial kidney is supplemented by the generation of a negative, or 'pulling', pressure in the dialysate compartment. Together they generate the total transmembrane pressure. Ultrafiltration has an action the same as convection in that it improves solvent removal through 'solvent drag'.

Osmosis facilitates the movement of plasma water as the dialysate is of a higher concentration than the blood. This difference in osmotic pressure is created by the presence of dextrose within the dialysate fluid. While this does not add in any significant way to the forces in haemodialysis, it does ensure that the movement of fluid will always be from the blood to the dialysate and never the reverse.

Haemodiafiltration

Haemodiafiltration applies the principles of convection as in CVVH and those of diffusion in haemodialysis. Thus it has the advantage of both systems in terms of fluid and electrolyte control with the effective removal of waste products. The process can be instigated using basic CVVH equipment but with the introduction of dialysate fluid, in a continuous, pumped supply to the filtrate compartment of the filter.

Alternately, the most sophisticated tehnique of CVVHDF, using a specialized haemodialysis machine, can be used in either a continuous or intermittent therapy regimen. The isotonic replacement fluid, at the high level of purity required, is generated by the machine itself from the ultrafiltrate which is passed through specialized filters in the machine.

Use of vascular catheters

The common requirement for effective renal replacement therapy in the acute situation is adequate access to the patient's circulation that allows a blood flow of at least 200 mL/min and up to 500 mL/min. Therefore the use of a temporary vascular access catheter is vital, and this makes care demands that are of prime importance.

There are two commonly used vascular catheters, the tunnelled cuffed and uncuffed. Both have double lumens and are inserted percutaneously. The three most common sites of insertion are the femoral, the internal jugular or the subclavian veins.

The insertion is usually swift and can enable therapy to commence within minutes of a check X-ray confirming the catheter's position (which is mandatory in the case of the subclavian or internal jugular approaches) to exclude potential complications associated with the insertion. These include haemorrage from damage to the vessels involved, puncture of the subclavian artery, puncture of the superior vena cava and mediastinal haemorrage. Other forms of damage can occur due to involvement of the surrounding tissue, including pneumothorax, haemothorax, brachial plexus injury and pericardial tamponade. Also, the catheter tip can irritate the right atria, leading to arrhythmias.

Any symptoms of respiratory distress, cardiac tamponade or extrasystole must be investigated and catheter involvement ruled out.

In the event of atrial perforation resulting in haemothorax, emergency procedures for severe respiratory distress must be instigated and an underwater sealed chest drain inserted. The catheter must be removed and repositioned, probably in the femoral vein for the continuation of therapy.

There are distinct advantages in the use of such catheters for dialysis or filtration, such as immediate availability with minimal patient discomfort, little danger of acute thrombosis, and ease of removal. However, the potential problems in their use must be considered when planning care.

Infection

Localized infection of the catheter exit site, especially in the femoral site, may occur, as may infection of the catheter tunnel with subsequent septicaemia or subacute bacterial endocarditis.

The use of occlusive dressings and strict aseptic technique will greatly reduce the incidence of infection. However, any symptoms must be treated swiftly with narrow-spectrum specific antibiotics, and possibly the removal and resiting of the catheter.

Thrombosis

Subclavian vein occlusion may occur owing to the restriction of blood flow around the catheter, and may result in swelling of the arm. Thrombosis within the catheter and subsequent embolism is a very rare occurrence. Any occlusion of the blood flow must be treated by the removal of the catheter, elevation of the arm and possibly the use of systemic anticoagulation.

Catheter patency

The catheter is literally the patient's 'lifeline'. It should be used only for the haemodialysis treatment and not for any other infusion purpose. Between dialysis sessions the catheter is 'heparin locked'; that is, a volume of heparin equal to the volume of each catheter lumen is inserted.

Air embolism

Any breach in the catheter integrity can result in air embolism owing to the 'vacuuming' effect of blood flow through the vein and heart. The security of the connections, caps and line itself must be monitored. The catheter should be 'double clamped' at all times between dialysis sessions; that is, clamped by the in-line clamps and by independent clips. The caps on each arm of the catheter must be Luer locked and the restraining suture secure.

Anticoagulation

Anticoagulation is essential for all forms of extracorporeal renal replacement therapy. It can range from continuous dosage in CVVH to intermittent in the case of haemodialysis.

Cautions on clotting

Potential clotting of the circuit means that it needs continual monitoring and care by the nursing staff. Problems can arise from the patient's blood coming into contact with the foreign materials of the dialysis/filter circuit, which activates platelet activity. This in turn activates the protein cascade, leading to clot formation. Increased blood viscosity, especially at the exit of the filter where large convection volumes have been removed, also predisposes to clotting.

The way in which the therapy is run can also have an impact on clotting. A low temperature increases the blood's viscosity. In haemodialysis the dialysate is run slightly cooler in order to promote vasoconstriction and so maintain the blood pressure throughout the session, but this can promote clotting (as can a slow blood pump rate).

Targets for anticoagulation

The aim is to maintain a clotting time that is as short as possible without endangering the circuit. Usually the target is between 120 and 150 seconds as measured by the activated clotting time (ACT) method. Alternatively, the laboratory established clotting time measured by activated partial thromboplastin time (APTT or PTT) will give more accurate results but with the disadvantage of not providing the results in 'real time'.

The goal is to maintain the ACT or APTT at a baseline value plus 80 per cent during the therapy, and at plus 40 per cent at the end of therapy.

Anticoagulation regimens

A variety of regimens are available to suit the individual patient's needs.

- Low-molecular-weight or sodium *heparin* is the most convenient short-term measure with a predictable half-life and clotting time.
- *An antiplatelet agent* such as a prostaglandin is an alternative where heparin is contraindicated, or where there is a need to minimize heparin dosage.
- A *protease inhibitor*, which inhibits platelet aggregation and the fibrinolysis cascade, can be used where heparin anticoagulation is inadvisable.

Other agents such as citrate, aspirin or hirudin are generally not used.

CASE STUDY 3.1

Phillip McHeany is a 48-year-old man who presented with oedema, breathlessness and oliguria. The RIFLE assessment shows a GFR reduced by 75 per cent and a creatinine three times raised from the baseline. His urine output is 0.3 mL/kg an hour over the next 24h. The urinalysis shows proteinuria +++ and the urine contains glomerular casts and red cells. His blood biochemistry indicates an elevated serum urea and creatinine, hyperkalaemia, hypernatraemia and a reduced bicarbonate level.

- What would be the immediate therapeutic interventions to preserve life?
- What difficulties to fluid removal would a poor nutritional status add?
- How would a diagnosis of acute rather than chronic renal failure be established?

Chronic kidney disease

Approaches to care

In the context of high-dependency nursing of patients with existing CRF requiring mechanical renal replacement therapy, attention will need to be paid to the care needs generated by the specific pathophysiology (Box 3.10) as well as the continuing care needs generated by the effects of CRF. In some cases these needs will be the same. What is important is the impact the disease will have on the person's ability to recover and achieve the optimum healthcare goal.

Continuity of treatment is the key, with modifications made to address specific problems in the light of the effects of CRF, and so a multidisciplinary approach incorporating good communication is essential.

The patient in chronic renal failure requiring high-dependency nursing for any reason will present

Box 3.10 Causes of chronic renal failure

- Glomerulonephritis
- Hypertension
- Obstructive uropathy
- Reflux nephropathy
- Pyelonephritis: with structural abnormality
- Toxic nephropathy
- Drugs (e.g. paracetamol and aspirin, and antibiotics such as tetracycline, the cephalosporins and amphotericin)
- Myeloma
- Polycystic disease
- Vasculitic disease

certain difficulties associated with the long-term effects of their renal problem. These effects will impact on the assessment and care planning and can present problems that need to be taken into consideration in addition to those associated with the pathology giving rise to their care needs. First and foremost will be the continuing need for mechanical renal replacement therapy. There are two principal long-term renal replacement therapies available:

- continuous ambulatory peritoneal dialysis (CAPD);
- intermittent haemodialysis.

Continuous ambulatory peritoneal dialysis

CAPD is based on the simpler, but now little used, temporary peritoneal dialysis (Fig. 3.5).

The large, highly vascular, semi-permeable surface of the patient's peritoneum is used as the dialysis membrane. A permanent catheter is placed through the abdominal wall, by which a hypertonic dialysis solution is instilled into the peritoneal cavity. A volume of 2 L is usually used, but this can be modified according to the size of the patient. After a number of hours the solution is drained, taking with it excess fluid, electrolytes and waste products that have moved from the patient's circulation through the forces of osmosis and diffusion.

Four exchanges of dialysate fluid per day achieves adequacy of dialysis, provided the hypertonic solution is continuously in contact with the peritoneum.

The high-dependency nurse's role may be confined to care of the CAPD catheter, ensuring adequate nutritional support for the patient, and control of the patient's fluid and electrolyte balances. However, as the system is designed for ease of use, there is no reason why the nurse should not undertake the exchange procedure for the patient following the specific steps described by the system's manufacturer. All systems are slightly different, but each follows the principles of asepsis during the exchange.

Potential complications in CAPD

The nurse will need to monitor the patient for potential complications associated with the treatment.

Peritonitis due to bacterial or fungal infection of the peritoneum will result in cloudy and turbid effluent and abdominal pain. A leukocyte count of greater than $100/mm^3$ in the dialysate will confirm the diagnosis, and a culture of Gram-positive or Gram-negative organisms will require the specific antibiotic to be administered via the dialysate fluid. Intravenous antibiotics may also be administered, but care must be taken to allow for the requirement of a renally adjusted dosage.

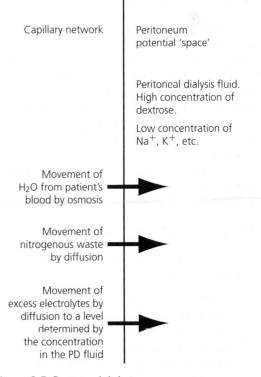

Capillary network | Peritoneum potential 'space'

Peritoneal dialysis fluid. High concentration of dextrose.

Low concentration of Na^+, K^+, etc.

Movement of H_2O from patient's blood by osmosis

Movement of nitrogenous waste by diffusion

Movement of excess electrolytes by diffusion to a level determined by the concentration in the PD fluid

Figure 3.5 Peritoneal dialysis

Another potential infection site is the exit of the catheter from the abdomen. These *tunnel infections* are a result of infection tracking back along the insertion site between the internal securing cuffs on the catheter. They can prove extremely difficult to eradicate. Characteristics of exit-site infection are tenderness, redness and inflammation with exudate. The catheter should be anchored at two sites to prevent pulling and potential exposure of the first 'cuff'. Cleaning of the site daily or every two days with soap and water, as well as the use of a sterile non-occlusive dressing, will help to avoid infections.

Treatment of infection will often start with broad-spectrum oral antibiotics to cover both Gram-positive and Gram-negative bacteria until a specific organism can be identified. Then the appropriate antibiotic can be given for 10–14 days.

Nutrition in CAPD

Nutrition is a particular problem because the CAPD process 'flushes' protein from the patient's body. This can result in hypoproteinaemia, with a corresponding hypercatabolic state, as well as fluid loss to the tissues, intractable oedema and circulatory collapse as described earlier. Adequate nutritional support either orally, nasogastrically or via TPN will be required to supply sufficient protein and calories to prevent hypercatabolism.

Accurate assessment of fluid balance is of paramount importance in the use of such feeds, but it is less critical than in other forms of mechanical replacement therapy (e.g. haemodialysis) because fluid balance is being controlled by the dialysate exchanges on such a regular basis. The use of stronger hypertonic fluids will assist in the removal of any excess fluid intake given that the serum protein level can be maintained.

Another problem associated with protein loss via the dialysate is the formation of fibrin in the fluid, appearing as either 'strings' of white fibres or as 'clouds' of milky white matter in the clear fluid. These collections of fibrin can block the catheter, so heparin 500 iu per exchange is added to the dialysate fluid to correct this if necessary.

Rapid exchanges of fluid will also assist in the removal of any potential blockages, but in the event of non-draining fluid the specialist renal personnel will have to be called to carry out system flushing.

If the patient becomes severely hypercatabolic it may be necessary to replace the CAPD treatment with the more aggressive haemodialysis, or even continuous venovenous or arteriovenous haemofiltration (CVVH or CAVH), and to treat the patient as an 'acute' renal failure until stabilized.

Haemodialysis

A patient requiring regular haemodialysis as the means of mechanically replacing the renal function will need to continue this treatment at his or her usual or more regular dialysis times during the current pathophysiological problems. The high-dependency nurse's role may be confined to general care of the patient in the resting period, with the renal personnel providing the dialysis treatment as an 'outreach' service. However, the success of the dialysis will depend on the high-dependency nursing that the patient receives, specifically consisting of care of the venous access, dietary and fluid modification and electrolyte control, as well as the specific care required due to the patient's specific condition.

Venous access

The venous access for a patient receiving long-term haemodialysis will usually be a Brescia–Cimino fistula, which consists of a permanent anastomosis of the patient's radial artery to the cephalic vein. The high-pressure blood being 'shunted' across the fistula into the low-pressure venous system results in distension of the veins of the forearm. This provides sites for cannulation which will allow the rapid removal and replacement of blood during haemodialysis.

The appearance of the patient's arm will be quite distinctive, having long areas of scar tissue along the distended veins from previous repeated cannulation for treatment. There will be a strong pulse at the fistula site, and a buzzing sensation (known as a bruit) on palpation. This is the actual flow of arterialized blood into the venous system and on auscultation will give a whooshing sound.

This fistula is the patient's 'life-line' and so great care must be taken to ensure its survival. Blood pressures must not be measured on the fistulated arm, nor should tight strapping of any kind be applied as this will result in restriction of the blood flow through the fistula and clotting of the anastomosis and veins. Venous cannulation for any purpose other than haemodialysis (such as IV drug administration, blood taking for investigations, or central pressure lines) should not be allowed in the fistulated arm. An unconscious patient should not be left to lie on the arm.

An alternative form of access, especially in patients who have arterial disease, is the synthetic graft. These grafts form a loop in either the forearm or more usually in the thigh where the graft joins to the femoral vein. The major problem here is the danger of infection and secondary bleeding following treatment. Any evidence of infection, redness, inflammation or exudate from the puncture sites

must be reported immediately. Evidence of secondary bleeding, with blood leakage or spurting from the needle sites, or swelling of the thigh, must also be reported immediately and pressure applied to the site until the bleeding ceases.

Dietary and fluid modification

Usually the patient in CRF will care for his or her own diet and fluids. However, people requiring high-dependency nursing will have very different requirements from those they are used to, and so additional instruction and care should be given.

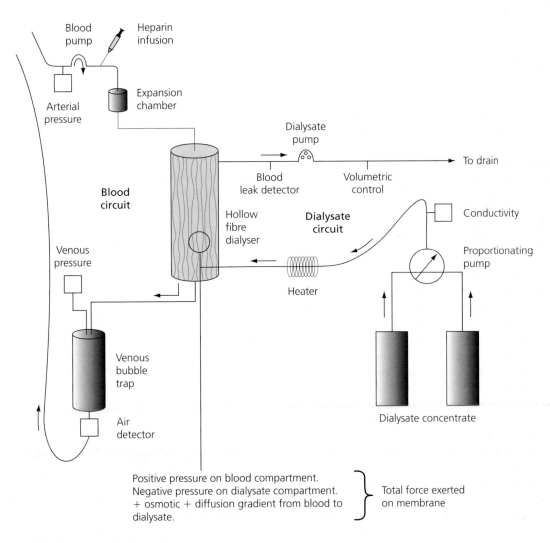

Figure 3.6 The circuit for haemodialysis

The principle of ensuring a nutritional input sufficient to prevent catabolism remains the same; but, as the patient may well be in a catabolic state due to their current condition, restriction of protein intake is contraindicated. The approach described in the section on acute renal failure applies (see page 88).

Fluid intake also has to be modified according to the patient's residual renal function, incidental loss and the volume that can be comfortably removed mechanically via dialysis. In other words, the mechanical renal replacement therapy creates 'space' that is filled during the intradialytic period.

During acute episodes of illness the usual intakes and losses may well be disrupted and so will need careful monitoring and control. The 'standard' approach of a 500 mL fluid allowance to account for incidental losses, plus the volume of the output from the previous 24 h with an additional allowance for volumes to be removed by dialysis, should be supplemented by a more thorough assessment of the patient. This assessment should be based on a previous history of body weight changes in order to form a 'baseline' of normal fluid balance for comparison to his or her present status. If possible the patient should be weighed daily; however if the patient is too ill then accurate intake and output records, taking into account fluid from all sources, should be used, comparing them with evidence of fluid retention.

Electrolyte control

As with fluids, dialysis creates 'space' that is then filled by dietary or metabolic production of electrolytes, the two of most concern being sodium and potassium. A familiarity with those foods containing high levels of these electrolytes will help the high-dependency nurse to regulate their intake.

Potassium is of particular concern because it poses a direct threat to life in levels exceeding 6 mEq/L owing to its effect on myocardial excitability. In patients with tissue damage, potassium will be shifting from the intracellular compartment and so a restriction of dietary intake may be insufficient to control hyperkalaemia. In such patients, regular assessment of the serum electrolytes is required as well as attention to any arrhythmias. In the presence of such irregularities, intravenous glucose and insulin provides an emergency treatment, driving the potassium back into the cells and providing time for mechanical renal replacement therapy to commence.

Care planning and prognosis

Problems associated with chronic renal disease can complicate any care planning for a patient's current condition and so will need to be taken into consideration. These include:

- hypertension dependent on renal artery disease, or salt and water retention;
- anaemia due to failure of erythropoietin production and complicated by blood losses due to dialysis or surgery;
- acidosis associated with the failure of the kidneys to excrete hydrogen ions and the failure to conserve bicarbonate;
- renal bone disease due to the failure of the kidneys to convert vitamin D into an activated form, thus allowing the absorption of calcium from the gut and so activating the demineralization of bone.

As symptoms associated with CRF will be present, it can be expected that the patient's current condition will exacerbate them. Infection, respiratory disorders, surgery, fractures or any condition may give rise to the need for high-dependency nursing. In such cases the effects of treatment and potential outcomes must be assessed in the light of what would be 'normal' for a renal patient; that is, what can be achieved through direct intervention for the current illness and what via mechanical renal replacement therapy. Good communication must exist between the high-dependency nurse, renal nurse and dietician in the care planning for the patient.

Ultimately the aim of the care is to return the patient to the same level of independence that was experienced within his or her long-term treatment regimen. As more nurses become aware of the special needs of such patients, then a favourable outcome of treatment becomes more likely. The sophistication of treatment offered to renal patients requiring high-dependency nursing is an example of two specialist branches of nursing working in harmony to produce the best possible care goals.

ACTIVITY   ?

Under what circumstances would a patient benefit from:

- peritoneal dialysis
- haemodialysis
- haemofiltration?

Conclusion

Caring for a patient in renal failure is complex and challenging owing to the multiple system problems that occur. For the patient in ARF the primary cause will complicate care and management and may itself be life-threatening. A sound understanding of the relationship between the underlying pathophysiology and the clinical features is essential to effective care so that deterioration and complications can be detected early and managed effectively. It must be recognized that patients in renal failure, particularly ARF, may have a poor short-term prognosis, which will be distressing for both patient and family and which will require excellent communication skills to communicate complex problems in ways that can be understood.

References

Bellomo R *et al.* (ADQI workgroup, 2004). Acute renal failure: definitions, outcome measures, animal models, fluid therapy and information technology needs, *Critical Care* **8**; R204–12.

Caimi G, Carollo C, LoPresti R (2005). Pathophysiological and clinical aspects of malnutrition in chronic renal failure, *Nutritional Research Reviews* **18**; 89–97.

Donald R (2003). The renal system. In: Bassett (ed.) *Essentials of Nursing Care*. New York: Whurr.

Fry AC, Farrington K (2006). Management of acute renal failure, *Postgraduate Medical Journal* **82**; 106–16.

Kellum JA, Bellomo R, Ronco C (2008). Definition and classification of acute kidney injury, *Nephron Clinical Practice* **109**; 182–7.

Krenitsky J (2004). Nutrition in renal failure: myths and management. In: *Nutritional Issues in Gastroenterology*, Series 20, September. pp. 40–59. www.healthsystems.virginia.edu/internet

Lameire NH, Devriese AS, Vanholder R (2003). Prevention and nondialytic treatment of acute renal failure. *Current Opinion in Critical Care* **6**; 481–90 (abstract).

Lewis JL (2009). *Disorders of Fluid Volume: Fluid and Electrolyte Metabolism*. Merck Manual Medical Library. Available at www.merck.com/mmpe (accessed July 2009).

McMillan JI (2007). *Acute Renal Failure*. Merck Manual Medical Library. Available at www.merck.com/mmpe (accessed August 2009).

Renal Association (2008). *Clinical Practice Guidelines: Module 5, Acute Kidney Injury*, 4th edn.

Ronco C (2005). Acute Dialysis Quality Initiative (ADQI): the PASSPORT project. *International Journal of Artificial Organs* **28**; 438–40.

Sweeney P, Rubin R, Tolkoff-Rubin N (eds) (2003). *Infectious Complications of Renal Disease*. London: Oxford University Press.

Thomas N, Smith T, Jeffrey C (2004). *Renal Nursing*. London: Baillière Tindall.

Wright SE, Bodenham A, Short AIK, Turney JH (2004). The revision and practice of renal replacement therapy on adult intensive care units in the United Kingdom. *Anaesthesia* **58**; 1063–9.

Vincente EG, Franco CA, Sordor V *et al.* (2008). Acute renal failure and renal replacement techniques, *Medicrit.org* **5**; 115–29. Available at www.medicrit.com/a/54115.php (accessed July 2009).

CHAPTER 4

NEUROLOGICAL ASSESSMENT AND MANAGEMENT

Catheryne Waterhouse

LEARNING OUTCOMES

Upon completion of this chapter the reader will:

1 have an understanding of the normal functioning of the neurological system and the impact pathophysiological changes through injury, disease or illness have on this system – and hence the patient

2 have an understanding of the assessment needs of a patient with a neurological disorder or head injury

3 be aware of the more common neurological disorders and injuries and the associated care and treatment of patients

4 appreciate the impact of neurological injury and/or disease on patients and their families.

Introduction

The aim of this chapter is to explore issues surrounding the care and treatment of patients exhibiting signs of neurological deterioration. Patients suffering from head injury, or other neurological episodes caused by disease or trauma, demand high levels of monitoring and observation, to decrease mortality and significantly reduce the likelihood of permanent brain injury and disability. This chapter focuses on some of the more common injuries and acute illnesses likely to be encountered.

The nervous system is divided into central and peripheral parts. The central nervous system (CNS) is made up of the brain, its cranial nerves and the spinal cord. The peripheral nervous system is composed of spinal nerves that connect to the spinal cord, and the autonomic nervous system divided into sympathetic and parasympathetic parts (Martini and Bartholomew 1997).

Anatomy and physiology of the nervous system

The brain is a hugely complex organ divided anatomically into the cerebrum, the cerebellum and the brainstem. Its primary functions are to monitor, integrate and process internal and external stimuli and respond appropriately.

The cerebrum

The cerebrum forms the major portion of the brain and is responsible for the higher functions, including control of conscious behaviour, intellect and integration of sensory stimuli to facilitate speech and understanding.

The cerebrum is divided into two hemispheres that are connected by a large bundle of 'white matter' (the corpus callosum) – myelinated axons that enable communication between the two hemispheres. The surface of the cerebrum (the cerebral cortex) is made

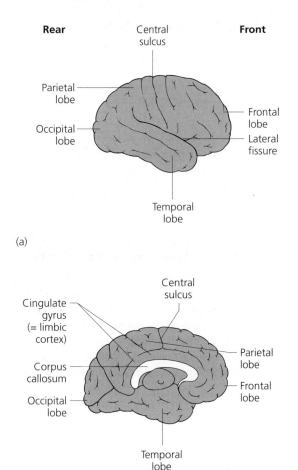

Rear   Central   **Front**
sulcus

Parietal
lobe

Frontal
lobe

Occipital
lobe

Lateral
fissure

Temporal
lobe

(a)

Central
sulcus

Cingulate
gyrus
(= limbic
cortex)

Parietal
lobe

Corpus
callosum

Frontal
lobe

Occipital
lobe

Temporal
lobe

(b)

Figure 4.1 Cerebral hemispheres of the forebrain: (a) external features, lateral view; (b) inner surface of the left hemisphere, with the right hemisphere removed

up of 'grey matter' or neurones, that form three main information processing areas – the motor, sensory and association areas. The surfaces or lobes of the cerebral cortex are named after the bones in the skull: frontal, temporal, parietal and occipital lobes (Bear *et al.* 2001; Fig. 4.1).

- The frontal lobes are responsible for the planning, execution and evaluation of actions. These include expressive speech, personality, behaviour, concentration and initiation of voluntary movement.
- The temporal lobes are the primary auditory receptive areas largely responsible for the understanding of speech but playing a major role

in integrating somatic, auditory and visual information.

- The parietal lobes are mostly responsible for sensory reception and perception and interpreting sensations such as touch and pain. This part of the brain is concerned with awareness and spatial orientation of the body and is also thought to be used in the creation of long-term memory.
- The occipital lobes are the primary receptive area for vision, receiving most of their input from the eyes, enabling visual interpretation.

The cerebral nuclei

Lying beneath the cortex are specialized processing areas known as the basal ganglia and the limbic system.

- The basal ganglia are involved with the control of movement and interact with the motor cortex.
- The limbic system consists of the hippocampus and the amygdala. This system has a role in long-term memory formation, behaviour and the control of emotions.

Deep within the forebrain lies the diencephalon, containing the thalamus and hypothalamus.

- The thalamus acts as the final relay centre for sensory input to the cortex. It also plays an important role in regulating consciousness, including sleep, awareness and alertness.
- The hypothalamus has multiple autonomic functions, linking with the endocrine system via the pituitary gland to regulate the release of a range of hormones (e.g. antidiuretic hormone, growth hormone, oxytocin and prolactin). In addition it is involved with the control of temperature, appetite, emotions and sexual behaviour (Guyton 2006).

The cerebellum

The cerebellum is a large structure at the back of the brain lying beneath the occipital lobe and separated from the cerebrum by the tentrium, a fold of the dura mater. It coordinates and 'fine tunes' voluntary muscle movements and activity to maintain posture, sense of balance and equilibrium.

The brainstem

The brainstem is located in front of the cerebellum and is composed of the midbrain, the pons varolii and the medulla oblongata.

- The midbrain lies deep within the brain and consists of the tectum and the tegtectum. The tectum forms the posterior part of the midbrain. The tectum receives input from the eyes, via the thalamus, and helps control eye movements. In addition to this it receives sound input from the ears. The tegtectum helps control skeletal movement via the substantia nigra and red nucleus (produces the neurotransmitter dopamine responsible for triggering Parkinson's disease). Functionally it contains the sensory spinal tracts connecting the cerebral hemispheres with the lower portion of the brain.
- The pons varolii is part of the relay system transferring information to the cerebellum and contains many of the control centres for respiratory function, eye and facial movement.
- The medulla oblongata links the brain with the spinal cord at the foramen magnum and is largely responsible for cardiac and respiratory regulation.

The cranial nerves

The cranial nerves form part of the peripheral nervous system. They connect directly to the brain rather than the spinal pathways (Fig. 4.2). There are 12 pairs of cranial nerves, each one responsible for a distinct activity (Table 4.1).

Blood supply of the brain

To maintain normal activity, the adult brain requires 20 per cent of the total amount of circulating blood volume, amounting to 750 mL of oxygenated blood per minute. Under normal conditions, cessation of blood flow to the brain for a short period (5–10 seconds) is sufficient to cause temporary changes in neural activity. Interruption of blood flow to the brain

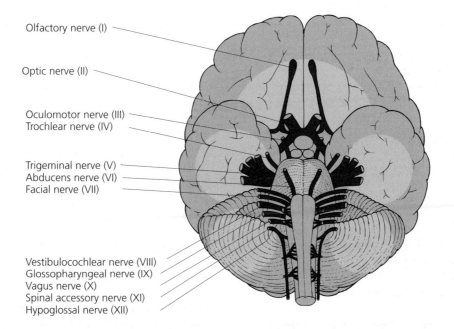

Olfactory nerve (I)

Optic nerve (II)

Oculomotor nerve (III)
Trochlear nerve (IV)

Trigeminal nerve (V)
Abducens nerve (VI)
Facial nerve (VII)

Vestibulocochlear nerve (VIII)
Glossopharyngeal nerve (IX)
Vagus nerve (X)
Spinal accessory nerve (XI)
Hypoglossal nerve (XII)

Figure 4.2 The cranial nerves

Table 4.1 Functions of the cranial nerves

	Cranial nerve	Branch	Function
I	Olfactory	Sensory	Sense of smell from the olfactory epithelium in the nose
II	Optic	Sensory	Arising from the retinal cells in the eye, it forms part of the visual pathways
III	Oculomotor	Motor	Controls a range of eye movements and accommodation for depth and distance appreciation
IV	Trochlear	Motor	Controls upward and downward eye movements using the superior oblique muscle
V	Trigeminal opthalmic mandibular maxillary	Mixed	Conveys sensations of pain, temperature and touch from the scalp, face, teeth, gums and palate Motor portion controls muscles of mastication, and the corneal reflex
VI	Abducens	Motor	Controls lateral eye movement via the lateral rectus muscles
VII	Facial	Mixed	Sensory – Innervates the anterior 2/3rds of tongue taste receptors Motor – controls muscles of facial expression, salivary and tear glands
VIII	Vestibulocochlear	Vestibular Sensory	Concerned with hearing, balance and maintenance of body posture
IX	Glossopharyngeal	Mixed	Sensory – innervates the pharyngeal muscles, conveys taste and sensation from tonsils and pharynx Includes visceral afferent impulses (ANS) from carotid arteries and aortic arch Motor – coordinates swallowing and visceral efferents (ANS) to the parotid salivary glands
X	Vagus	Mixed	Sensory – innervates the pharynx, larynx, oesophagus and organs in the thoracic and abdominal cavity Motor – involved with swallowing movements, controls the larynx, pharynx, and soft palate
XI	Accessory	Motor	Supplies the sternocleidomastoid and part of the trapezius muscle
XII	Hypoglossal	Motor	Innervates the tongue to provide normal speech and swallowing

for 5–10 minutes will result in irreversible brain damage.

The brain is supplied by two pairs of cerebral arteries. Two vertebral arteries supply the posterior portion of the brain, the brainstem and spinal cord, and two internal carotid arteries divide into internal and external branches. The external carotid arteries supply the pharynx, the larynx and the face, while the internal carotid arteries supply the root of the brain. All four vessels supply the posterior and anterior blood supply through the circle of Willis (Fig. 4.3), located at the base of the brain.

Intracranial pressure

The skull, along with the meninges, forms a rigid container that is filled to capacity with brain tissue (80 per cent of the total volume), blood (10 per cent) and cerebral spinal fluid (CSF; 10 per cent). It is therefore unyielding to any additional volume (Reilly and Bullock 2005). The intracranial pressure (ICP) is the pressure exerted by the normal brain components within this closed structure (Chudley 1994). In the adult human the ICP is maintained at between 5 and 15 mmHg. If any one of the components within it increases in volume, a decrease in the volume of one or both of the other two components must occur to maintain normal intracranial pressure (McNair 1996).

Raised intracranial pressure can occur as a result of the ventricular system becoming impeded by a blood clot or debris. It can also be due to a congenital malformation within the system, as in infantile hydrocephalus. It also occurs as a result of a space-occupying lesion such as a tumour or abscess, or subsequent oedema.

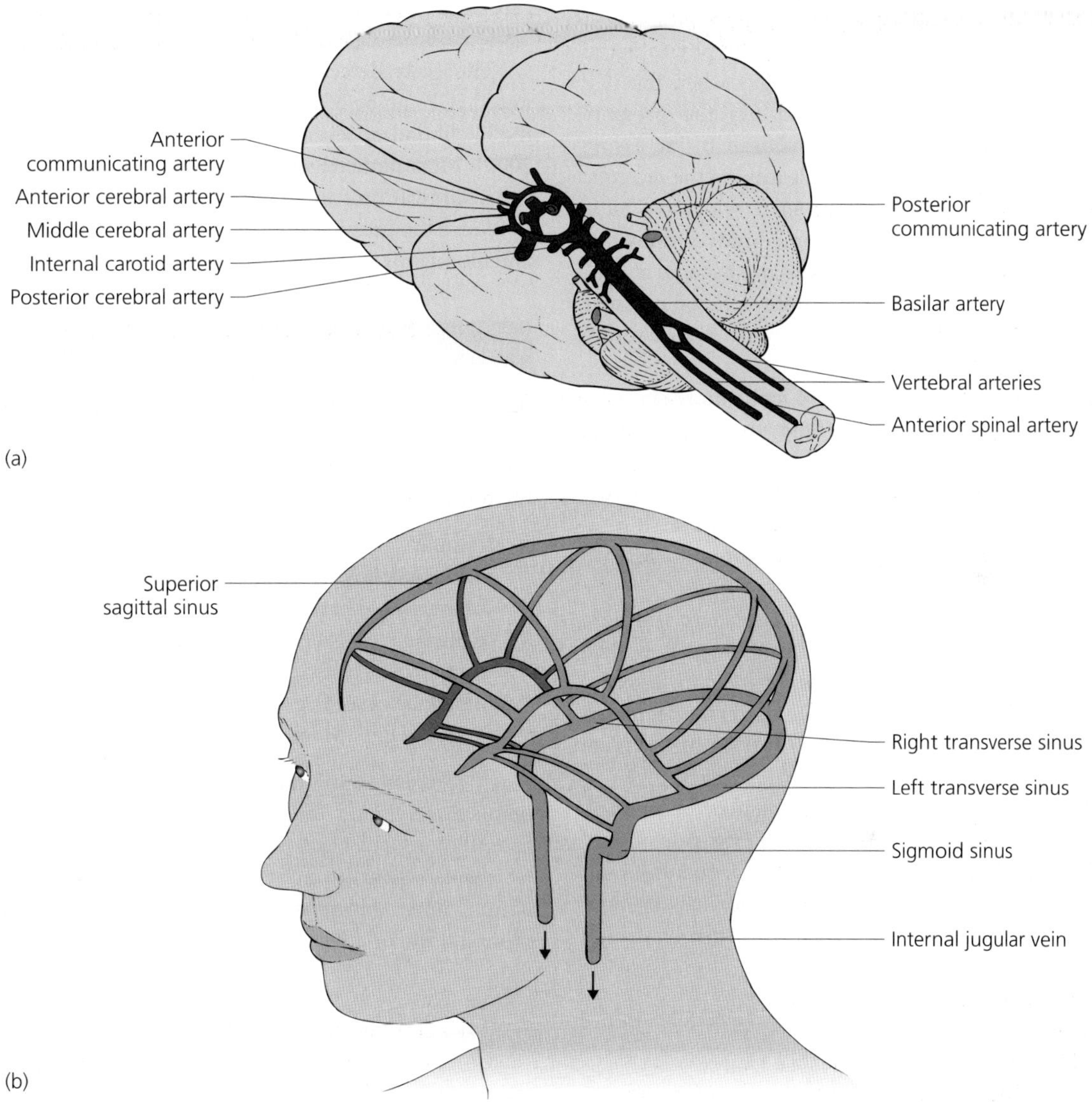

Figure 4.3 Blood flow to and from the brain. (a) The anterior and posterior communicating arteries join the three pairs of cerebral arteries to form the circle of Willis around the base of the brain. (b) Venous drainage

ACTIVITY ?

What are the signs of a rising intracranial pressure?

The compensation mechanism

The brain has certain protective mechanisms that allow it to adjust to small changes in volume, thereby maintaining cerebral blood flow and perfusion. This is referred to as the 'Munro–Kellie doctrine' (Garner 2007; Reilly and Bullock 2005).

The 'Cushing's reflex' refers to the physiological changes that occur in the vital signs when the ICP starts to rise within the brain. As the pressure increases, the brain tries to compensate by increasing the systolic blood pressure while leaving the diastolic largely unchanged, resulting in a widening *pulse pressure*. The patient will become bradycardic while the respiratory rate will also slow and become irregular. These classic signs of raised intracranial pressure are very late signs that occur just before brain herniation.

Initially the brain will try to make more space by displacing cerebral spinal fluid from the cranial subarachnoid space and basal cisterns to the spinal subarachnoid space and lumbar cisterns. As the ICP continues to rise, the CSF produced in the choroid plexus will reduce, and the reabsorption of CSF into the arachnoid villi will increase.

If the pressure continues to rise there will be a reduction in the volume of cerebral blood flow. The venous blood will be shunted away from the affected area into the distal venous sinuses. The decreased cerebral blood flow will lead to further brain tissue ischaemia, due to the reduced cerebral perfusion.

When the compensatory mechanisms reach their maximum capacity, intracranial hypertension occurs, and brain tissue moves from a compartment of high pressure to one of lower pressure, known as 'coning' or *cerebral herniation*. When this involves high sustained pressure upon the medulla and pons, cardiac arrest and death will result (Reilly and Bullock 2005).

The early detection of signs and symptoms of raised ICP can be life-saving, and will help to reduce the likelihood of severe brain damage (Bullock *et al.* 2000). Most patients will need to be transferred to a neurosurgical unit to facilitate surgical intervention to relieve the pressure and control cerebral perfusion and blood flow (Andrews *et al.* 1990).

Neurological assessment

Levels of consciousness

A patient can be *unconscious* for a number of reasons, including:

- trauma;
- a space-occupying lesion (e.g. tumour);
- subarachnoid haemorrhage;
- hypoxia;
- drug/alcohol intoxication;
- metabolic cause (e.g. hypo- or hyperglycaemia);
- renal and hepatic failure.

Full consciousness depends on the cerebral hemispheres being intact and interacting with the ascending reticular activating system (RAS; Fig. 4.4). This system runs through the brainstem, the hypothalamus and thalamus to the cerebral cortex. Stimulation of the RAS promotes wakefulness,

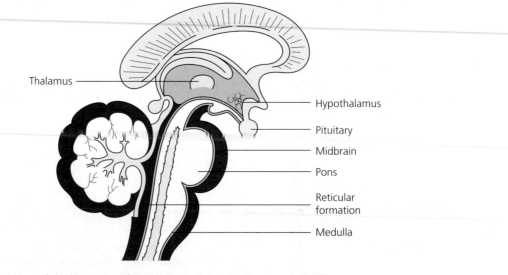

Figure 4.4 Lateral view of the brain, identifying the reticular activating system (RAS)

increasing attention, perception and alertness. Chipps *et al.* (1992) describe a person's state of consciousness as his or her degree of arousal and awareness. They describe arousal as the measure of being awake, whereas awareness involves the person being able to interpret incoming sensory data, and make sense of it by responding appropriately.

Locked-in syndrome describes a condition in which the patient can be aroused and is aware but, because of damage to the motor pathways in the brainstem, is unable to respond either verbally or through purposeful movement (Viney 1996).

A patient who is described as being in a *persistent vegetative state* (PVS) has no awareness, but demonstrates arousal that is not in response to any sensory stimuli.

One of the most important roles of the nurse caring for a seriously ill, neurologically impaired patient is the accurate assessment of neurological status, and correct interpretation of the observed data (Woodward 1997). The most widely used assessment tool is the Glasgow Coma Scale (GCS), developed by Teasdale and Jennett (1974). It allows the nurse to make rapid, repeated evaluations of the patient's neurological status in response to stimuli.

Glasgow Coma Scale observations

The patient's level of consciousness is evaluated by examining *three areas of behaviour* which directly correspond to an area of brain function; these are eye opening, verbal response and motor activity (Fig. 4.5).

Each response scores a numerical value that correlates with the patient's best level of responsiveness (or degree of deficit). The highest possible GCS score is 15. The lowest possible score is 3, indicating no eye opening (E1), no verbal response (V1) and no movement in response to a painful stimulus (M1).

Eye opening

Eye opening evaluates the patient's level of wakefulness by directly assessing the integrity of the ascending reticular activating system. Many severely head-injured patients will eventually open their eyes, but not be aware. They usually show signs of spontaneous blinking and their eyes will rove around; this must not be misinterpreted as the patient being aware (Table 4.2).

Verbal response

This test is performed to assess the language and interpretive centres in the temporal lobe of the cerebral cortex. It examines the transmission and understanding of verbal and also physical stimuli, and the person's ability to respond to questions appropriately (Waterhouse 2005; Table 4.3).

Motor activity

The nurse evaluates the integrity of the sensory and motor strip in the cerebral cortex. When carrying out this part of the assessment, the nurse must observe for the best level of response from the arms (Table 4.4).

Table 4.2 GCS scoring for eye opening

Score	Eye response	Explanation
4	Eyes open spontaneously	Patient is aware of the surroundings and opens eyes as the practitioner approaches
3	Eyes open to voice	Patient responds to a normal voice If this is insufficient, a greater verbal stimulus is required (hearing difficulties must be considered)
2	Eyes open to pain	In the first instance, touch or gently shake the patient If a deeper stimulus is required, a peripheral painful stimulus must be applied (i.e. pressure to the side of the finger distil to the last interphalangeal joint, applied with graduating intensity for 10–15 seconds, but may be repeated)
1	No eye opening	No response to verbal or painful stimulus This should be recorded when the nurse is satisfied that sufficient stimulus has been applied

Date:																										
Hour:																										
Minutes:																										
EYES OPEN C = eyes closed by swelling	Spontaneously	4																								
	To speech	3																								
	To pain	2																								
	None	1																								
BEST VERBAL RESPONSE T = ETT or Tracheostomy	Orientated	5																								
	Confused	4																								
	Inappropriate words	3																								
	Incomprehensible sounds	2																								
	None	1																								
BEST MOTOR RESPONSE Record best response from arms P = Paralysed	Obey commands	6																								
	Localises to pain	5																								
	Normal flexion	4																								
	Abnormal flexion	3																								
	Extension	2																								
	None	1																								
TOTAL GLASGOW COMA SCORE																										
PUPILS + = Reacts − = No reaction S = Sluggish	RIGHT	Size																								
		Reaction																								
	LEFT	Size																								
		Reaction																								
LIMB MOVEMENTS Record Right (R) and Left (L) separately if there is a difference	A R M S	Normal power																								
		Mild weakness																								
		Severe weakness																								
		Abnormal flexion																								
		Extension																								
		No response																								
	L E G S	Normal power																								
		Mild weakness																								
		Severe weakness																								
		Extension																								
		No response																								

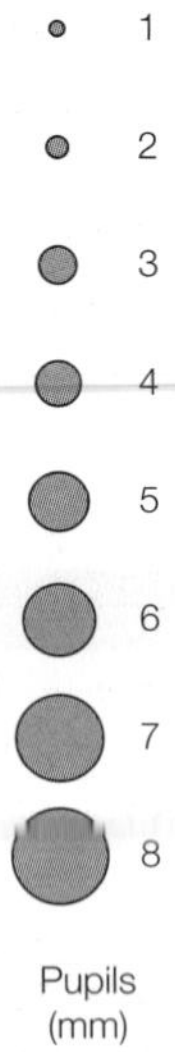

Pupils (mm)
1
2
3
4
5
6
7
8

Blood pressure (mmHg)	240 220 210 200 190 180 170 160 150 140 130 120 110	
Heart Rate (beats/min)	100 90 80 70 60 50 40 30	
Respiratory Rate		
Initials:		

TEMPERATURE °C
41 40 39 38 37 36 35 34 33 32 31 30

Figure 4.5 Glasgow Coma Scale (GCS) chart

Table 4.3 GCS scoring for verbal response

Score	Verbal response	Explanation
5	Orientation	Patient knows who he is, the year and the month, and where he is
4	Confusion	Patient answers one or more of the questions incorrectly
3	Inappropriate words	Patient answers, often in sentences but with no clear discernible words
2	Incomprehensible sounds	Patient moans or groans without any understandable words
1	No response	No verbal response to voice or a painful stimulus

Table 4.4 GCS scoring for motor activity

Score	Motor response	Explanation
6	Obeys commands	Patient is asked to carry out two different commands, establishing that the response is not a reflex movement (e.g. stick out tongue, lift up arms)
5	Localizes to pain	Patient localizes towards a central stimulus in an attempt to remove the source (e.g. supraorbital ridge pressure, trapezium muscle squeeze) The arm should move across the midline towards the level of the chin
4	Flexion to pain	Patient will flex or bend the arm at the elbow towards the pain but does not actually localize or try to remove the source
3	Abnormal flexion	Known as decorticate posturing, demonstrated by internal rotation, abduction of the shoulder and flexion of the elbow It is a much slower response than flexion and may be accompanied by spastic wrist flexion
2	Extension of limbs	Known as decerebrate posturing, characterized by extending the arms away from the body The patient will straighten the elbow joint, internally rotating the shoulder away from the source of the pain
1	No response	Recorded when there is no response to painful stimuli This may occur with disease, trauma, paralysing agents, spinal cord injury or from failure to apply sufficient painful stimulus

In addition, limb assessment provides a useful baseline for future assessments, noting any changes in range of movement, power and sensation.

Methods of applying a central painful stimulus

- *Trapezius pinch.* This involves pinching the trapezius muscle on the shoulder. Pressure should be increased in order to elicit the best response.
- *Supraorbital ridge pressure.* This method involves resting the hand on the patient's head, with the flat of the thumb placed underneath the supraorbital ridge or eyebrow, and the degree of pressure gradually increased. This cannot be used if there is any suspicion of facial damage or fractures.

In the past, other common sites for applying physical stimuli have been sternal rubbing, applying pressure to the nailbeds and pinching the ear lobes. These are known to cause excessive bruising and are generally not recommended.

Pupil reactions

Pupils should be round and equal in shape and size (2–5 mm). Changes in the size, shape or speed of pupil reaction can provide vital information about cerebral function.

To elicit the light response, move a torch beam across the eye from the outer aspect of the eye towards the nose so that the response of each pupil can be assessed individually for both direct and consensual light response. The pupil should react briskly and return to its original size immediately after the light beam is removed. Repeat the procedure for each eye, noting any differences.

A unilateral unreactive pupil may be the result of raising intracranial pressure from an expanding lesion such as a haematoma, compressing the third cranial nerve (occulomotor). Bilateral fixed and dilated pupils can be an indication of herniation of the medial temporal lobe through the tentorium cerebelli; this is a grave sign.

ACTIVITY ?

What are the contributory causes of raised intracranial pressure?

CASE STUDY 4.1

John is an 18-year-old man who has been assaulted while out with friends in town. He has reportedly been unconscious for 30 minutes. When he is admitted to the unit he can recall his personal details but is unaware of his surroundings. His Glasgow Coma Score is recorded as 12.

- What might be happening to John?
- What might be the long-term consequences of the head injury?

Subtle changes in behaviour such as vagueness, disorientation, agitation, uncharacteristic withdrawal, headache and vomiting are early subtle signs of neurological deterioration. Frequent neurological assessment is essential to identify signs of raised ICP. Box 4.1 summarizes good practice guidance for assessing the patient.

Caring for the unconscious patient

Unconscious patients are extremely vulnerable and need a high level of nursing care to address their activities of daily living, minimize the risk of developing long-term disabilities and maintain their personal dignity and safety.

Neurological observations must be carried out frequently and recorded on the patient's chart, as described on page 105.

The nurse should evaluate the effectiveness of interventions frequently to optimize the care the patient receives.

Box 4.1 Good practice guidance for the Glasgow Coma Scale

- A complete set of observations should be performed by the same person throughout the shift to maintain consistency of scoring.
- To maintain continuity of care, one set of observations should ideally be performed together on commencement of shift handover.
- Dots should be used in preference to lines or ticks to complete the GCS chart.
- Individual recording of each response is more useful to observe trends or alterations in neurological function (e.g E4/V5/M6 (Teasdale et al. 1983).
- A deterioration of **1 point** in the motor response or an overall deterioration of **2 points** in the GCS score must be reported immediately to the nurse in charge and to the medical staff, and the frequency of observations must be increased.
- The patient who scores **8 or less** on the scale is considered to be in a coma.

Airway management

The airway must be protected at all times, if necessary using an adjunct such as an oropharyngeal (guedel) or nasopharyngeal airway.

The importance of preventing hypoxia and hypercapnia cannot be over-emphasized. Oxygen therapy, or in some cases mechanical ventilation, may be required to achieve an oxygen saturation of 95–100 per cent or Pao_2 of >14.0 kPa and $Paco_2$ of 4.3–5.0 kPa (Garner and Amin 2007).

Humidification using a heated circuit is more comfortable for the patient and can reduce the incidence of tracheal and bronchiole congestion and infection.

Deep vein thrombosis prophylaxis

Immobile patients are prone to the development of DVT. The application of graduated compression stockings (Kolbach et al. 2004), or a pneumatic compression device, and low-dose subcutaneous unfractionated heparin are first-line measures aimed at prevention (Vincent and Berre 2005).

Patient positioning

The patient should be nursed with the head slightly elevated (15–30 degrees of tilt) to reduce the incidence of chest infection and assist venous drainage via the jugular and vertebral veins. Drainage can be inhibited by slight flexion or extension of the neck, so particular attention must be paid to ensuring that the patient maintains a neutral alignment at all times. This must include log rolling the patient when changing position, and using a small pillow to maintain the head's position when the patient is on his or her side. Hip flexion must be avoided as this has been shown to increase intrathoracic pressure (Brunner and Suddarth 1995; Ng *et al.* 2004).

Immobile patients are particularly vulnerable to developing pressure sores. Restless patients are prone to skin breakdown and excoriation.

Nutrition and fluids

The patient is at risk of aspiration and subsequent chest infection or pneumonia. Intravenous fluids should be maintained until the patient's ability to swallow safely has been established by the speech and language therapist. The dietician will assess the patient's nutritional and hydration needs. Early enteral feeding has been shown to improve recovery and long-term prognosis (Twyman 1997). Care should be taken to check the position of a nasogastric tube (NGT) before use (NPSA 2005).

Intravenous glucose is contraindicated in patients who are neurologically compromised. It can precipitate acidosis, triggering ischaemia and infarction. Isotonic saline is preferable and can be administered safely (Feldman *et al.* 1995).

Pain management

Pain assessment is a fundamental part of nursing activity. However, in the unconscious patient direct feedback is unavailable and the nurse must rely on the non-verbal cues such as grimacing, moaning or crying, and possibly changes in the cardiovascular observations.

Other nursing considerations

Personal hygiene needs

All hygiene requirements must be met by the nursing team. This will include at least a daily bed bath especially if the patient is sweating profusely. Particular care should be taken with the eyes; if the patient has lost the blink and corneal reflex the eyes will quickly become dry and damaged (Lloyd 1990).

Elimination

The patient may need to be catheterized in order to accurately record the hourly urine output. Other patients may manage with penile sheaths, incontinence pads or other aids and appliances.

Mild aperients, laxatives or suppositories may be required as part of the patient's daily bowel regime, to avoid the development of constipation.

Communication

Unconscious patients may still be able to hear, so it is important to continually reassure them by explaining all procedures and interventions. Similarly, it is important to remind relatives to be sensitive to any discussions or conversations they may have at the bedside (Hendrickson 1987; Mitchell and Habermann 1999).

Common neurological conditions

Subarachnoid haemorrhage

Clinical features

A subarachnoid haemorrhage (SAH) affects approximately 150 people per million population each year and can cause severe disability or death. It is caused by a bleed into the subarachnoid space from a weakness (aneurysm) or a congenital malformation in the cerebral arteries. The severity of symptoms depends on the extent of the bleed.

It produces a sudden, severe headache, described by some patients as 'the worst headache I have ever experienced'. Severe neck stiffness and a positive Kernig's sign (resistance to straight-leg raising) are further indications of meningeal irritability. Vomiting is almost always a feature and occurs as a result of increased pressure on the brain. Photophobia with alteration in consciousness is common. Blurred vision, photophobia and papilloedema develop over a few hours and seizures may occur as a consequence of the blood irritating the meninges. Patients do not die from the blood loss itself; rather they will succumb to the damage to the cerebral tissue caused by increased intracranial pressure and lack of oxygenation to cerebral tissue (Hickey 2003).

Diagnostic procedures

Early diagnosis and prompt intervention depends on obtaining and documenting a thorough history, taking into consideration the clinical presentation and symptoms. A computed tomography (CT) scan will confirm the diagnosis and extent of the damage. CT angiography (CTA) or invasive carotid angiography can identify the location of the bleed, as well as indicating whether it can be embolized endovascularly by implanting tiny coils into the aneurysm or whether direct clipping of the aneurysm through a craniotomy is more appropriate.

Nursing care

Hydrocephalus is a common complication following a subarachnoid haemorrhage (Hickey 2008). Consistent, repeated recordings of Glasgow Coma Scale observations will help to identify any changes in the patient's consciousness. This period should include pupil reaction tests and limb assessment. The frequency of the observations will depend on the patient's condition.

Regular analgesia and anti-emetics should be administered to try to minimize pain and control nausea caused by the meningeal irritation and raised ICP. Positioning the patient with the head slightly elevated will encourage cerebral venous drainage, thereby reducing pressure. The addition of a benzo diazepine is sometimes indicated to reduce anxiety and enhance the effects of the analgesia.

Constipation is a common side-effect of codeine-based analgesia. Regular aperients should be prescribed. If the patient is sufficiently conscious, assistance in using a commode is often less stressful than trying to use a bedpan.

A low-grade pyrexia is common following a cerebral bleed. This should be treated with antipyretic medication when sources of infection have been identified and eliminated.

Blood electrolyte levels must be monitored at least once daily. Observe particularly for signs of hyper- or hyponatraemia or diabetes insipidus caused by insufficient antidiuretic hormone, leading to the production of large quantities of dilute urine (Edwards 2001).

Vasospasm occurs as a direct response to the haemorrhage, causing increased cerebral ischaemia and infarction of cerebral tissue. A fluid intake of up to 3 litres in 24 hours, administered orally, via the enteral route or intravenously, will help to optimize the central venous pressure (CVP) and blood pressure, thereby minimizing the risk of vasospasm of the cerebral blood vessels. In some cases, colloids and vasoactive drugs such as noradrenaline will be necessary to maintain a good mean arterial blood pressure and cerebral perfusion. Calcium-channel blockers or calcium antagonists such as nimodipine act on the smooth muscle to help reduce the incidence of vasospasm, but the patient should be closely monitored for signs of hypotension (Cooke 2005).

Other routine nursing interventions such as pressure area care and hygiene needs should be coordinated with the physiotherapists to allow the patient sufficient time to rest.

Psychological support for the patient and his or her family is paramount. They need constant reassurance and opportunities to discuss results from investigations or the proposed management plan. Ward visitors should ideally be restricted to family and close friends to avoid unnecessary stress to the patient.

The patient will have to be transferred to a specialist neurosurgical unit to instigate any treatment. Treatment options will depend on the underlying pathology. If there is a confirmed aneurysm, for example, the treatment will depend on the location, size, shape and accessibility to the lesion. Endovascular treatment is now considered to be an important first-line intervention, but a small number of patients will still require a surgical approach whereby the aneurysm is directly visualized to allow placement of a clip around the neck of the aneurysm (Molyneux et al. 2005).

For several weeks following a subarachnoid haemorrhage the person is at risk of further acute haemorrhages. Unfortunately, other than the measures already outlined, little can be done to prevent further rebleeds (Cooke 2005). Nuchal rigidity, severe headache, a deteriorating level of consciousness, focal neurological signs and changing pupil reactions are commonly observed. Patients will need a CT scan to confirm the diagnosis and probable transfer to an intensive care unit.

Head injury

Causes

Brain injury can be the result of a sudden, violent and traumatic event. It requires close monitoring and frequent assessment of neurological status to detect any signs of deterioration and allow prompt treatment of complications (Hickey, 2003). Following even a minor head injury there is a risk of raised intracranial pressure as a result of damage to the dura or cerebral tissue.

Irreversible structural brain damage occuring at the moment of injury (primary injury) can result from:

- acceleration/deceleration incidents such as a road traffic accident or falling from a height;
- direct localized trauma such as from a weapon or assault;
- a crush injury;
- a high-velocity injury from a gun shot;
- a penetrating injury from falling on a sharp object;
- a skull fracture that crosses vascular structures to produce a space-occupying haematoma, or a CSF leak due to a dural tear.

Complications

Possible complications (secondary injuries) that emerge shortly after or several hours after the initial injury include cerebral oedema, hydrocephalus, seizures, electrolyte disturbance, cranial nerve damage, hypoxia and hypercarbia. Haematomas are classified as in Box 4.2.

Morbidity can be reduced and the long-term prognosis improved with early neurosurgical intervention. Surgical removal of the haematoma can help reduce the mass effect (Bullock *et al.* 2000). A decompressive craniectomy involving the removal of a portion of the skull makes additional space for the swollen brain (Chibbaro and Tacconi 2007).

Box 4.2 Classification of haematomas in head injuries

- **Intracerebral** haematoma – contusion and laceration to the cortical surface of the brain, resulting in microscopic haemorrhages and necrosis to brain tissue.
- **Subdural** haematoma – bleeding from the cortical vessels between the dura and the brain, causing direct pressure on the cerebral tissue.
- **Extradural** haematoma – bleeding occurring under the skull between the dura mater, triggering an acute increase in the intracranial pressure.

CASE STUDY 4.2

Florence is a 72-year-old woman with dementia. She is frail but fairly mobile. She has been admitted to the ward following a fall at home. According to her husband she has become more confused and has now become incontinent of urine. On admission her blood pressure is 130/90 mmHg, pulse rate 80 beats/min and respiration 12/min. During the evening she becomes increasingly drowsy. Her blood pressure rises to 180/100 mmHg and pulse rate decreases to 60 beats/min.

- What is the likely underlying diagnosis following the head injury?
- Following surgery, outline the care she will require?
- What possible complications or problems could Florence develop in the future?

Nursing care

Therapeutic goals when managing a patient with raised ICP is to support body functions, attempt to treat the underlying cause, and prevent the development of secondary complications. All nursing interventions are aimed at controlling or reducing intracranial pressure (Andrus 1991).

Care of an unconscious patient is discussed on page 108. In addition, a patient who has sustained a head injury should be managed as if he or she potentially has an underlying spinal cord injury – until the spine has been cleared radiologically or the patient has been observed to move normally. An unconscious patient should be nursed in a neutral position, keeping the spine in alignment when attempting to 'log roll' or move the person to attend to hygiene needs (Williams 1993). Bolus doses of sedation prior to repositioning can decrease the risk of exacerbating a raised ICP.

Restless and agitated patients are at risk of injury. The use of padded cot sides may be helpful with this in mind.

Airway management includes continuous recording of oxygen saturation levels as there may be a need to intubate and commence mechanical ventilation. Oral pharyngeal suction is known to increase ICP (Gemma *et al.* 2002), so suctioning should be performed only following a clinical assessment of the patient's respiratory function, and ideally when the ICP is below 20 mmHg. Hyperoxygenation for 1–3 minutes can help to minimize hypoxia. Prophylactic analgesia or a bolus dose of sedation may help blunt the expected rise in ICP associated with the procedure.

Meticulous neurological assessment and observations should follow the principles outlined on page 105. Once the nurse has assessed the patient and established a sound baseline, then any alterations will be quickly identified and the delivery of care can be planned.

The head injury may affect the functioning of the endocrine system, in particular the pituitary gland. Urinary output should be monitored every hour and the specific gravity measured to identify early signs of diabetes insipidus.

Analgesia must be used cautiously. Opioid analgesia and benzodiazepines will calm agitation but can also mask neurological changes and make assessment ambiguous.

Calorific requirements are dramatically increased following major trauma, caused by an induced state of hypermetabolism and hypercatabolism. Early enteral feeding (within the first 24 hours) should be commenced as soon as practicable to maintain the integrity of the gut and reduce the likelihood of bacterial spread (Bhardwaj *et al.* 2004; Twyman 1997).

Any activity that might involve the patient holding his or her breath, such as straining when defecating, will increase intracranial pressure. Constipation must be avoided, so a bowel regime that includes daily rectal examination and the use of stool softeners, laxatives or suppositories may be necessary.

Clustering of nursing activities – such as attending to personal hygiene, repositioning, physiotherapy or exposure to noxious stimuli – should be coordinated to allow a break of at least 10 minutes between procedures to reduce the adverse effect on ICP (Lee 1989; Mestecky 2007; McGuinness 2007).

Communication and gentle therapeutic touch have been reported to reduce the ICP of patients following a head injury (Viney 1996). Even if the patient is unconscious, speaking quietly while explaining what you are doing and providing constant reassurance can be beneficial.

Relatives will be anxious, especially if their loved one is either unconscious or extremely confused. It is important for the nurse to ensure that they are fully informed regarding the diagnosis, and the possible complications such as short-term memory and concentration difficulties, neurological deficits such as hemiparesis, personality changes and fatigue. Referral to a social worker is a priority as many head-injured patients have difficulty returning to their previous occupation and most families will have additional financial concerns.

Documentation of the information that relatives have received is important, as they may well require reinforcement of the information given earlier. Documenting what has already been told to them helps to avoid confusion and reduces the risk of conflicting information being given.

Meningitis

Causes

Meningitis is inflammation of the meninges (dura, arachnoid and pia mater) that cover the brain and spinal cord. It may develop as a result of:

- viral infection;
- bacterial infection;
- fungal infection;
- chemical toxins;
- tubercle bacillus (TB);
- carcinoma.

Bacteria can enter the brain and central nervous system via an open skull fracture due to trauma, or through the nasal sinuses. Infection may be transmitted to the meninges from an infection elsewhere in the body via the blood circulation.

Clinical features and diagnosis

Common signs and symptoms of meningitis include severe headache and neck stiffness, pyrexia and photophobia. Patients with a meningococcal meningitis have a characteristic rash that does not blanche when compressed by a drinking glass. Life-threatening complications include circulatory collapse, coagulopathy hydrocephalus, raised ICP and seizures – all requiring urgent medical intervention.

In the first instance, a CT scan or magnetic resonance imaging (MRI) and routine X-rays can aid diagnosis and exclude a space-occupying lesion. A lumbar puncture and blood cultures may help determine the original site of the infection.

ACTIVITY   ?

A 19-year-old man complains of headaches, flu-like symptoms, neck stiffness and photophobia. He has a pin-prick rash on parts of his body and is diagnosed with meningitis. What assessment and observations would you undertake to support his care on your ward?

Nursing care

Baseline observations must include temperature, respiration and pulse rate. There is a potential risk of developing hydrocephalus due to the intracranial inflammatory processes, which may result in blockages in the choroid plexus, impeding the flow of cerebrospinal fluid. Repeated consistent Glasgow Coma Scale observations should be used to ascertain the level of consciousness and detect any signs of neurological deterioration, including motor and sensory function.

Patients should be nursed in a single room, applying barrier nursing principles to minimize the risk of cross-infection. Intravenous antibiotic therapy must be commenced without waiting for the results from cultures. Once the causative organism and

sensitivity has been identified, the choice of antibiotic can then be adjusted (Garner 1996).

The patient will be sensitive to noise and light and, while it is not easy to modify the environment on a busy ward, the patient will benefit from being nursed in a quiet room avoiding bright lights until symptoms have improved.

In severe cases, airway support and management will be required with the use of airway adjuncts. Positioning, postural drainage and physiotherapy will help reduce the likelihood of a chest infection. Oral and tracheal suction will aid removal of excess secretions, and oxygen therapy will help maintain adequate oxygenation and O_2 saturation.

The head of the bed should be slightly raised to promote venous drainage to reduce cerebral oedema. High-dose dexamethasone may help reduce swelling and improve some of the symptoms.

Nausea and vomiting are common in these patients. Anti-emetics and analgesia must be prescribed as soon as possible to reduce discomfort. Fluid replacement will be required either orally or intravenously. Close monitoring of fluid intake and output must be carefully documented. The patient will be pyrexial, so therapeutic cooling with regular doses of antipyretics and parecetamol, fanning or the use of cooling blankets should be instigated.

Pressure area care is important. Although the patient may be restless and able to change position frequently, friction may soon cause red areas to develop, especially if the skin is moist through sweating. All other basic hygiene needs must be implemented as previously discussed.

The patient is at risk from seizures resulting from cerebral irritation. It is essential to document the time, duration and pattern to the seizures (i.e. factors that might have triggered the event).

Safety measures such as one-to-one supervision and the use of padded cot sides will avoid the patient injuring themselves if they are restless.

Epilepsy

Causes and types

Epilepsy is the name given to an intermittent, stereotyped disturbance of consciousness, behaviour, emotions, motor function, perception or sensation (which may occur singly or in any combination), that on clinical grounds results from cortical neuronal discharge (Appleton and Gibbs 2004).

Anyone can develop epilepsy. It occurs in all age groups and social classes and affects approximately 1 in 120 of the UK population. Some people will develop epilepsy because of structural damage to the brain (symptomatic epilepsy). Others can identify factors such as stress, lack of sleep, alcohol consumption or hypoglycaemia that trigger their seizure. Still others suffer from what is referred to as ideopathic epilepsy where there is no known cause (Boxes 4.3 and 4.4). Figure 4.6 shows a classification of seizure types.

People are admitted to hospital for various reasons. They may have status epilepticus (see below) and require control of their seizures. Others require a review of their medication or observation of their seizure pattern in order to attempt to clarify the diagnosis.

Status epilepticus is described as serial seizures without recovering full consciousness between the fits. It is classed as a medical emergency because the condition has a mortality of about 30 per cent (Cascino 1996). The main cause of status epilepticus is the abrupt withdrawal of treatment; compliance is well-documented as being a problem with some sufferers. Other fairly common causes are alcohol withdrawal, brain tumour or brain assault. Patients suffering from status epilepticus will require intensive care and medical intervention in an attempt to reverse the crisis and avoid permanent brain damage.

Sudden unexplained death in epilepsy (SUDEP) accounts for 17 per cent of epilepsy-related deaths in patients where no other cause of death is found (www.epilepsy.org.uk).

Box 4.3 Some causes of epilepsy

Acute symptomatic seizures

- Fluid, electrolyte imbalance
- Alcohol or alcohol withdrawal

Remote symptomatic seizures

- Hypoxic, ischaemic cerebral insults
- Head injury
- Intracranial tumour
- Cerebral vascular disease
- Central nervous system infection
- Neurodegenerative disease

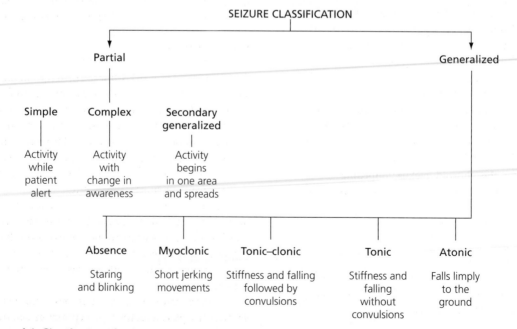

Figure 4.6 Classification of seizures

Box 4.4 Types of seizure

Partial

This type usually arises from the temporal lobe of the brain.

- **Simple partial**. Patients rarely require hospitalization unless it progresses to a prolonged tonic–clonic seizure. Many patients only experience an aura, and consciousness and normal awareness are usually maintained.
- **Complex partial**. The patient often adopts purposeless activity such as lip-smacking or other bizarre behaviour and memory disturbances, including déjà vu.
- **Secondary generalized**. The abnormal electrical activity may spread to involve other areas of the brain to cause a tonic–clonic seizure.

Generalized seizures

- **Absence**. These seizures are particularly common in children. The person experiences a sudden brief interruption in consciousness sometimes with fluttering of the eyelids or nodding of the head.
- **Myoclonic**. This is characterized by an abrupt involuntary jerking usually involving the arms and trunk.
- **Atonic**. This involves a complete loss of muscle tone, and head and facial injuries are common.
- **Tonic**. The person usually falls backwards, and the body will go stiff and rigid.
- **Tonic–clonic**. The patient experiences the tonic (rigid) phase, becoming cyanosed due to spasm of the respiratory muscles. This is followed by the clonic phase when the muscles relax and there are rapid uncontrolled movements of the limbs, often accompanied by incontinence of urine. This stage lasts for several minutes, followed by a period of relaxation and unconsciousness (postictal).

First aid

Box 4.5 has some basic guidance on dealing with an epileptic episode. When the first aid has been administered, document details as follows.

- Record the time and duration of the seizure.

Box 4.5 First aid measures for an epilepsy attack

DO

- Loosen clothing and move any objects that are likely to cause harm.
- Place in the recovery position to prevent the patient from obstructing or aspirating.
- Allow time for the patient to recover. The person may become confused and remain drowsy before falling into a deep sleep. Upon awakening there is often no recollection of the preceding events.

DON'T

- Try to restrain convulsive movements.
- Try and put anything into the patient's mouth.
- Try to move the patient unless he or she is in immediate danger.

- Record the pattern of the seizure. For example, did the person experience an aura? Did the jerking start in one part of the body and progress? Remember that the diagnosis of epilepsy often relies on witness accounts of the seizure. An electroencephalogram (EEG) cannot prove or refute the diagnosis unless the patient is actually having a seizure at the time of the investigation.

Nursing care

Once the person has stopped convulsing, an airway adjunct such as a guedel airway may be required. It is usual for the patient to become severely cyanosed during the seizure due to tonic contraction of the muscles inhibiting respiration. Administration of oxygen therefore will have little benefit. However, intravenous access will be required to enable administration of anticonvulsant medication.

The patient will require nursing in a safe environment, with access to oxygen and suction. The person may bite the tongue and produce excess saliva during the seizure. It is important to avoid trying to place anything between the teeth as this often results in broken teeth.

Cot sides must be in situ at all times and pillows strategically placed to try to prevent injuries during any subsequent seizures.

The patient will require constant reassurance. The nurse must remain with the patient throughout a seizure, making observations of the duration and any special focal signs that may assist with diagnosis. Neurological assessment is not practicable while the patient is in a clonic phase.

Referral to an epilepsy specialist nurse is recommended to titrate medication and review patient education regarding medication compliance once the patient's condition has been stabilized.

Guillain–Barré syndrome

Causes and clinical features

Guillain–Barré syndrome (GBS, also known as acute inflammatory polyneuritis) is relatively rare, occurring in 1.7 per 100 000 people. It is an acute illness that develops following widespread inflammation and demyelination of peripheral and some cranial nerves (Marsden and Fowler 1988).

The aetiology of GBS is not fully understood. It is considered to be an abnormal autoimmune response to a viral infection. Patients often experience a non-specific infection – such as an upper respiratory or gastrointestinal infection – between one and three weeks prior to the onset of their current symptoms (Box 4.6).

The person experiences ascending weakness, sensory loss and complete flaccid paralysis, beginning in the fingers and toes and graduating towards the trunk, sometimes quite rapidly. In severe cases patients suffer acute neuromuscular respiratory failure, autonomic dysfunction (including postural hypotension, arrythmias and tachycardia) and dysphagia.

Nursing care

Most patients with GBS are conscious and acutely aware of what is happening to them. They feel vulnerable, frightened and isolated. Once the diagnosis has been confirmed, the patient and relatives will require psychological support and must be prepared for the possibility of the patient requiring artificial ventilation.

Frequent monitoring (every 15–30 minutes) of respiratory function using forced vital capacity (FVC) is essential to detect any further deterioration and facilitate elective ventilation in a calm, planned

Box 4.6 Features of Guillain–Barré syndrome

Ascending type
- This is the most common type.
- Weakness and numbness start in the lower extremities and progress upwards to the trunk and arms, and then affect the cranial nerves.
- The patient may present with either paresis or, in extreme cases, quadriplegia.

Descending type
- There is initial cranial nerve involvement affecting cranial nerves VII, IX, X, XI and XII. Weakness develops in a downwards progression.
- Sensory deficits include numbness, most often in the hands and feet.
- Reflexes are diminished or absent.
- There is rapid respiratory involvement.
- Once the weakness reaches the level of the diaphragm, the need for ventilatory support becomes inevitable.

manner rather than as an emergency when the patient has a respiratory arrest. Ventilation is normally indicated if FVC falls below 1.5 L.

Long-term ventilation support is not unusual and may be as long as 6 months. As a consequence, depression and low morale are prevalent. The support of family and friends is crucial, and the nurse can advise and encourage them to become involved in the patient's care.

There is a high level of fatigue both in the acute stage and during recovery. Spacing of interventions, ensuring adequate rest periods and sleep and optimizing visiting, can be useful strategies.

Many patients experience a hypersensitivity to pain especially when touched or when flaccid joints and muscles are moved. Pain assessment must be a priority with regular effective analgesia administered, often in the form of opioids (e.g. a fentanyl patch).

Patients with GBS require intensive support from all members of the multidisciplinary team. This includes prophylaxis against deep vein thrombosis (DVT), supporting limbs in a functional position to reduce the incidence of hyperextension injuries, foot drop and spasticity, assessment of the involvement of the cranial nerves, and nutritional support.

Myasthenia gravis

Cause

Myasthenia gravis (MG) is an autoimmune neurodegenerative disorder caused by defective neurotransmission of nerve impulses at the synapse between the axon at the lower motor neurone and the muscle at the motor end-plate. Antibodies block the acetylcholine receptors on the postsynaptic membrane, inhibiting the propagation of the nerve impulse along the axon.

Clinical features and diagnosis

The most prominent clinical symptom is progressive muscular fatigue and weakness upon exertion, usually improving after a period of rest. The severity of the condition varies from a mild facial weakness, ptosis and diplopia to dysphagia, dysarthria and then incapacitating muscular weakness involving the respiratory muscles – which is life-threatening (Box 4.7).

A myasthenic crisis is often triggered by a change to medication, an adverse reaction or an acute infection. Patients usually require intubation and ventilation to support their respiratory failure. A similar level of support is required for patients experiencing a cholinergic crisis, although this is due to the toxic effects of anticholinesterase medication (Box 4.7).

In the first instance a CT scan is required to exclude a tumour of the thymus gland. A detailed clinical history, presentation and examination will usually help to confirm the diagnosis, aided by EMG (electromyographic conduction) studies and a positive response to edrophonium chloride (Tensilon®) test. The latter is an anticholinesterase inhibitor that is given intravenously (resuscitation equipment must be available as the patient can become profoundly bradycardial during the test). The myasthenic patient will experience an immediate but temporary improvement in muscle strength.

Treatment

Some patients have benefited from the removal of the thymus gland, which produces T lymphocytes, intensifying the autoimmune response. Anticholinesterase medication (e.g. pyridostigmine) is prescribed to

Box 4.7 Signs and symptoms of myasthenic and cholinergic crises

Myasthenic crisis

- Increased blood pressure and tachycardia
- Muscle weakness, resulting in dysarthria and dysphagia
- Excessive salivation, bronchial secretions and sweating
- Lack of cough reflex
- Restlessness and apprehension

Cholinergic crisis

- Decreased blood pressure and bradycardia
- Respiratory distress including dyspnoea and wheezing
- Abdominal cramps including nausea and vomiting
- Excessive salivation, bronchial secretions and sweating
- Vertigo
- Restlessness and apprehension
- Blurred vision
- Dysarthria
- Dysphagia

increase neuromuscular transmission at the synaptic junctions. Tablets must be given in a timely manner to optimize physical activities, including eating and work commitments. Steroid and immunosuppressant therapy may be helpful to reduce the effects of the symptoms. Plasmaphoresis (plasma exchange) with or without immunoglobulin therapy may be used in the acute stages or to manage crisis events.

Nursing care

Assessment of the patient's physical needs must be made upon admission. The patient will usually be able to tell the nurse when he or she feels least fatigued, and these times should be incorporated into the nursing care plan to accommodate the activities requiring most exertion, such as eating and washing.

Patients admitted to the high-dependency unit with deteriorating MG symptoms will be extremely weak, dependent and frightened. Frequent observations should be undertaken to observe for an increase in weakness using regular FVC measurements. Oxygen saturation levels must be observed as these may decrease due to weakness of the respiratory muscles. Any deterioration in observations must be urgently referred to the anaesthetist.

It is essential that medication be administered on time at regular intervals, often outside of normal drug times, to optimize patient function and mobility.

A swallowing assessment must be performed by a speech and language therapist or a dysphagia trained nurse before the patient is given any fluid or food orally. Enteral feeding prescribed by the dietician can supplement nutrition until the patient has regained function. Some patients will benefit from having a percutaneous endoscopic gastroscopy (PEG) tube sited to support nutritional requirements.

Conclusion

It is important that nurses caring for patients with long-term progressive diseases or for those who have suffered acute trauma of the brain and central nervous system understand some of the neuropathophysiology and evidence base for the interventions used in the care and management of these patients. Diseases of the neurological system are often very challenging for the nursing team to deal with. For the patients and their families, both acquired and traumatic brain injury presents daily challenges for nearly every aspect of daily life, from mobility problems to memory, concentration and emotional problems. In addition, financial difficulties resulting from loss of employment and the loss of their own caring position in the family is an added burden. A unified team approach, involving the patients and their families, ensures that they can be cared for in a sensitive and focused way.

This chapter has explored the most commonly seen neurological diseases and provided essential information on caring for and supporting the patient and his or her family through this difficult time.

References

Appleton R, Gibbs J (2004). *Epilepsy in Childhood and Adolescence*, 3rd edn. London: Taylor & Francis.

Andrews PJD, Piper IR, Deardon NM, Miller JD (1990). Secondary insults during interhospital transport of head-injured patients, *Lancet* **335**; 327–30.

Andrus C (1991). Intracranial pressure: dynamics and nursing management, *Journal of Neuroscience Nursing* **23**(2); 85–91.

Bhardwaj A, Mirski M, Ulatowskin J (eds) (2004). *Handbook of Neurocritical Care*. New Jersey, Humana Press.

Bear M, Connors B, Paradiso M (2001). *Neuroscience: Exploring the Brain*, 2nd edn. London: Lippincott Williams & Wilkins.

Bullock RM, Chesnut R, Clifton GL *et al.* (2000). Management and prognosis of severe traumatic brain injury, *Journal of Neurotrauma* **17**; 451–553.

Brunner LS, Suddarth DS (1995). *Textbook of Adult Nursing*. London: Chapman & Hall.

Cascino GD (1996). Generalized convulsive status epilepticus, *Mayo Clinic Proc* **71**; 787–92.

Chibbaro S, Tacconi L (2007). Role of the decompressive craniectomy in the management of severe head injury with refractory cerebral oedema and intractable intracranial pressure: our experience with 48 cases. *Surgical Neurology* **68**; 632–8.

Chipps E, Clanin N, Campbell V (1992). *Neurological Disorders*. Baltimore: Mosby.

Chudley S (1994). The effect of nursing activities on intracranial pressure. *British Journal of Nursing* **3**; 454–9.

Cooke NF (2005). Fundamentals of fluids and hydration in the nursing of the neuroscience patient. *British Journal of Neuroscience Nursing* **1**(2); 61–4.

Edwards S (2001). Regulation of water, sodium and potassium: implications for practice, *Nursing Standard* **15**(22); 36–44.

Feldman Z, Zachari S. Reichenthal E, Artu A. Shapira Y (1995). Brain oedema and neurological status with rapid infusion of Ringers or 5% dextrose solution following head trauma, *Journal of Neurosurgery* **83**; 1060–6.

Garner A, Amin Y (2007). The management of raised intracranial pressure: a multidisciplinary approach, *British Journal of Neuroscience Nursing* **3**; 516–21.

Garner JS (1996). Guideline for isolation precautions in hospitals. *Infect Control Hosp Epidemiol* **17**; 53–80. Available at www.cdc.gov/ncidod/hip/INFECT/isolation.htm.

Gemma M, Tommasino C, Cerri M *et al.* (2002). Intracranial effects of endotracheal suctioning in the acute phase of head injury, *Journal of Neurosurgery and Anesthesiology* **14**; 50–4.

Guyton AC, Hall JE (2006). *Textbook of Medical Physiology*, 11th edn. Philadelphia: Elsevier Saunders.

Hendrickson S (1987). Intracranial pressure changes and family presence, *Journal of Neuroscience Nursing* **19**(1); 14–17.

Hickey J (2008). *Neurological and Neurosurgical Nursing*, 6th edn. London: Lippincott Williams & Wilkins.

Kolbach DN, Sandbrink M, Hamulyak K *et al.* (2004). Non-pharmaceutical measures for prevention of post-thrombotic syndrome. *Cochrane Database Syst Rev* 2004, (1):CD004174.

Lee S (1989). Intracranial pressure changes during positioning of patients with severe head injury, *Heart Lung* **18**; 411–14.

Lloyd F (1990). Eye care for ventilated or unconscious patients, *Nursing Times* **86**; 36–37.

Marsden CD, Fowler TJ (1988). *Clinical Neurology*, 2nd edn. London: Arnold.

Martini F, Bartholomew E (1997). *Essentials of Anatomy and Physiology*. New York: Prentice-Hall.

McGuinness A (2007). Role of the nurse in managing patients with hepatic cerebral oedema, *British Journal of Nursing* **16**; 340–3.

McNair ND (1996). ICP monitoring. In JM Clochesy, C Breu, S Cardin, AA Whittaker & EB Rudy (Eds), Critical Care Nursing (pp 289–307). WB Saunders Company.

Mestecky AM (2007). Management of severe traumatic brain injury: the need for the knowledgeable nurse, *British Journal of Neuroscience Nursing* **3**; 7–13.

Mitchell P, Habermann B (1999). Rethinking physiologic stability: touch and intracranial pressure, *Biological Research for Nursing* **1**(1); 12–19.

Molyneux A, Kerr R, Ly Mee Yu *et al.* (2005). International subarachnoid aneurysm trial (ISAT) of neurosurgical clipping versus endovascular coiling in 2143 patients with ruptured intracranial aneurysms: a randomised comparison of effects on survival, dependency, seizures, rebleeding, subgroups, and aneurysm occlusion, *Lancet* **366**; 809–17.

Ng I, Lim J, Wong H (2004). Effects of head posture on cerebral hemodynamics: its influences on intracranial pressure, cerebral perfusion pressure and cerebral oxygenation, *Neurosurgery* **54**; 593–7.

NPSA (2005). Reducing the harm caused by misplacement of nasogastric feeding tubes. Patient safety alert 0180. Available at www.npsa.nhs.uk/advice.

Reilly P, Bullock R (2005). *Head Injury: Pathophysiology and Management*, 2nd edn. Oxford: Hodder Arnold.

Spratt P, Cooke NF, Gillespie M (2007). Emergency care of the patient with subarachnoid haemorrhage, *British Journal of Neuroscience Nursing* **3**; 210–16.

Teasdale G, Jennett B (1974). Assessment of coma and impaired consciousness: a practical scale, *Lancet* **2**, 81–4.

Teasdale G, Jennett B, Murray L, Murray G (1983). Glasgow Coma Scale: to sum or not to sum, *Lancet* **2**; 678.

Twyman D (1997). Nutritional management of the critically ill neurologic patient, *Critical Care Clinics* **13**; 39–49.

Vincent J, Berre J (2005). Primer on medical management of severe brain injury, *Critical Care Medicine* **33**; 1392–9.

Viney C (1996). *Nursing the Critically Ill Patient*. London: Baillière Tindall.

Waterhouse C (2005). The Glasgow Coma Scale and other neurological observations, *Nursing Standard* **19**; 55–64.

Williams A (1993). Effects of neck position on intracranial pressure, *American Journal of Critical Care* **2**; 68–71.

Woodward S (1997). Neurological observations. 1: Glasgow Coma Scale, *Nursing Times* **93**(45); suppl. 1/2.

CHAPTER 5

INFECTION CONTROL AND SEPSIS

Mick Ashman

LEARNING OUTCOMES

On completion of this chapter the reader will:

1   have an understanding of basic immunology and the possible causes of infection arising from hospital care

2   have an understanding of the principles of infection control and infection control measures

3   have an appreciation of the distinction between sepsis, severe sepsis and septic

shock, and the importance of clinical observations

4   have an understanding of pathophysiology involved in the development of septic shock

5   have an understanding of the appropriate evidence-based therapies when treating patients with septic shock.

Introduction

This chapter presents an overview of basic immunological principles and considers the organisms and conditions that pose a risk to acutely ill patients. The chapter will review the problem of healthcare-associated infection and examine why it presents such a challenge. The principles of infection control will be reviewed before sepsis and severe sepsis are defined and the pathophysiology of these conditions discussed. Finally, the chapter considers septic shock.

An overview of immunology

Micro-organisms

Our environment contains an incredible variety of micro-organisms that are capable of causing infections. These microscopic single-celled organisms

– bacteria, viruses, fungi and protozoa – are found everywhere, including in plants and animals. There are more micro-organisms on and inside the human body than there are individual cells that comprise the body.

These organisms can cause pathological damage to the infected host and if unchecked they will eventually kill the host organism. In normal health this does not happen because most infections are of limited duration and we have defence mechanisms that allow us to fight infectious diseases.

Physiological defence mechanisms

The human immune system comprises two intrinsic defences:

● the innate or non-specific immune system;
● the adaptive or specific immune system.

The innate or non-specific immune system is always prepared and is able to respond immediately to protect from foreign substances. The first line of defence is the barrier provided by intact skin and mucous membranes that prevent the entry of micro-organisms. The second line of defence responds when the external barrier is breached and relies on our ability to produce antimicrobial proteins and phago-cytes, white blood cells that are able to ingest harmful foreign particles including bacteria (a process known as 'phagocytosis'). The second line of defence is enabled by the process of inflammation, which is discussed later in this chapter.

The adaptive or specific immune system, as its name suggests, attacks specific or particular foreign substances and provides the third line of defence.

The immune system is considered to be a functional system rather than an organ-based system because it is made up of many millions of cells – primarily macrophages and lymphocytes – which are found in all body fluids and not located in a particular organ.

An effective immune system is capable of providing protection against most infectious micro-organisms, but it also offers protection against cancer cells and foreign tissues such as those found in trans-planted organs.

Surface membrane barriers

While they are intact and unbroken, the skin and mucous membranes provide an effective first line of defence against disease-causing micro-organisms. Mucous membranes line all the tissues that open to the exterior, including the respiratory tract, gastroin-testinal tract and urinary tract.

There will be occasions when the skin and mucous membranes are breached. A tiny cut to the skin, for example, will allow micro-organisms to enter the body. When this happens the non-specific mecha-nisms come into play.

Non-specific mechanisms

Physiologically there are myriad non-specific cellular and chemical mechanisms that provide protection.

Phagocytes are cells that are able to engulf particu-late matter. They do this by extending themselves around the foreign particle or debris before pulling it inside. Once inside the cell the particle is surrounded by a membrane-lined vacuole which fuses with a lysosome – a spherical structure within the cell that contains enzymes that are able to break up the engulfed particles.

The most common type of phagocyte is the *macrophage*. Macrophages develop from monocytes (white cells) that have moved from the circulation into surrounding tissues in search of foreign micro-organisms. Other examples of phagocytes are the *Kupffer cells* (or stellate reticuloendothelial cells) that are found in the blood vessels (or sinusoids) of the liver, and *alveolar macrophages* that are present in the alveoli of the lungs.

Neutrophils, the most abundant type of white blood cell (comprising around 60 per cent of the white cell population), also become phagocytic on encountering infectious material. However, eosinophils (1–6 per cent of white cells) are weakly phagocytic and mainly target larger parasites and some viral infections.

Natural killer cells (NK cells) are types of lymphocyte. They can recognize cell surface changes that occur on some tumour cells and cells infected by viruses. They bind to these target cells and kill them by releasing small cytoplasmic granules of proteins that cause the target cell to die.

The inflammatory response

The inflammatory response is triggered when tissues are injured. Usually it is a localized response that occurs, for example, in response to trauma or exposure to intense heat (burns) or irritating chemical substances. It is triggered also in response to infec-tions from bacteria, fungi and viruses.

Just as the blood supply to muscles is increased during exercise, to provide additional glucose and oxygen, so it is necessary to improve the perfusion of local tissues when they are injured or infected.

The inflammatory process begins with a chemical 'alarm' (Marieb 2003), whereby a host of powerful chemicals are released into the extracellular fluid. Phagocytes, lymphocytes, mast cells and various blood proteins are all sources of inflammatory media-tors. These include histamine, kinins, prostaglandins and complement proteins all of which have slightly different roles yet they all give rise to localized vasodilation.

There are three major events that occur during the inflammatory response:

- increased blood supply to the infected or injured area;
- increased capillary membrane permeability, allowing larger molecules to move from the circulation to reach the site of infection (or injury);
- migration of leucocytes and macrophages from capillaries to the surrounding tissue.

These physiological changes give rise to the four classic signs of inflammation – swelling, redness, heat and pain – that are seen at the site of infection or injury. When inflammation occurs in response to a systemic infection, the resulting physiological changes are dramatic because they occur on a much greater scale. The result can be septic shock, which is discussed later.

Immunity

It has long been known that individuals who contract and survive certain diseases tend not to have those illnesses again. In the fifth century BC the Greek historian Thucydides recorded that, when a plague was raging in Athens, the sick and dying would have received no nursing at all had it not been for the devotion of those who had already recovered from the disease. What Thucydides did not appreciate was the concept of immunity.

Understanding of the mechanism of immunity developed in the late 1800s when it was demonstrated that animals surviving a serious bacterial infection retained protective factors in their blood. Those factors are now known to be *antibodies* capable of proving defence against attack by the same micro-organism. It was also shown that, if serum containing antibodies was taken from surviving animals and injected into animals that had not been exposed to the pathogen, this immunity could be transferred and they would now be protected. These experiments revealed three key features of the immune response:

- *antigen specificity* – it recognizes and targets against particular pathogens or foreign substances that trigger the inflammatory response;
- *systemic function* – immunity is not restricted to the site of infection;

- *memory* – after initial exposure the immune system recognizes and can attack previously encountered pathogens and foreign substances.

It was later discovered that there were two mechanisms involved, each capable of using a variety of other mechanisms depending on the precise nature of the intruding pathogen.

Organisms and sources of infection

Micro-organisms are ubiquitous in the environment. Practically every area of the Earth is inhabited by a microscopic ecosystem of life forms that are uniquely adapted to their environments. An overview of specific organisms in relation to sites of infection in a human is given in Fig. 5.1.

Bacteria

Bacteria are in a large group of single-celled organisms that contain a nucleus. They are invisible to the naked eye because they are usually no more than a few micrometres across (one micrometre is equal to one-thousandth of a millimetre). They grow in soil, in water and in inhospitable conditions such as acidic hot springs, but they also grow on organic matter and will live on the bodies of both living and dead animals and plants.

There are many thousands of species of bacteria and for more than 200 years attempts have been made to classify them based on their similarities. The processes that microbiologists use to this end have become increasingly complicated, encompassing techniques to determine the extent to which they share their genes. Precise identification is particularly important in healthcare because appropriate treatment is determined by the bacterial species causing an infection.

The Gram staining technique was developed in 1884 by Hans Christian Gram. It classifies bacteria based on the structure of their cell walls – which stain differently depending on their chemical composition. By looking at the shape of the bacterium under the microscope and using the Gram staining technique, most bacteria can be classified as belonging to one of four groups: Gram-positive cocci, Gram-positive bacilli, Gram-negative cocci and Gram-negative bacilli. Other bacteria, particularly mycobacteria, are better identified with other staining techniques.

Samples of blood, urine or secretions are taken from patients and then microbiologists use techniques to promote the growth of particular bacteria, while restricting the growth of other micro-organisms in the sample. Usually these techniques are designed for specific specimens. For example, a sputum sample will be subjected to techniques that identify organisms that are able to cause pneumonia, whereas stool specimens are cultured on selective media that will allow the identification of organisms that cause diarrhoea, while preventing growth of other non-pathogenic bacteria.

Blood samples, which would normally be expected to be sterile, are cultured under conditions that will promote the growth of all possible organisms.

Viruses

Viruses are ubiquitous companions of cellular life forms. Virologists now believe that every cellular organism studied – including, animals, plants and bacteria – has its own viruses or, at least, 'virus-like selfish genetic elements' (Koonin *et al.* 2006).

Viruses are companions of cellular life forms because they can replicate only inside living cells. They do, however, possess genes and can evolve but they do not have a cellular structure. Some virologists have therefore questioned whether viruses can be described as a true life form or whether they are simply organic structures that interact with living organisms. Viruses consist of two or three parts: DNA or RNA (the molecules that carry their genetic information), a protein coat that protects these genes, and in some cases a lipid envelope that offers a further protective coating.

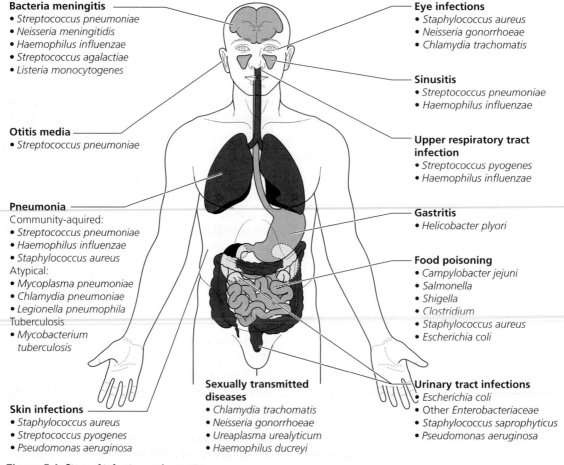

Bacteria meningitis
- *Streptococcus pneumoniae*
- *Neisseria meningitidis*
- *Haemophilus influenzae*
- *Streptococcus agalactiae*
- *Listeria monocytogenes*

Otitis media
- *Streptococcus pneumoniae*

Pneumonia
Community-aquired:
- *Streptococcus pneumoniae*
- *Haemophilus influenzae*
- *Staphylococcus aureus*
Atypical:
- *Mycoplasma pneumoniae*
- *Chlamydia pneumoniae*
- *Legionella pneumophila*
Tuberculosis
- *Mycobacterium tuberculosis*

Skin infections
- *Staphylococcus aureus*
- *Streptococcus pyogenes*
- *Pseudomonas aeruginosa*

Sexually transmitted diseases
- *Chlamydia trachomatis*
- *Neisseria gonorrhoeae*
- *Ureaplasma urealyticum*
- *Haemophilus ducreyi*

Eye infections
- *Staphylococcus aureus*
- *Neisseria gonorrhoeae*
- *Chlamydia trachomatis*

Sinusitis
- *Streptococcus pneumoniae*
- *Haemophilus influenzae*

Upper respiratory tract infection
- *Streptococcus pyogenes*
- *Haemophilus influenzae*

Gastritis
- *Helicobacter plyori*

Food poisoning
- *Campylobacter jejuni*
- *Salmonella*
- *Shigella*
- *Clostridium*
- *Staphylococcus aureus*
- *Escherichia coli*

Urinary tract infections
- *Escherichia coli*
- Other *Enterobacteriaceae*
- *Staphylococcus saprophyticus*
- *Pseudomonas aeruginosa*

Figure 5.1 Sites of infection and organisms

Viral infections are capable of triggering the immune response in humans and animals, and usually this will over the course of a few days eliminate the infecting virus. These immune responses can also be produced by administering vaccines (usually made from dead or inactivated viruses) which confer the acquired immunity described earlier to the specific viral infection. Some viruses, such as the human immunodeficiency virus (HIV) and viral hepatitis, can evade these normal immune responses and lead to chronic infections. Antibiotics have no effect on viruses, but antiviral drugs such as oseltamivir and aciclovir have been developed.

In humans, illnesses caused by viruses include the common cold, influenza, chickenpox and cold sores. Many life-threatening diseases such as avian influenza (bird flu) and severe acute respiratory syndrome (SARS) are also caused by viruses. The relative ability of a particular virus to causing disease is described in terms of its *virulence*.

Fungi

Fungal infections (mycoses) arise when fungal material crosses the normal physiological resistance barriers. These infections are more prevalent when the environment is warm and humid, and when people live in crowded conditions. Most fungi reproduce by releasing tiny spores into the air. These spores are either inhaled or they land on the surface of the skin. For this reason, fungal infections tend to originate in the lungs or on the surface of the skin.

Individuals are at greater risk of developing a fungal infection when they are receiving antibiotic therapy for a long period. This is because antibiotics kill not only the bacteria causing an infection but also healthy commensal bacteria. This alters the normal balance of micro-organisms in the mouth or gut, allowing an overgrowth of the fungus. Immunocompromised patients are also vulnerable.

One example of a fungal infection is aspergillosis (caused by *Aspergillus*). This most commonly affects the respiratory tract, giving rise to bronchopulmonary aspergillosis with cough, fever, chest pain and breathlessness. Most of us will inhale *Aspergillus* spores on a regular basis, but unless we are immunocompromised an infection is unlikely to develop. Patients with leukaemia are particularly vulnerable to

this type of fungal infection. The infection is usually treated with amphotericin or voriconazole.

Candidiasis (thrush) is a fungal infection by any *Candida* species, although C. albicans is the most common. Candidiasis infections, such as oral thrush, tend to be localized and superficial. However, systemic candidiasis can be a life-threatening condition; as with other fungal infections it is usually confined to severely immunocompromised persons, such as those with cancer, a transplant or AIDS.

Nosocomial infections

Healthcare-associated infections cost the NHS more than £1 billion per year and can lead to serious disability and in some cases death. ... it is disappointing that the Department of Health still has not taken on board a number of key recommendations.

Parliamentary Public Accounts
Committee (2009)

Nosocomial infections are defined as infections that are neither present nor incubating when a patient begins receiving treatment in a hospital or a healthcare service unit. The term 'hospital-acquired infection' (HAI) is sometimes used when referring to infections arising from hospital admission, although the term 'healthcare-associated infection' (HCAI) is increasingly preferred because this applies to all patients receiving healthcare.

Nosocomial infections are common in the United Kingdom, affecting around 9 per cent of the patient population. This figure was arrived at in studies published in 1981 and 1996 and translates to over 300 000 patients. In 2000, the Public Accounts Committee concluded that the NHS did not have a grip on the extent and costs of hospital-acquired infections and argued that, without robust data, it was difficult to see how activity and resources could be targeted to best effect. Five years later, progress in improving infection prevention and control was described as patchy.

A more concerted approach since then has been credited with reducing the rates of infection of two micro-organisms that contribute to nosocomial infection rates – methicillin-resistant *Staphylococcus aureus* (MRSA) and *Clostridium difficile*. It is felt that hospital cleanliness has improved and the priority given to reducing the two targeted infections has begun to have a wider impact on hospital-acquired infection prevention and control in general.

Basic measures for infection control

Infection control is concerned with the prevention of acquired infections and is an essential consideration in healthcare delivery. For someone to become infected while in hospital there has to be a source of the infective agent and a means of transmission. However, there are recognized risk factors that are associated with the increased likelihood of a patient acquiring an infection.

Risk factors

The known risk factors fall into three broad categories.

General state of health

Acutely ill patients in hospital are often in chronic poor health, which reduces the effectiveness of their normal immune response. They may have immuno-deficiency resulting from the illness itself, drugs, irradiation or simply advanced age. Certain conditions will also increase their vulnerability; for example chronic obstructive pulmonary disease (COPD) can increase the probability of a respiratory tract infection.

Hospital procedures

Invasive hospital procedures are associated with increased infection risk because they frequently lead to the bypassing of normal defence mechanisms. For example, endotracheal intubation, intravenous catheters, urinary catheters and surgical drains will all provide a potential conduit for infective micro-organisms. For this reason the clinical justification for invasive procedures needs to be balanced against the associated risk.

Treatment or therapy

The actual treatment a patient receives can also leave him or her vulnerable to infection. For example, treatment resulting in immunosuppression will undermine the defence mechanisms discussed earlier in the chapter, while antimicrobial therapy can eradicate commensal bacterial populations allowing potentially resistant organisms to proliferate.

Control measures

Hand hygiene

The most important measure for preventing the spread of pathogens is effective handwashing. Hands should be decontaminated prior to direct contact with patients and after every contact with patients, or potentially contaminated equipment. Alcohol hand gels and rubs are increasingly being used but, while they are a practical alternative to soap and water, alcohol is not a cleaning agent. Therefore hands that are visibly dirty or potentially grossly contaminated must be washed with soap and water and dried thoroughly.

Drying is an essential part of the hand hygiene process. Studies comparing the bacteria levels present after the use of paper towels and various types of hand dryer have shown that only paper towels reduce the total number of bacteria on hands, with 'through-air dried' towels that have a greater absorbency being the most effective.

Personal protective equipment

Personal protective equipment (PPE) is defined by the Personal Protective Equipment at Work Regulations (HSE 1992) as all equipment that is intended to be worn or held by a person at work and which protects against one or more risks to his or her health or safety. It includes eye protection, high-visibility clothing, safety footwear, safety harnesses and safety helmets. For healthcare worker, examples of PPE include gloves, gowns and face masks.

In the clinical setting the hazards can be biological. This will include exposure to blood or other bodily fluids or aerosols that may carry infectious materials including viruses such as hepatitis C, and other microbiological pathogens found in blood or bodily fluids. Personal protective equipment creates a physical barrier to prevent contact. Because the protective equipment can be discarded after a procedure it is an important mechanism for reducing the risk of cross-contamination between patients. Personal protective equipment can also protect healthcare workers from chemical hazards such as cleaning agents, disinfectants and certain medicines.

Decontamination of medical devices

Adequate decontamination of medical devices is another important factor in the prevention of health-care-associated infections. Decontamination involves three processes – cleaning, disinfection and sterilization – which can be adopted to ensure that a reusable medical device is safe for second use. The proportion of HAIs that could be prevented by more effective decontamination practices is very difficult to estimate, but it has been known for some time that decontamination failures of equipment, such as endoscopes, can result in a serious spread of infection (Spach *et al.* 1993).

Each instrument or piece of medical equipment that comes into contact with a patient can present a potential source of infection. However, the level of risk depends on what the equipment is used for and will fall into one of three recognized risk categories.

- *High-risk category*. In this category is equipment that comes into close contact with a break in the skin or mucous membranes or is introduced into a normally sterile body area. Examples include surgical instruments, needles, and intravenous and urinary catheters. Sterilization is an absolute requirement for these items although, because of the cost involved, many high-risk items are disposable.
- *Intermediate-risk category*. This includes equipment that comes into close contact with mucous membranes, such as items of respiratory equipment (e.g. laryngoscope blades, endotracheal and tracheostomy tubes, oropharyngeal and nasal airways). Disinfection is required for this group.
- *Low-risk category*. This equipment comes into contact only with normal intact skin (e.g. a washing bowl). Cleaning and drying with soap and water is usually considered adequate for this group.

Cleaning is the process that removes contaminants including dust, large numbers of micro-organisms, blood, vomit etc. It is an essential prerequisite to disinfection and sterilization because otherwise debris on the surface of the equipment will prevent these processes from being effective. Cleaning will also remove any residual organic matter on which micro-organisms might subsequently thrive.

Disinfection is any process used to reduce the number of micro-organisms and involves using liquid chemicals on surfaces at room temperature. The process does not necessarily kill or eradicate all micro-organisms, but it will reduce their number to a level that is not harmful to health. Examples of commonly used chemical disinfectant solutions are hypochlorites, aldehydes and alcohols (Box 5.1).

Box 5.1 Common chemical disinfectant solutions

- **Hypochlorites** (e.g. bleach) have a wide range of activity against bacteria, fungi, viruses and bacterial spores. They are therefore appropriate for decontaminating any area with blood spillage. However, they are potentially corrosive to metals and must be applied at the correct concentration.
- **Aldehydes** (e.g. glutaraldehyde) are active against bacteria, viruses and fungi. However, they are particularly irritant to skin and eyes and require appropriate measures to minimize such risk.
- **Alcohols** (e.g. ethanol and isopropanolol) have good activity against bacteria and viruses and are used increasingly in clinical settings. To work effectively they should be applied only after thorough cleaning has ensured that all visible surface debris has been removed from the area to be disinfected.

Sterilization processes remove or destroy all forms of microbial life including more resistant bacterial spores. This can be achieved by steam, steam plus formaldehyde, or hot air. Irradiation or ethylene oxide can be used to sterilize heat-sensitive equipment. In the hospital setting, autoclaving is the most reliable way to sterilize instruments: using pressurized steam at a temperature of 134°C for 3 minutes or 121°C for 15 minutes is recommended.

Cleaning the environment

The NHS Plan published in 2000 (DH 2000) set out a reform agenda for the National Health Service. Included in the document and subsequent publications was a clear statement of intent to improve standards of cleanliness in hospitals. This included the introduction of new investment to support immediate improvements to cleanliness with the aim of ensuring that higher standards were maintained in future years.

The National Standards of Cleanliness were first published in 2001 and involved hospitals across the country undertaking a baseline audit using a standards framework to measure the 'technical cleanliness' of their establishments. The importance of clean hospitals was further emphasized with the publication of the *NHS Healthcare Cleaning Manual* (NHS Estates 2004) which set out to provide guidance and advice to healthcare organisations in order for them to meet their obligation to deliver effective and safe healthcare in clean premises. Subsequent revisions to the *Cleaning Manual* included an increasing emphasis on best practice and research evidence to promote the clean hospital agenda and minimize patient risk.

Sepsis: the problem of overwhelming infection

Despite the current structured and evidence-based approach to infection control measures the problem of healthcare-associated infection remains. The fact that patients will also be admitted to hospital having acquired an infection in the community means that many patients in acute and high-dependency areas will display the classic signs of acute infection, including pyrexia and tachycardia.

These clinical signs represent the first stages of the physiological response to infection that was discussed earlier in the chapter. This physiological response can cause dramatic changes and may result in the development of *septic shock*, a condition with an overall mortality of up to 50 per cent. Indeed, in the United States sepsis arising from a nosocomial or community-acquired infection was reported as the tenth most common cause of death (Hoyert *et al.* 2001). The actual number of deaths associated with the condition may be even higher than current estimates suggest because many sepsis patients have at least one other co-morbidity and deaths are often attributed to these rather than to sepsis.

What prevalence studies can reveal

Studies can provide valuable information regarding disease prevalence and demographics. The European Prevalence of Infection in intensive Care (EPIC) report demonstrated how international collaboration can succeed in providing such information. Although the study was conducted as long ago as 1992, the number of patients in the sample makes the study highly significant. Data were collected on all patients present in the participating ICUs. On the nominated day:

- there were 10 037 patients in 1472 European intensive care units;
- 44.8 per cent of them were being treated for infection with antimicrobial drugs;
- 47 per cent of these were acquired following admission to the critical care area and, of these, nearly a half were pneumonias.

The authors identified a number of risk factors that were associated with increased likelihood of ICU acquired infection:

- length of stay in the critical care environment;
- use of central venous, pulmonary artery and urinary catheters (i.e. invasive monitoring);
- mechanical ventilation;
- patients who were admitted with a diagnosis of trauma;
- use of stress ulcer prophylaxis (which results in an alteration to normal gut flora).

The study also identified that many of the organisms responsible for these infections were resistant to commonly used antibiotics. In 1992, 60 per cent of the *Staphylococcus aureus* isolated were resistant to methicillin, and 46 per cent of *Pseudomonas aeruginosa* were resistant to gentamicin.

More recent prevalence studies using smaller patient samples in both intensive care and other settings concur with the findings of the EPIC study. Length of hospital stay and extent of invasive monitoring are risk factors regardless of the clinical setting.

The importance of clear definitions

The need for precise and clear definitions of sepsis and septic shock, in order to promote effective clinical investigations and management, was recognized some 20 years ago (Parker and Fink 1991).

In 1991, a joint American College of Chest Physicians and Society of Critical Care Medicine conference was held with the goal of agreeing on a set of universal definitions that could be applied to patients with sepsis and its related conditions. The conference came up with new definitions for some terms, while other terms were discarded. Broad definitions of sepsis and the systemic inflammatory response syndrome were proposed, together with precise physiological parameters that could be used to catagorize patients. The use of severity scoring methods when dealing with septic patients was also recommended as an adjunctive tool to predict mortality. Since then the definitions have gained near-universal acceptance (Box 5.2).

Many individuals will experience these clinical signs, perhaps caused by influenza and other viral infection; and, while they will feel unwell, few will require hospital treatment. The term *uncomplicated sepsis* is sometimes used to describe this condition.

Box 5.2 also defines severe sepsis. This is sepsis as previously defined, but associated with:

- organ dysfunction;
- hypoperfusion;
- hypotension.

Hypoperfusion and perfusion abnormalities may include (but are not limited to) lactic acidosis,

---

Box 5.2 Definitions

Infection

A microbial phenomenon characterized by the presence of micro-organisms or the invasion of normally sterile host tissue by those organisms.

Bacteraemia

The presence of viable bacteria in the blood.

Hypotension

Systolic blood pressure of <90 mmHg or a reduction of >40 mmHg from the patient's own baseline in the absence of other causes for hypotension.

Systemic inflammatory response syndrome (SIRS)

Systemic inflammatory response to a variety of severe clinical insults, including infection, burns, multiple trauma and pancreatitis. The response is manifested by *two or more* of the following conditions:
- temperature >38 or <36°C
- heart rate >90 beats/min
- respiratory rate >20 breaths/min or $Paco_2$ < 32 mmHg (4.3 kPa)
- white blood cell count >12 000 or <4000 mm^3, or >10% band forms (immature white blood cells).

Sepsis

Systemic response to infection, manifested by *two or more* of the following conditions as a result of infection:
- temperature >38 or <36°C
- heart rate >90 beats/min
- respiratory rate >20 breaths/min or $Paco_2$ < 32 mmHg (4.3 kPa)
- white blood cell count >12 000 or <4000 mm^3, or >10% band forms (immature white blood cells).

Severe sepsis

Sepsis as previously defined, but associated with:
- organ dysfunction
- hypoperfusion
- hypotension.

Septic shock

Sepsis with hypotension, despite adequate fluid resuscitation, along with the presence of perfusion abnormalities that may include (but are not limited to):
- lactic acidosis (serum lactate greater than 4 mmol/dL)
- oliguria (urine output <1 mL/kg/h in infants, <0.5 mL/kg/h in children, and <400 mL/day in adults)
- acute alteration in mental status.

oliguria, or an acute alteration in mental status. Patients are considered to have septic shock if they have sepsis (as defined) plus hypotension after aggressive fluid resuscitation – typically upwards of 6 L or 40 mL/kg of crystalloid.

Micro-organisms that cause sepsis

All the micro-organisms discussed earlier in the chapter are capable of causing sepsis and initiating the inflammatory response; these include bacteria, fungi, viruses and protozoa. However, severe sepsis (as defined above) is primarily associated with bacterial infections by Gram-negative and Gram-positive bacteria, with Gram-negative organisms most commonly responsible for sepsis and septic shock (Table 5.1).

Table 5.1 Organisms responsible for severe sepsis

Gram-negative organisms	Gram-positive organisms

Primarily respiratory infections:
   Haemophilus influenzae
   Klebsiella pneumoniae
   Legionella pneumophila
   Pseudomonas aeruginosa
	Cocci (sphere-shaped bacteria):
	   Enterococci
	   Staphylococci
	   Streptococci

Primarily urinary tract infections:
   Enterobacter cloacae
   Escherichia coli
   Proteus mirabilis
   Pseudomonas
	Bacilli (rod-shaped bacteria):
	   Clostridia
	   Listeria

Primarily gastrointestinal infections:
   Helicobacter pylori
   Salmonella enteritidis
 	
 Others:
   Acinerobacter
   Neisseria gonorrhoeae	

Exotoxins

Exotoxins are the toxins released by micro-organisms (bacteria, fungi, protozoa) that are harmful to the host. Some bacteria produce only one significant toxin, which is the principal determinant of the disease process (e.g. tetanus). Such exotoxins may exert their effect locally or produce systemic effects. Examples of exotoxins include the botulinum toxin produced by *Clostridium botulinum* and the *Corynebacterium diphtheriae* exotoxin which is produced during life-threatening diphtheria. Most exotoxins are sensitive to raised temperatures and are antigenic, making them susceptible to antibodies produced by the immune system. However, some exotoxins are so toxic that they may be fatal to the host before the immune system has been able to effectively respond to them. Gram-positive bacteria tend to produce exotoxins.

Endotoxins

Endotoxins are part of the outer membrane of the cell wall of bacteria and are more typically associated with Gram-negative bacteria whether the organisms are pathogens or not. The term 'endotoxin' dates back to the discovery that portions of Gram-negative bacteria, although no longer viable, could still give rise to adverse clinical symptoms.

Although the term 'endotoxin' is occasionally used to refer to any cell-associated bacterial toxin, it actually refers to the lipopolysaccharide (LPS) complex associated with the outer membrane of Gram-negative bacteria. LPS consists of a polysaccharide (sugar) chain and a lipid portion known as lipid A.

Humans are able to produce antibodies to endotoxins after exposure but these are generally directed at the polysaccharide (sugar) chain and not the lipid A group. The presence of a small amount of endotoxin in humans will lead to the inflammatory response – fever, a fall in blood pressure, and activation of inflammatory mechanisms. Endotoxins are therefore considered to be responsible for the dramatic systemic inflammatory response associated with infections by pathogenic Gram-negative bacteria. The relationship of endotoxins to the bacterial cell surface is illustrated in Fig. 5.2.

It is thought that in the clinical situation Gram-negative bacteria release very small amounts of endotoxin while they are growing. However, for the most part, endotoxins remain associated with the cell wall until disintegration or destruction of the bacteria. In patients, this might result from autolysis of the bacteria, external lysis mediated by complement proteins and lysozyme, and phagocytic digestion of bacterial cells.

The lipid part of the molecule (lipid A) serves to anchor the molecule in the bacterial membrane and is

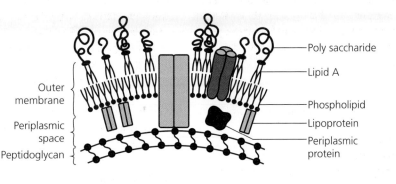

Figure 5.2 Structure of the cell surface of a Gram-negative bacterium

not exposed to the environment in intact bacteria. However, treatment with antibiotics and our own host defence mechanisms can damage the bacterial membrane, causing exposure of this normally embedded lipid A molecule. It appears that it exerts its toxic effects (triggering the inflammatory response) only when released from multiplying cells in a soluble form, or when the bacteria are ruptured (lysed) as a result of autolysis, or killing by phagocytes or antibiotics.

Mechanism of the inflammatory response

Sepsis, severe sepsis and septic shock represent progressive stages on a continuum of the systemic inflammatory response to an infection. We can appreciate how dramatic this is if we consider the profound changes that occur at the site of localized infection. If the tip of our finger becomes infected we see the classic signs of reddening, swelling and pain. Here the localized inflammation occurs because of the release of powerful hormones or vasoactive mediators. We produce these chemical substances as part of a physiological reaction to improve the blood supply to an affected area and to increase the permeability of capillaries. This is an appropriate response because the dilation of blood vessels improves blood flow to the affected area, therefore enabling the targeting of proteins and immunoglobulins that can fight infection. The increase in capillary permeability allows the white cells and proteins to move easily out of the blood vessels to the site of infection.

As the term suggests, in the systemic inflammatory response arising from sepsis, these local changes occur throughout the circulatory system. When the inflammatory response is localized it is focused and specific: it improves perfusion and tissue oxygenation. However, when the inflammatory response is systemic the consequences are dramatic.

The inflammatory response is summarized in Fig. 5.3. It is actually an extremely complicated process involving numerous biochemical mediators and cytokines. Cytokines are small secreted proteins that regulate immunity, inflammation and haematopoiesis. They are produced in response to an antigenic stimulus such as bacterial endotoxin. They usually act over short distances, a short time frame and exert their effects at very low concentration. A list of some of the groups of biochemical mediators released is provided in Table 5.2.

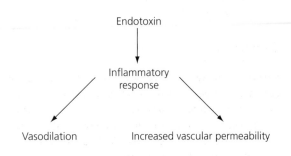

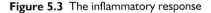

Figure 5.3 The inflammatory response

Table 5.2 Mediators of the inflammatory response

Mediator	Source	Main effect
Histamine	Mast cells, especially numerous at sites of potential injury (oropharynx, nose, blood vessels) Basophils or basophil granulocytes, the least common granulocyte, comprising 0.01–0.3% of circulating white blood cells	Acts on one of four types of histamine receptor (H1–H4) Vasodilatation Increased vascular permeability
Serotonin	Platelets	Increased vascular permeability Platelet aggregation
Prostaglandins	All leucocytes, platelets, endothelial cells	Most cause vasodilatation (although thromboxane is a vasoconstrictor)
Leukotrienes	All leucocytes	Vasoconstriction Bronchospasm Increased vascular permeability
Platelet activating factor (PAF)	All leucocytes, platelets, endothelial cells	Platelet aggregation Vasodilatation Increased vascular permeability Leukocyte adherence
Nitric oxide (NO)	Endothelial cells, macrophages, platelets	Vasodilatation
Cytokines (interleukin, tumour necrosis factor)	Macrophages, lymphocytes	Vasodilatation Fever Lethargy Attracts leucocytes
Kinin system (bradykinin)	Circulates in plasma (normally inactive)	Increased vascular permeability Vasodilatation
Complement system	Cascade of inactive plasma proteins	Leucocyte activation Phagocytosis Proteins C3a and C5a cause increased vascular permeability and vasodilatation

Haemodynamic changes and altered tissue perfusion

In the past, septic shock has been described in terms of a *warm* phase and a *cold* phase. These terms are no longer used but they do help us understand the impact of the physiological changes on the patient's appearance. Initially the vasodilation will be met by a corresponding but brief baroreceptor reflex-generated increase in cardiac output. The 'cold' stage that follows arises from the onset of perfusion abnormalities when cardiac output is no longer sufficient to generate an adequate perfusion pressure. The phases are better viewed as points on a continuum rather than discrete phases.

It is important to appreciate that the haemodynamic changes that characterize septic shock are not determined by the nature of the infecting organism but by the response of the host to that infection.

The extensive peripheral vasodilation that is a consequence of the inflammatory response gives rise to a decrease in systemic vascular resistance (SVR) and the initial increase in cardiac output, achieved primarily by increased heart rate. However, cardiac output is only increased up to a point. When there is failure to achieve or to maintain an appropriately augmented cardiac output, the resulting hypotension will lead to inadequate tissue perfusion and failing tissue oxygenation.

Failing tissue oxygenation

The vasodilation and consequent poor tissue perfusion can give rise to the 'bypassing' of metabolically active tissues with ineffective tissue oxygen extraction and utilization.

This will lead to increased anaerobic metabolism in tissues and a resulting metabolic acidosis (evident in raised lactate levels). Current literature suggests that the redistribution of blood flow and volume in septic shock patients can vary, which suggests that not all tissues will be subjected to the same deterioration in perfusion. Therefore some organs are more at risk of ischaemia (and possible failure) than others.

Another significant change is myocardial dysfunction. It is widely accepted that most patients with septic shock develop abnormalities in cardiac function, and it has been shown that myocardial dysfunction is already present in patients early on when cardiac output is briefly increased. Signs of myocardial dysfunction include diminished left and right ejection fractions and suggestions of a deterioration in myocardial contractility.

CASE STUDY 5.1

Mrs James is a 68-year-old woman who has returned from theatre following surgery consisting of a right hemicolectomy. For the first two hours on the ward her condition is stable: temperature 37.5°C; heart rate 80/min; blood presure 135/85 mmHg; respiratory rate 12/min; oxygen saturation on air 94 per cent.

Six hours after returning to the ward her observations are: temperature 38.2°C; HR 95/min; BP 120/75 mmHg ; respiratory rate 14/min; oxygen saturation on air 94 per cent.

- Would you be concerned about these observations? If so, why?
- What clinical signs would you look for that might suggest any further change in her condition?

Management of septic shock

The Surviving Sepsis Campaign (SSC) is an initiative of the European Society of Intensive Care Medicine (ESICM), the International Sepsis Forum (ISF) and the Society of Critical Care Medicine. It was established in 2008 with the aim of improving the management, diagnosis and treatment of sepsis. The multi-point strategy of the Surviving Sepsis Campaign (www.survivingsepsis.org) aims to reduce mortality from sepsis primarily by:

- building awareness of sepsis;
- improving diagnosis;

- increasing the use of appropriate treatment;
- educating healthcare professionals;
- improving post-ICU care;
- developing guidelines of care;
- facilitating data collection for the purposes of audit and feedback.

The following overview of therapeutic interventions followed the establishment of a working group by Vincent *et al.* (2002). They selected the five clinical interventions that had been shown in randomized controlled trials to reduce mortality: early goal-directed therapy; tight control of blood sugar; use of low tidal volumes in ventilated patients; use of activated protein C; and use of moderate doses of steroids.

Early goal-directed therapy

Early goal-directed therapy (EGDT) has been identified as a key intervention in septic shock patients (Rivers *et al.* 2001). The therapy is an attempt to adjust the cardiac preload, afterload and contractility to balance systemic oxygen delivery with oxygen demand, and this approach has been the mainstay of treatment for these patients for the past 25 years.

Edwards *et al.* (1989) claimed to show a reduced mortality when goals of cardiac index above 4.5 L/min/m^2, Do_2 above 600 mL/min/m^2 and Vo_2 equal to 168 mL/min/m^2 were used (Box 5.3). However, Vincent *et al.* (2002) stated that, in the intensive care setting, supranormal and normal approaches have met with little or no success. They suggested one

Box 5.3 Therapeutic goals

- Cardiac index > 4.5 L/min/m^2
  Cardiac output taking into account the size of the patient (i.e. per square metre of body surface area)
- Do^2 > 600 mL/min/m^2
  Oxygen delivery (or dispatch), the amount of oxygen in the blood leaving the left ventricle per minute taking into account the surface area of the patient
- Vo_2 = 168 mL/min/m^2
  Oxygen consumption: the amount of oxygen consumed per minute taking into account the surface area of the patient

explanation might be that, by the time these therapies are applied in the setting, any such intervention could be too late. Hence the focus has shifted towards delivering EGDT earlier, such as in the A&E department.

A prospective, randomized, predominantly blinded study was initiated by the Early Goal-Directed Therapy Collaborative Group to examine the results of haemodynamic interventions in the emergency department (Rivers *et al.* 2001). Patients were randomly assigned to either 6 hours of EGDT or to standard therapy prior to admission to the ICU. The in-hospital mortality was 30.5 per cent in the group assigned to EGDT and 46.5 per cent in the group assigned to standard therapy. This indicates that EGDT provides significant benefits in improving outcomes in patients with severe sepsis and septic shock.

In the 1990s it was recognized that the number of critically ill patients presenting to, and being treated in, emergency departments was increasing (Nguyen *et al.* 2000). Vincent *et al.* (2002) thought that this may give rise to significant resource challenges in the emergency department environment seeking to administer EGDT.

Tight control of blood sugar

Raised serum glucose (hyperglycaemia), caused by insulin resistance in the liver and muscle, is a common finding in critically ill patients. It can be considered an adaptive response, to make more glucose available for the brain, red cells and wound healing, and in the past hyperglycaemia has been treated only when blood glucose exceeds 12 mmol/L.

However, Vincent *et al.* (2002) cited studies showing that high levels of insulin-like growth factor-1 (ILGF-1: a very good marker of lack of hepatic insulin effect) predict mortality. Patients with high levels of this factor also tend to have the lowest insulin levels, indicating that the activity of their pancreatic beta cells is impaired and as a result not enough insulin is being produced. These findings suggest that hyperglycaemia may not always be adaptive, so it should be treated to avoid the onset of specific complications.

So the conventional wisdom that hyperglycaemia in critically ill patients is beneficial (and that hypoglycaemia should be avoided) has been challenged and this has been borne out in some important randomized trials (Van den Berghe 2001).

Acute lung injury and respiratory distress syndrome

The conventional approach to the management of critically ill patients with acute lung injury and acute respiratory distress syndrome (ALI /ARDS) has been to ventilate them using tidal volumes between 10 and 15 mL/kg of body weight, which is almost twice the tidal volume of healthy individuals at rest. However, these higher volumes lead to high inspiratory airway pressures and to excessive stretch of the aerated lung. Stretching lung tissue in this way releases inflammatory mediators, which is undesirable in patients already showing clinical signs of the systemic inflammatory response. It is therefore recommended that, when mechanical ventilation is indicated for treatment of patients with ALI /ARDS, the tidal volume should be limited to about 6 mL/kg of ideal body weight.

Activated protein C

Protein C (also known as autoprothrombin IIA) is an inactive serum protein. However, in its activated form it plays an important role in regulating inflammation, blood clotting, cell death and the permeability of blood vessel walls. A number of studies have shown that patients with sepsis have severe depletion of protein C (Yan *et al.* 2001), and the association of protein C depletion with high mortality in sepsis has also been established (Vincent *et al.* 2002).

The findings of the PROWESS trial (Protein C Worldwide Evaluation in Severe Sepsis; Bernard *et al.* 2001) confirmed that treating patients using an artificially manufactured form of protein C could reduce mortality by over 6 per cent. The treatment carries the risk of severe bleeding and is expensive. This has led some authors to suggest that measurement of disease severity – such as using the 'APACHE II' score – may be used to decide which patients would benefit most from the therapy (Vincent *et al.* 2002).

Moderate-dose corticosteroids

The value of steroids in the treatment of patients with severe sepsis or septic shock has been debated for some time (Vincent *et al.* 2002). While high-dose therapy carries risks there is strong evidence supporting the use of low-dose therapy in patients with refractory septic shock (defined as septic shock lasting more than one hour, that does not respond to fluid resuscitation or pharmacological therapy). This is because adrenal insufficiency appears to be common in patients with refractory septic shock (50–75 per cent of patients). It is now suggested that moderate-dose corticosteroids should be considered in cases of refractory septic shock following an ACTH test to determine whether adrenal gland function is normal.

Guidelines for the management of severe sepsis and septic shock

The Surviving Sepsis Campaign recently published guidelines (Dellinger *et al.* 2008). The SSC states that its guidelines do not cover every aspect of management of patients with septic shock, and that the guidelines should be supplemented by 'generic best practice and specific treatment as required'.

The SSC has chosen to rank its interventions as 'recommended' or 'suggested'. The recommended interventions are underpinned by a stronger evidence base and are summarized below. The detailed guidelines can be found at www.survivingsepsis.org.

As the research evidence base supporting these and other interventions changes they will be subject to revision. However, the fundamental principle of prompt assessment and decision-making will remain unchanged.

ACTIVITY ?

The approach to patient assessment will depend on the clinical area in which you work. As you read through the SSC guidelines below, consider your own area of clinical practice and which of the guidelines involve assessment by the nurse. For each intervention, identify whether the nurse will have direct, indirect or limited responsibility.

Initial resuscitation: the first six hours

- Begin resuscitation immediately in patients with hypotension or elevated serum lactate (>4 mmol/L). Do not wait for the patient to be admitted to intensive care.
- Resuscitation goals are: central venous pressure (CVP) 8–12 mmHg; mean arterial blood pressure (MAP) ≥65 mmHg; and urine output ≥0.5 mL/kg/h.

Diagnosis

- Obtain appropriate cultures before starting antibiotics, provided that this does not significantly delay administration of antibiotics.
- Perform imaging studies to confirm and sample any source of infection, if safe to do so.

Antibiotic therapy

- Begin intravenous antibiotics as early as possible, and always within the first hour of recognizing severe sepsis and septic shock.
- Use broad-spectrum antibiotics.
- Reassess the antimicrobial regimen daily to optimize efficacy, prevent resistance, avoid toxicity and minimize cost.
- Therapy usually limited to 7–10 days (longer if the response is slow, if there is an undrainable focus of infection or if the patient has immunological deficiencies).
- Stop antimicrobial therapy if the cause is found to be non-infectious.

Source identification and control

- The specific site of infection should be established as rapidly as possible and within the first 6 hours of presentation.
- Formally evaluate the patient for a focus of infection amenable to source control measures, such as abscess drainage or tissue debridement.
- Implement the source control measures as soon as possible following successful initial resuscitation (except in infected pancreatic necrosis).
- Choose a source control measure with maximum efficacy and minimal physiological upset.
- Remove intravascular access devices if they are potentially infected.

Fluid therapy

- Fluid resuscitation should be performed using crystalloids or colloids.
- Aim for a CVP of ≥8 mmHg (≥12 mmHg if the patient is mechanically ventilated).
- A fluid challenge technique is used for as long as it is associated with haemodynamic improvement. Give fluid challenges of 1000 mL of crystalloid or 300–500 mL of colloid over 30

minutes. More rapid and larger volumes may be required in sepsis-induced tissue hypoperfusion.

- The rate of fluid administration should be reduced if cardiac filling pressures increase without a concurrent haemodynamic improvement.

Vasopressors

- Maintain MAP ≥65 mmHg.
- Noradrenaline or dopamine (administered via a central line) are the initial vasopressors of choice.
- Do *not* use low-dose dopamine for renal protection.
- In patients requiring vasopressors, insert an arterial catheter as soon as possible.

Inotropic therapy

- Use dobutamine in patients with myocardial dysfunction as indicated by the presence of elevated cardiac filling pressure and low cardiac output.
- Do *not* increase cardiac index to predetermined supranormal levels.

Steroids

- Hydrocortisone dose should be <300 mg/day.
- Corticosteroids should *not* be used to treat sepsis in the absence of shock unless the patient's endocrine or corticosteroid history warrants it.

Recombinant human activated protein C (rhAPC)

- Adult patients with severe sepsis and low risk of death (e.g. single organ failure) should *not* receive recombinant human activated protein C.

Blood product administration

- Give red blood cells when haemoglobin decreases to <7.0 g/dL (<70 g/L) to target a haemoglobin of 7–9 g/dL in adults.
- A higher haemoglobin level may be required in special circumstances (e.g. myocardial ischaemia, severe hypoxaemia, acute haemorrhage, lactic acidosis).
- Do *not* use erythropoietin to treat sepsis-related anaemia. Erythropoietin may be used for other accepted reasons.
- Do *not* use antithrombin therapy.

Mechanical ventilation of sepsis-induced ALI/ARDS

- Target a tidal volume of 6 mL/kg body weight.
- Target an initial upper limit plateau pressure ≤30 cmH$_2$O.
- Allow $Paco_2$ to increase above normal, if needed, to minimize ventilator plateau pressures and tidal volumes.
- Positive end-expiratory pressure (PEEP) should be set to avoid extensive lung collapse at the end of expiration.
- Maintain mechanically ventilated patients in a semi-recumbent position unless this is contraindicated.
- Use a weaning protocol and a spontaneous breathing trial (SBT) regularly to evaluate the potential for discontinuing mechanical ventilation.
- Do *not* use a pulmonary artery catheter for the routine monitoring of patients with ALI/ARDS.
- Use a conservative fluid strategy for patients with established ALI who do not have evidence of tissue hypoperfusion.

Sedation, analgesia, and neuromuscular blockade

- Use sedation protocols with a sedation goal for critically ill mechanically ventilated patients.
- Use either intermittent bolus sedation or continuous infusion sedation to predetermined end-points (using sedation scales), with daily interruption/lightening to produce awakening and re-titrate sedation if necessary.
- Avoid using neuromuscular blockers where possible. Monitor the depth of block when using continuous infusions.

Glucose control

- Use intravenous insulin to control hyperglycaemia in patients with severe sepsis following stabilization in the intensive care unit.
- Provide a glucose calorie source and monitor blood glucose values every 1–2 hours (4-hourly when stable) in patients receiving IV insulin.
- Interpret with caution low glucose levels obtained with point-of-care testing (BM sticks), as these techniques may overestimate arterial blood or plasma glucose values.

Bicarbonate therapy

- Do *not* use bicarbonate therapy for the purpose of improving haemodynamics or reducing vasopressor requirements when treating hypoperfusion-induced lactic acidaemia with pH ≥ 7.15.

Deep vein thrombosis (DVT) prophylaxis

- Use heparin (either low-dose unfractionated heparin or low-molecular-weight heparin) unless contraindicated.
- Use a mechanical prophylactic device, such as compression stockings or an intermittent compression device, when heparin is contraindicated.

Stress-ulcer prophylaxis

- Provide prophylaxis using an H_2 blocker or proton-pump inhibitor. The benefits of prevention of upper gastrointestinal (GI) bleeding must be weighed against the potential for possible development of ventilator-acquired pneumonia.

Consideration for limitation of support

- Discuss advance care planning with patients and families. Describe likely outcomes and set realistic expectations.

Conclusion

The increasing challenge posed by healthcare-associated infections has been discussed. Crucial to the management of HAIs is the effective implementation of basic evidence-based control measures, including effective hand hygiene, appropriate use of personal protective equipment, and cleaning and decontamination of equipment and environments. Regardless of the clinical setting the nurse has a crucial role in the implementation of effective control measures.

The main clinical focus of the chapter has been on sepsis and septic shock, which studies have shown carries a mortality of up to 50 per cent. We have seen how sepsis can develop into severe sepsis and then septic shock, and that it is important to have clear and precise definitions of the various stages of sepsis in order to assist the management of the condition.

A fundamental principle in the treatment of patients with septic shock is prompt decision making to allow early intervention using evidence-based therapies. The nurse has a critical role in undertaking assessment that helps this decision-making, including routine observations of temperature, heart rate and blood pressure (undertaken with the appropriate frequency) together with assessment of urine output, to detect oliguria, and acute alteration of mental status – both early indicators of perfusion abnormalities. Early-warning scoring (EWS) tools are increasingly used to formalize this assessment process.

The chapter has outlined the interventions that have been shown to reduce mortality, together with guidelines for the management of severe sepsis and septic shock produced by the Surviving Sepsis Campaign. Nurses in clinical practice have a key role in this management and there should be clear protocols established in order to enable prompt intervention.

Suggested further reading

Bone RC, Balk RA, Cerra FB *et al.* (1992). Definitions for sepsis and organ failure and guidelines for use of innovative therapies in sepsis, *Critical Care Medicine* **101**; 1644–55.

Bridges E J, Dukes MS (2005). Cardiovascular effects of septic shock, *Critical Care Nurse* **25**; 14–40.

Daniels R (2007). Pathophysiology of sepsis (NHS evidence: emergency and urgent care). Available at www.library.nhs.uk/emergency/ViewResource.aspx?resI D=269238&tabID=290&catID=1870 (accessed December 2010).

Pittet D, Hugonnet S, Harbarth S *et al.* (2000). Effectiveness of a hospital-wide programme to improve compliance with hand hygiene, *Lancet* **356**; 1307–12.

Price S, Anning PB, Mitchell JA, Evans TW (1999). Myocardial dysfunction in sepsis: mechanisms and therapeutic implications, *European Heart Journal* **20**; 715–24.

Vincent JL (2000). Microbial resistance: lessons from the EPIC study. *Intensive Care Medicine* **26**(Suppl. 1):S3–8.

Websites

Guideline for Hand Hygiene in Health-Care Settings (Recommendations of the Healthcare Infection Control Practices Advisory Committee and the HICPAC/SHEA/APIC/IDSA Hand Hygiene Task Force): www.cdc.gov/mmwr/preview/mmwrhtml/rr5116a1.htm.

National Resource for Infection Control (NRIC): www.nric.org.uk/.

References

Bernard GR, Vincent JL, Laterre PF *et al.* (2001). Recombinant Human Protein C Worldwide Evaluation in Severe Sepsis (PROWESS) Study Group: efficacy and safety of recombinant human activated protein C for severe sepsis, *New England Journal of Medicine* **344**; 699–709.

Dellinger RP, Levy MM, Carlet JM *et al.* (2008). Surviving Sepsis Campaign: guidelines for the management of severe sepsis and septic shock, *Intensive Care Medicine* **34**; 17–60.

Department of Health (2000). The NHS Plan: a plan for investment, a plan for reform. See www.dh.gov.uk/en/Publicationsandstatistics/Publications/PublicationsPolicyAndGuidance/DH_4002960 (accessed December 2010).

Edwards JD, Brown GCS, Nightingale F, Slater RM, Faragher EB (1989). Use of survivors' cardiorespiratory values as therapeutic goals in septic shock, *Critical Care Medicine* **17**; 1098–103.

Health and Safety Executive (1992). *The Personal Protective Equipment at Work Regulations.*

Hoyert DL, Arias E, Smith BL, Murphy SL, Kochanek KD (2001). *National Vital Statistics Reports (serial online).* Available at www.cdc.gov/nchs/data/nvsr/nvsr49/nvsr49_08.pdf (accessed December 2010).

Koonin EV, Senkevich TG, Dolja VV (2006). The ancient Virus World and evolution of cells, *Biology Direct* **1**; 29.

Marieb EN (2003). *Human Anatomy and Physiology.* London: Pearson.

National Patient Safety Agency (2009). *The Revised Healthcare Cleaning Manual.*

NHS Estates (2004). *The NHS Healthcare Cleaning Manual.*

Nguyen HB, Rivers EP, Havstad S, *et al.* (2000). Critical care in the emergency department: a physiologic assessment and outcome evaluation, *Academic Emergency Medicine* **7**; 1354–61.

Parker MM, Fink MP (1991). Septic shock. In: Rippe *et al.* (eds) *Intensive Care Medicine*, 2nd edn. Boston: Little, Brown.

Parliamentary Public Accounts Committee (2009). Available at www.parliament.uk/business/news/2009/11/report-on-healthcare-associated-infections/ (accessed December 2010).

Rivers E, Nguyen B, Havstad S *et al.* (2001). Early goal-directed therapy in the treatment of severe sepsis and septic shock, *New England Journal of Medicine* **345**; 1368–77.

Spach DH, Silverstein FE, Stamm WE (1993). Transmission of infection by gastrointestinal endoscopy and bronchoscopy, *Annals of Internal Medicine* **118**; 117–28.

Van den Berghe G, Wouters P, Weekers F *et al.* (2001). Intensive insulin therapy in the critically ill patients, *New England Journal of Medicine* **345**; 1359–67.

Vincent JL, Abraham E, Annane D *et al.* (2002). Reducing mortality in sepsis: new directions, *Critical Care* **6**(Suppl. 3); S1–18.

Yan SB, Helterbrand JD, Hartman DL, Wright TJ, Bernard GR (2001). Low levels of protein C are associated with poor outcomes in severe sepsis, *Chest* **120**; 915–22.

CHAPTER 6

ACUTE CARE AND MANAGEMENT OF DIABETES

Paul Swainsbury

LEARNING OUTCOMES

On completion of this chapter the reader will:

1 understand normal and abnormal blood sugar control

2 be able to present an overview of diabetes, contrasting types 1 and 2

3 be able to discuss blood sugar control for seriously ill patients

4 be aware of the management of diabetes emergencies

5 be aware of the management of hyperglycaemia in a critically ill non-diabetic patient

6 be able to outline the management of a patient with diabetes requiring surgery.

Introduction

This chapter will provide knowledge and understanding of the management of diabetes in the acute care setting. Patients with diabetes occupy one in ten hospital beds, and generally admissions are a result of diabetes or its complications (Page and Hall 1999). The overall aim here is to provide the reader with the underpinning knowledge and confidence to care and treat this group of patients in the most effective way possible.

The chapter will describe essential background information about diabetes and its treatment, mainly focusing on blood glucose control in relation to the seriously ill patient. Diabetic emergencies including ketoacidosis, hyperosmolar hyperglycaemic state and hypoglycaemia are considered in detail. The management of hyperglycaemia in the non-diabetic seriously ill patient is reviewed. Finally the management of the diabetic patient before, during and after surgery is discussed. These patients can often be prevented from deteriorating with effective and appropriate care.

The seriously ill diabetic patient constitutes a medical emergency requiring intensive nursing care in order to restore metabolic equilibrium.

Overview of diabetes mellitus

Diabetes mellitus is a group of metabolic diseases characterized by hyperglycemia resulting from defects in insulin secretion, insulin action, or both.
(American Diabetes Association 2009)

This means either that the amount of insulin being produced by the pancreas is low, or that there is insufficient insulin or insulin action to meet the body's needs (i.e. the needs of the body may exceed the supply). Both states lead to an elevated blood glucose concentration (hyperglycaemia) and glycosuria (Dunning 2003).

Diabetes is usually a permanent condition and a lifelong diagnosis for patients, although acute derangement of blood glucose can occur as a temporary pathology following physiological stress.

Normal blood sugar control

Box 6.1 shows the normal plasma levels of glucose. At any point in time plasma glucose concentration reflects the net balance between:

- the rate of appearance of glucose in the circulation;
- the rate of disappearance from the circulation (Krentz 2000).

Box 6.1 Normal plasma glucose levels

- Fasting or pre-prandial plasma glucose is usually between 3.8 and 5.5 mmol/L.
- The level rises to 5–7 mmol/L about 30–90 minutes after a meal.
- The level falls again within 2–3 hours to a base level of 4–5 mmol/L.

The level is controlled by several interacting systems, of which hormone regulation is the most important. There are two types of mutually antagonistic metabolic hormones affecting blood glucose levels (Fig. 6.1):

- catabolic hormones (such as glucagon, growth hormone, cortisol, thyroxine and catecholamines) which increase blood glucose;
- anabolic hormone (insulin) which decreases blood glucose by increasing glucose uptake and utilization by the muscles and reducing glucose formation and release by the liver.

Under normal circumstances insulin is produced in regions of the pancreas called the Islets of Langerhans. Adults secrete approximately 40–50 units of insulin per day. The rise in insulin begins about 8–10 minutes after the ingestion of food (known as stimulated insulin secretion); this peak is primarily in response to plasma glucose levels. When the glucose concentration in the system is increased suddenly, an initial short-lived burst of insulin is released: the early phase. If the glucose stays at this level the insulin production falls and then begins to rise again, this time at a steadier rate: the late phase. Insulin and glucagon together regulate blood glucose levels.

Insulin is an anabolic hormone synthesized by the β-cells of the pancreatic islets. It is secreted chiefly in response to rising blood glucose and amino acids. Insulin has the following functions:

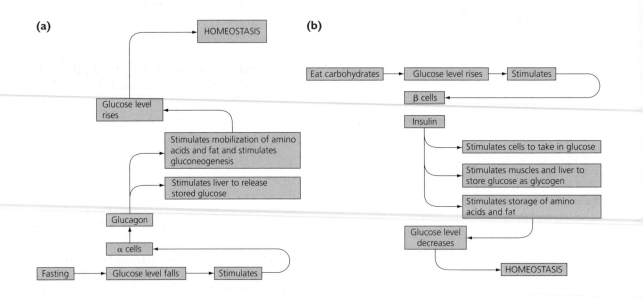

Figure 6.1 Glucose regulation by (a) glucagon and (b) insulin

- It facilitates the uptake of glucose by the cells.
- It promotes glycogenesis, which is the conversion of glucose to glycogen for storage in the liver and skeletal muscle.
- It promotes protein synthesis.
- It promotes the conversion of glucose to triglycerides for ultimate storage as body fat.
- It inhibits production of certain enzymes by binding to the insulin receptor.

These actions lower blood sugar and help to keep glucose within normal parameters, so preventing hyperglycaemia after meals. Insulin secretion peaks after meals and is lowest in fasting states.

Insulin is the only hormone capable of lowering plasma glucose and its major metabolic effects are in skeletal muscle, adipose tissue and the liver.

Glucagon is a catabolic hormone secreted by α-cells of the Islets of Langerhans in response to a falling blood sugar and certain amino acids. It is the most potent hyperglycaemic hormone. Glucagon has the following functions.

- The major target of glucagon is the liver and it promotes conversion of stored glycogen to glucose in the liver (glycogenolysis).
- It promotes fat and protein breakdown to provide an alternative source of glucose (lipolysis and gluconeogenesis).
- It influences the generation of ketone bodies (ketogenesis). In total or near-total insulin lack, these weak acids are produced as a result of chemical processes involved in the breakdown of fat.

Glucagon secretion increases (and insulin secretion decreases) whenever the sympathetic branch of the autonomic nervous system is activated, particularly in stressful situations in the form of disease, physical injury or emotional anxiety.

With increasing age, regulation of normal blood sugar control becomes less effective as there is decreased sensitivity to insulin and a reduction in the number of insulin receptors on the body cells. Some individuals maintain normal blood glucose by increasing their secretion of insulin. Others will be unable to do this and will show impaired glucose homeostasis entering *a pre-diabetic state.*

Epidemiology

Diabetes mellitus (DM) is the most common endocrine disorder and is a global disease affecting people of all ages. The World Health Organization estimated that at least 171 million people worldwide suffered from diabetes in 2006, and that by 2030 this number is projected to rise to 366 million (WHO 2006). An estimated 2.6 million people have diabetes in the United Kingdom, with up to half a million having undiagnosed diabetes. In the UK the prevalence of DM is about 2 per cent (Diabetes UK 2010). The prevalence increases with age, and the number of older people with diabetes in the UK is expected to grow as their population increases.

Life expectancy is reduced by at least 15 years for someone with type 1 diabetes. In type 2 diabetes, which is preventable in two-thirds of people who have it, life expectancy is reduced by up to 10 years. Approximately 90 per cent of people with diabetes have type 2.

Incidence and prevalence of diabetes are greater in areas of higher deprivations. Mortality rates from diabetes are higher in people from lower socioeconomic groups. People from minority ethnic communities have up to a six times higher than average risk of developing diabetes. The greatest increase in prevalence is, however, expected to occur in Asia and Africa, where most patients will probably be found by 2030 (WHO 2006).

Around 5 per cent of total NHS spending (and up to 10 per cent of hospital inpatient spending) is used for the care of people with diabetes. Diabetes UK in 2000 stated that about 40 per cent of this was used to manage preventable complications of diabetes.

Diagnosis

Detection of glycosuria may suggest the possibility of DM, but a diagnosis of DM must never be based simply on urine tests. It cannot be diagnosed from the presence of glycosuria alone; accurate measurement of blood glucose is necessary.

The World Health Organization (2006) state that there are three ways to diagnose diabetes. Each, in the absence of *unequivocal hyperglycemia*, must be confirmed on a subsequent day by any one of the three methods given in Box 6.2.

Classification

The classification of disordered glucose homeostasis continues to evolve. The latest categories suggested by the WHO (2006) are:

- type 1 diabetes (formerly 'insulin-dependent diabetes'): β-cell destruction, usually leading to absolute insulin deficiency;
- type 2 diabetes (formerly 'non-insulin-dependent diabetes'): may range from predominantly insulin resistance with relative insulin deficiency to a predominantly secretory defect with insulin resistance;
- impaired glucose tolerance/impaired fasting blood sugar: may be the first stage in developing DM, and associated with increased risk of becoming diabetic and increased risk of coronary heart disease (CHD);
- gestational diabetes;
- other rare forms: genetic, endocrine, infections affecting the pancreas.

The principal features of types 1 and 2 disease are summarized in Table 6.1, and their aetiologies and pathophysiologies are explained in detail below.

Type 1 diabetes

Aetiology

Type 1 diabetes is a chronic autoimmune disease caused by the destruction of insulin-producing β-cells of Islets of Langerhans. The majority of patients have antibodies in their serum. By the time the classical symptoms develop, over 90 per cent of β-cells have been destroyed, leading to a lack of insulin and hyperglycaemia. In addition the hyperglycaemia causes glucose toxicity, preventing the remaining β-cells from functioning normally (Malloch and Allwinkle 2006).

Classically it is a disease of the young, with a rapid onset, but it can occur at any age with one-third of patients presenting over the age of 30. In genetically susceptible people, environmental agents may trigger the autoimmune response. Possible triggers include viruses such as Coxsackie and mumps viruses or toxins. Dietary constituents have also been explored, for example vitamin D deficiency and cow's milk exposure in infancy.

Table 6.1 Characteristics of diabetes types 1 and 2

	Type 1	Type 2
Typical age	Child to young adult	Middle age to elderly
History	A few weeks	Months or years
Typical weight	Lean or normal and history of weight loss	Overweight or obese
Symptoms	Intense thirst, polyuria, frequency, weight loss	May be asymptomatic or mild thirst, nocturia, tiredness
Urine	Heavy glycosuria, often ketones	Glycosuria but no ketones
Treatment	Diet Insulin	Diet Exercise Oral hypoglycaemic drugs

Pathophysiology

In type 1 disease insulin production is totally (or almost totally) absent. Although the destruction of the β-cells may be a gradual process, the signs and symptoms can appear to occur quite suddenly. This seemingly sudden onset is usually linked to a sudden increased demand for insulin – such as the response to a physical or psychological stress due to illness, trauma, surgery, pregnancy or bereavement. At such times, the additional metabolic demands posed by the body's stressed state can no longer be met by the failing pancreas and symptoms of diabetes become apparent (Malloch and Allwinkle 2006).

The signs of diabetes are really the effects of the lack of insulin. The flow chart in Fig. 6.2 shows the relationship between the altered metabolism and the signs and symptoms.

Patients with type 1 disease may visit their general practitioner complaining of thirst and polydipsia, polyuria, nocturia and weight loss: these are the 'classic signs' of diabetes. Patients may also complain of feeling tired or lethargic. Traditionally, urine testing which showed glucose and ketones, coupled with a high blood sugar, triggered referral to a diabetes consultant. In recent years, many newly diagnosed people are managed in partnership with a diabetes healthcare team provided in different settings depending on the patient's specific needs, such as a GP surgery or local hospital. However, some newly diagnosed people may require admission to hospital; if dehydrated and severely ketoacidotic the patient may be unconscious (Malloch and Allwinkle 2006).

Type 2 diabetes

Aetiology

Type 2 diabetes accounts for 90 per cent of diabetes worldwide. It is multifactoral and more complex than type 1 but is particularly associated with lifestyle factors such as diet, obesity and inactivity. The following seem to influence susceptibility to the disease (Box 6.3).

Genetic factors

There is a strong inheritable genetic component in type 2 diabetes, with a high incidence among identical twins and familial clustering.

Hyperglycaemia
(Unable to enter cells glucose accumulates in the blood)

Glycosuria (Level of glucose passes through renal threshold)

Increased osmotic pressure within tubules

Polyuria

Polydipsia

Body compensates
(release of glucagon and other stress hormones)

Glucose not utilized

Body tries to gain energy by converting proteins and fats to glucose

Use of body proteins
(Leading to muscle weakness, tiredness and lethargy)

Use of body fats (fat metabolism)

Ketonuria (leading to pear-drop breath)
Ketoacid Accumulation
Bicarbonate excreted
Kussmaul's respirations (Hydrogen ions removed from body)

Metabolic Acidosis
(Nausea, vomiting and abdominal pain)

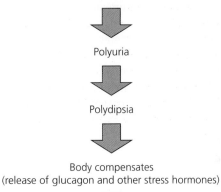

Figure 6.2 Signs and symptoms of lack of insulin (Malloch and Allwinkle 2006)

Box 6.3 Risk factors for groups at higher risk of developing type 2 diabetes

- First degree relative with DM parent or sibling
- Ethnic origin S. Asian, W. African, Peninsular Arab
- Middle age to elderly (earlier in high-risk groups)
- Pre-diabetes evident: impaired glucose tolerance (IGT) or impaired fasting glucose (IFG)
- Obesity and/or sedentary lifestyle
- Some drugs (e.g. steroids)
- Endocrine disorders
- Low birthweight
- History of gestational diabetes
- Cigarette smoking

Age

Prevalence increases with age, being 1 in 20 in the over-65s rising to 1 in 5 in the over-85s. Glucose metabolism becomes less efficient from around the fourth decade, but it is only a problem if other factors co-exist (e.g. obesity).

Insulin resistance

In type 2 disease, tissue sensitivity to insulin can decline. Even when circulating levels of insulin are normal or raised, hyperglycaemia can still occur. Several theories have been proposed, including resistance in peripheral tissues if obese, the effects of ageing, and the presence of anti-insulin antibodies. Whatever the cause, although insulin is present, it does not work as efficiently (Malloch and Allwinkle 2006).

Beta-cell deficiency

There is markedly reduced insulin secretion in response to glucose.

Obesity

This is increasingly recognized as a risk factor, particularly central obesity. According to Diabetes UK, statistics show that over 80 per cent of people diagnosed with type 2 disease are overweight. Increase in obesity in children is linked to the increased prevalence of type 2 in younger people. It is thought to be due to increased insulin resistance as weight increases,

which significantly improves when the person loses weight.

Physical inactivity

Activity seems to increase the body's sensitivity to insulin. It does not simply reduce obesity, as those who are overweight but active are less likely to be diabetic.

Ethnic and environmental factors

There are wide geographical variations in the prevalence of type 2 diabetes. In Western Europe it is about 3 per cent. In the UK, type 2 disease is particularly common among certain ethnic groups: 20 per cent of Asians and 17 per cent of Afro-Caribbean people over the age of 40 are known to have the disease, roughly four times the rate in the Caucasian population.

Pathophysiology

Signs, symptoms and clinical features, although still marked, are less severe than those with type 1 disease. This is related to the more gradual onset and the fact that some insulin is still being secreted. Hyperglycaemic patients with type 2 diabetes are less likely to be ketoacidotic and dehydrated.

The effects of a relative insulin lack include hyperglycaemic-related symptoms such as nocturia, polyuria and thirst. Genital or oral fungal infections such as thrush are common owing to the presence of sugar-rich urine providing a suitable environment for yeast organisms to multiply. This leads to symptoms such as pruritus vulvae in 40 per cent of women and balanitis in men. Staphylococcal skin infections commonly result in boils and abscesses, which may be the reason a patient presents to a GP. Visual disturbances – such as the development of myopia at the outset of diabetes (caused by osmotic change in the lens of the eye) – are diagnosed by an optician.

Non-specific symptoms such as tiredness, lethargy, excessive somnolence and a tendency to fall asleep are often reasons for a patient's first visit to a GP. There may be evidence of retinopathy, sexual dysfunction, or ischaemic heart disease on diagnosis. Indeed, diabetes may be diagnosed secondary to an admission or consultation for a related complication such as chest pain. Secondary pathology associated with type 2 diabetes, such as coronary heart disease, may develop before the diagnosis of diabetes is made as the individual may have had undiagnosed diabetes with hyperglycaemia for a number of years (Malloch and Allwinkle 2006).

Diabetic ketoacidosis

Diabetic ketoacidosis (DKA) is a potentially life-threatening complication of diabetes mainly associated with type 1 disease (Williams and Pickup 2004). It is the result of severe insulin deficiency (Moore 2004). This deficiency inhibits the metabolism of proteins, carbohydrates and fats, resulting in hyperglycaemia, metabolic acidosis, ketoacidosis and volume depletion (Lewis 2000). DKA can affect a person of any age.

The National Service Framework for Diabetes (DH 2003) asserts that protocols for rapid and effective treatment of diabetic emergencies by appropriately trained healthcare professionals should be implemented. Protocols will include the management of acute complications and procedures to minimize the risk of recurrence.

Epidemiology

In 2000, DKA represented 14 per cent of all diabetic-related hospital admissions (Lewis 2000). Watkins *et al.* (2003) estimated that 25 per cent of these patients would have undiagnosed diabetes. Merinac and Mesa (2000) stated that DKA was the highest cause of death for a patient with diabetes under 20 years of age, and this mortality rate increases with age. Despite advancements in recognition, treatment and implementation of guidelines, this is still the case.

Precipitating factors

DKA may be precipitated by a stressful situation such as infection (usually urinary tract or pneumonia), trauma, surgery or myocardial infarction. Emotional stress, errors in insulin management and newly diagnosed diabetes are other factors.

Symptoms and signs

Patients with DKA present with the following: thirst and polyuria, both due to osmotic diuresis; flushed appearance; Kussmaul breathing (sighing respirations) due to metabolic acidosis; smell of ketones on the breath due to ketones being excreted via the lungs; dehydration; and drowsiness. In severe cases, life-threatening signs include coma, severe acidosis (pH < 6.8) and severe hypotension unresponsive to intravenous (IV) fluids.

Investigations

The patient should be assessed carefully with regard to hydration, cardiovascular status and respiration. There may be signs of underlying pathology (infection, myocardial infarction or cerebrovascular accident). Some patients are mentally alert at presentation, but confusion and stupor are common. Up to 5 per cent present in coma, so if the patient is comatose it is important to consider causes other than metabolic derangement (see Chapter 4). The patient may also be in acute retention of urine.

A venous blood sample for serum creatinine, electrolytes and ketones should be obtained as well as a blood glucose (laboratory, not just BM stick) and an arterial sample for blood gases, particularly to ascertain the degree of acidosis. If clinical features suggest haematological abnormality, a full blood count should be taken as well as a urine sample for ketones and bacteriological examination. Hypokalaemia and cardiac ischaemia can be a clinical finding, so a 12-lead ECG should be recorded.

Assessment

Assessment of the patient should be structured, for example using an ABCDE approach and using early-warning scoring tools (see Chapter 10). The first priority in the treatment of diabetic ketoacidosis, as in the treatment of any life-threatening illness, is protection and maintenance of the airway. If there is accompanying respiratory pathology, intubation and ventilation may be required.

The level of consciousness should be assessed and, if impaired, the nursing care will be that for an unconscious patient (see Chapter 4). Deterioration in level of consciousness may signify cerebral oedema requiring referral to intensive care. Oxygen saturation should be monitored with an aim to maintain saturations at above 92 per cent, and high-flow oxygen using a non-rebreathing mask may be necessary to maintain adequate oxygenation. A chest X-ray may be required to exclude possible infection. Cardiovascular status is monitored including heart rate and rhythm, via a cardiac monitor, and blood pressure. It should be noted that persistent hypotension is a poor prognostic sign.

Initial management

Intravenous fluids

Rehydration is the first priority because the patient may be in a critical state of fluid depletion amounting to between 4 and 6 litres. Fluid replacement helps to lower blood glucose by dilution and improving glomerular filtration thereby encouraging glucose loss in the urine (Page and Hall 1999). In all cases careful monitoring of blood pressure and pulse is essential. As patients will require large amounts of fluid rapidly they will need careful monitoring of input and output to prevent fluid overload. This is critical in the first few hours after admission. Typically a patient with severe DKA may not pass urine for the first hour or two of rehydration; if this persists he or she may need catheterization and even a central venous line, particularly in the elderly, those in heart failure and those in severe shock.

Provided the BM stick reading is above17 mmol/L, treatment should begin while awaiting the results of laboratory blood tests. First give IV fluids starting with sodium chloride 0.9% over 30 minutes; however, if the serum sodium is above 155 mmol/L, sodium chloride 0.45% rather than 0.9% should be considered initially. If the blood glucose is above 17 mmol/L, administer 1 L of sodium chloride 0.9% solution over the first hour. In the event that the patient is hypotensive it is vital that a plasma expander be considered.

The rate of fluids after the first 30 minutes depends on factors such as age and co-morbidities, but it would typically be 1 L in the next two hours, 1 L in the following four hours, then 1 L six-hourly. The exception to this is if the patient is elderly, has cardiac disease or is mildly acidotic (HCO3 > 10) as a more rapid infusion increases the risk of respiratory distress syndrome. Switch to dextrose 5%, 1 L eight-hourly once the blood glucose is at or below 15 mmol/L; continue saline 0.9% if still volume-depleted. If the serum sodium rises above 155 mmol/L, switch to saline 0.45%, or dextrose 5% if blood glucose is below 15 mmol/L.

Increase the rate if:

- there is persistent hypotension (systolic blood pressure below 90 mmHg;
- the urine output is very high.

Reduce the rate if:

- the patient is elderly and frail;
- there is a risk of heart failure.

Potassium

Although serum potassium is often normal or even increased, total body potassium is low. Potassium should *not* be given until the serum creatinine and electrolytes are known. Potassium should be added to the infusion according to the serum potassium measurement:

- < 3.5 mmol/L, add 40 mmol of KCl per litre of fluid;
- 3.5–5 mmol/L, add 20 mmol of KCl per litre of fluid;
- > 5 mmol/L, add no potassium.

If the initial serum potassium is low, larger doses of potassium chloride will be required. Commence continuous ECG monitoring as hypokalaemia can cause life-threatening cardiac arrhythmias (see Chapter 3).

Insulin

It is critical that there be no delay in initiating the insulin infusion. Commence an insulin infusion of 50 units of actrapid in 50 mL of normal saline infused through a syringe driver infusion pump at a rate of 6 units an hour.

Monitor capillary blood glucose (by BM) hourly: it should fall at a rate of 5 mmol/L per hour. Once blood glucose is below 15 mmol/L, reduce the insulin infusion to 3 units an hour and change the IV fluid to glucose 5%.

Continuing management

Intravenous fluids

Continue to replace fluids according to the pulse, blood pressure, degree of dehydration and age of the patient. The total fluid deficit will be at least 3 L and in severe cases 6–7 L. Rehydration should continue with normal saline until the blood glucose is 11 mmol/L or less or the serum sodium is above the upper limit of normal. Once the blood glucose is 11 mmol/L or less, give glucose 5% in place of normal saline. If during rehydration with normal saline the serum sodium rises above the upper limit of the normal range (>150), rehydration should continue with saline 0.45% until blood glucose reaches 11 mmol/L.

Potassium

Adjust potassium chloride replacement according to the serum level. An average patient will require 20 mmol/L of KCl per litre of IV fluid.

Insulin

Continue with the IV insulin regimen set out earlier until the acidosis is reversed and the patient is eating and drinking. Discontinue the insulin therapy one hour after the first subcutaneous injection of insulin and when the patient has eaten the subsequent meal.

Before the patient is stable, infusion should never be switched off for more than one hour, unless the patient has persistent hypoglycaemia. In rare resistant cases the infusion rate may have to be increased; in such cases, specialist diabetologist opinion should be sought. If progress is not satisfactory, ensure that insulin is being infused and that all connections are satisfactory before increasing the insulin dose. If the patient is failing to respond to the measures taken, then specialist diabetology assistance should be sought.

Follow-up

Once the patient is stable a complete history and physical assessment can be undertaken. If no obvious cause of DKA has been found, further investigations are warranted. The patient should be referred to the diabetes specialist nurse to discuss any changes to his or her diabetic self-management to prevent future DKA episodes. Patient education is important as 50 per cent of DKA admissions are preventable (Kearney and Dang 2007).

Factors adversely affecting outcome are:

- advanced age;
- shock;
- low pH;
- hypokalaemia;
- myocardial infarction (MI).

Hyperosmolar hyperglycaemic state

Hyperosmolar hyperglycaemic state (HHS) is a clinical emergency in patients with type 2 diabetes. Patients develop severe hyperglycaemia without ketosis. There is no ketonuria as occurs in ketoacidosis, which explains why it was previously referred to as

---

CASE STUDY 6.1

Sarah is 19 years old and has had type 1 diabetes for two years. She has recently returned from a holiday abroad and has suffered from nausea and vomiting for 24 hours. Sarah has omitted her insulin injections because she thought her blood glucose levels might drop too far without food. Despite having no food for 24 hours, her morning blood glucose was 28 mmol/L. Sarah arranged an emergency appointment with her GP, but when her mother arrived home from work she found Sarah difficult to rouse, breathless and unable to get out of bed, so called for an ambulance. On admission to MAU her blood glucose is 32 mmol/L and her urine shows +++ ketones and +++ glucose. Her sodium is 127 mmol/L and her potassium 8.6 mmol/L. Her Glasgow Coma Score is 9/15.

- What are the immediate priorities for Sarah following admission?

HONK (hyperglycaemic hyperosmolar non-ketotic coma) as in type 2 diabetes mellitus there is sufficient insulin available to prevent the formation of ketone bodies but not hyperglycaemia (Moore 2004).

The clinical picture is usually one of an insidious onset (unlike the acute presentation of DKA) and an erroneous provisional diagnosis of stroke is not uncommon. Patients may present with general deterioration, dehydration and diffuse or focal neurological signs. The blood glucose is usually very high (above 40–50 mmol/L) and the blood urea and serum sodium are also high, producing a very high serum osmolarity. Mortality is 30–35 per cent and increases with age, medical co-morbidity, severity of metabolic derangement and the degree of impairment of consciousness.

It is usually restricted to middle-aged or elderly patients who suffer type 2 diabetes, though a significant number have previously undiagnosed diabetes. Often these patients may have some degree of congestive heart failure or renal failure and the prognosis is worse if this is found to be the case. There may be an event or trauma such as CVA that precipitates the event. Drugs implicated in the development of HHS are thiazide diuretics, phenytoin and glucocorticoids.

Symptoms and signs

Patients with HHS present with a similar picture to those with DKA, with the following signs and symptoms:

- intense thirst;
- fatigue and weakness;
- polyuria;
- decreased level of consciousness and confusion;
- dry skin resulting from dehydration.

The similarities between HHS and DKA include hyperglycaemia, dehydration and electrolyte losses. Although the treatment is very similar to DKA, the conditions do differ in a number of important respects (Table 6.2).

Management

Treatment in the acute phase is similar to DKA (see earlier) and is aimed at replenishing intravascular volume and correcting hyperosmolarity without precipitating circulatory overload (Lewis 2000). Investigations to elucidate a precipitating cause for the hyperosmolar state should include an ECG, mid-stream urine (MSU), chest X-ray and blood cultures. Appropriate treatment should be commenced if a precipitating cause is identified.

The patient may be comatose. He or she may be suffering from concurrent respiratory problems such as a respiratory infection (Lewis 2000).Treatment will depend on the patient's consciousness level.

If the patient fails to respond to the following measures, specialist support should be sought.

Intravenous fluids

The patient (usually elderly) will be very dehydrated. As much as 25 per cent of the total body water (which is 50 per cent of body weight in this age group) may have been lost. It is generally advised to replace half of this loss in the first 12 hours and the rest in the ensuing 24 hours. Thus a significant volume of fluid (1–2 L) may be required to be infused initially over a short period (Moore 2004). Give IV fluids starting with sodium chloride 0.9% over eight hours. If serum sodium is above 155 mmol/L, sodium chloride 0.45% rather than 0.9% should be considered initially. Insert a bladder catheter if the patient is anuric or unconscious, to monitor urine output.

Insulin

Lower rates of insulin infusion may be required as patients are often insulin-sensitive (Moore 2004). Soluble insulin at a strength of 1 unit/mL in sodium chloride 0.9% via a syringe pump is administered at a rate of 3 units/h. Capillary blood glucose should be monitored hourly (by BM). If blood glucose does not fall after two hours, double the dose of insulin infusion to 6 units/h. Once the blood glucose is below 15 mmol/L, change the IV fluid to glucose 5%. A laboratory blood glucose, serum creatinine and electrolytes are checked after two hours and then three-hourly until blood glucose is below 11 mmol/L.

Table 6.2 Comparison of the important features of DKA and HHS

	DKA	HHS
Age	Any	Usually > 60 years
Prodromal development	Days	Weeks
Type of diabetes	Type 1	Type 2
Abdominal pain/vomiting	Often present	Rare
Neurological abnormalities	Usually absent	Usually present
Plasma glucose	Usually below 40 mmol/L	Usually above 40 mmol/L
Plasma ketones	Strongly positive	Absent or weakly positive
Serum sodium	Normal or low	Normal or high
Osmolarity	Variable	Above 340 mOsmol/L
pH	Low (usually < 7.3)	Normal
Bicarbonate	Low (usually < 15 mmol/L)	Normal

Potassium

Unless the initial serum potassium is high (>6 mmol/L), give 10 mmol of KCl per litre of fluid. If the serum potassium is above 6 mmol/L, omit potassium replacement from the first litre of fluid replacement. If the initial serum potassium is low, larger doses of potassium chloride will be required (e.g. 40 mmol potassium in subsequent bags of IV fluid). Monitor serum potassium every time the IV fluid is changed. An ECG monitor will be required particularly if the patient is hypo- or hyperkalaemic. If there is renal failure, potassium chloride may not be required initially; if it is given, very careful monitoring will be necessary.

Anticoagulation

There is a high frequency of thromboembolic complications in patients with HHS, resulting from dehydration and hyperosmolarity. A subcutaneous anticoagulant will be administered, provided there is no contraindication, to reduce the risk of thromboses.

Follow-up

Once the patient is stable, a complete history and physical assessment can be undertaken. If no obvious cause of HHS has been found as yet, further investigations are required. In some cases the patient is a newly diagnosed diabetic and will require relevant education. After recovery some patients will be able to discontinue insulin and maintain good glycaemic control with oral diabetic agents or even dietary measures.

Factors adversely affecting outcome are the same as for DKA:

- advanced age;
- shock;

- low pH;
- hypokalaemia;
- myocardial infarction (MI).

Hypoglycaemia

In 2004/5 there were 8000 admissions to hospitals due to hypoglycaemia in England (Kearney and Dang 2007). Although A&E departments treat most episodes of hypoglycaemia, an understanding of causes, diagnosis and treatment is important for nurses working in all clinical areas.

Hypoglycaemia can affect people with either type 1 or type 2 diabetes. It can mimic any neurological presentation and the possibility of hypoglycaemia must always first be considered where the patient presents with behavioural disturbance whether or not they are diabetic. Hypoglycaemia occurs when the serum glucose concentration falls below the normal range.

Symptoms and signs

The symptoms of hypoglycaemia are conventionally described as either *autonomic* (usually present first when the blood glucose is 3.3–3.6 mmol/L and adrenaline is released) or related to *neuroglycopenia* (usually present when the blood glucose is below 2.6 mmol/L). Symptoms and signs of both are given in Table 6.3.

Hypoglycaemia in type 2 diabetes occurs more frequently when the patient is taking long-acting sulphonureas, especially in those with impaired liver or renal function. In older patients or those with frequent hypoglycaemic attacks, autonomic responses may be blunted and the presentation is more neuroglycopenic (confusion and loss of cognitive ability). Signs and symptoms may vary from patient to patient, as may time of onset; however one particular patient

Table 6.3 Symptoms and signs of hypoglycaemia

Autonomic symptoms	Autonomic signs	Neuroglycopenic symptoms	Neuroglycopenic signs
Sweating Shaking Feeling hot Feeling anxious Nausea Palpitations Vomiting	Pallor Tremor Perspiration Tachycardia or bradycardia	Difficulty speaking Loss of concentration Drowsiness Dizziness	Slurred speech Irritability Confusion Lethargy

may tend to follow a similar pattern to previous hypoglycaemic attacks.

In type 1 diabetes, the normal ability to counter-regulate hypoglycaemia by releasing a surge of glucagon is lost a few years after developing diabetes, so for many hypoglycaemia is the most frequent complication. From the time of losing the ability to secrete glucagon, the patient is solely reliant on autonomic adrenal responses to counteract a hypoglycaemic crisis, and to alert him or her of impending crisis. However, as individuals age the responses to this crisis become blunted and a potentially life-threatening scenario emerges of neuroglycopenic convulsions or coma.

Assessment

Patient assessment is initially aimed at ensuring an adequate airway, breathing and circulation through the ABCDE approach, including assessment of level of consciousness (see Chapter 10). Specific assessment requires identifying the blood glucose initially via capillary blood glucose (BM). A wide-bore IV cannula is inserted and venous blood taken for urea and electrolytes (U&E) and liver function tests (LFTs). A full cardiac assessment can be undertaken when the patient has been stabilized.

Management

If the patient's level of consciousness allows safe eating and drinking, give 20 g of quick-acting carbohydrate, for example:

- 100 mL of Lucozade; or
- 3 or 4 glucose tablets; or
- 4 teaspoonfuls of sugar; or
- a glass of fruit juice.

Gluco gel (Hypostop) can be administered via the buccal mucosa and repeated after 10 minutes if necessary.

If the patient is unconscious or not responding it is clearly unsafe to give anything by mouth. In this case administer 25–50 mL of glucose 50%, followed by a normal saline 0.9% flush (as the glucose solution is hypertonic and may cause thrombophlebitis). If there is no improvement in blood glucose, or the patient remains unconscious, or there is difficulty gaining intravenous access, glucagon 1 mg intramuscular injection is administered (Krentz 2004).

The BM should be checked at 5 and 30 minutes to ensure it has risen above 4 mmol/L. The patient's consciousness level and response to treatment is monitored and, once the patient regains consciousness, oral glucose and carbohydrate can be given. As the patient is already depleted of glucose these sugars may be utilized instantly; therefore it is important to follow this with carbohydrates to prevent hypoglycaemia recurring; for example a sandwich, fruit or biscuits and milk.

Follow-up

The patient should be monitored for at least 36 hours. A detailed history and physical assessment can be undertaken once the patient is stable. The precipitating cause for hypoglycaemia should be established so that appropriate measures can be put into place to minimize future episodes.

CASE STUDY 6.2

Roy, a 29-year-old man, has had type 1 diabetes for 12 years. He is insulin-controlled and is currently being treated with oral antibiotics by his GP for tonsillitis. Fearing that he may lose his job if he takes sick leave, he is on a very busy shift missing his mid-morning snack and unable to go for lunch. In the afternoon he finds it increasingly difficult to concentrate, suffering a persistent headache, trembling and sweating profusely. Roy is unable to communicate coherently and his work colleagues drive him to hospital.

- Describe Roy's initial management and nursing care on the medical assessment unit.

Hyperglycaemia

Hyperglycaemia in the critically ill patient is defined as a blood glucose above 12 mmol/L in any patient who is unwell for whatever reason. The patient does not have to be known previously to be diabetic (Mesotten and Van den Berghe 2003). Acute hyperglycaemia frequently occurs during a critical illness such as heart attack, stroke or sepsis as a result of the metabolic and hormonal changes that accompany the so-called stress response. This physiological response can be harmful, including increased susceptibility to infections and detrimental effects on the cardiovascular system leading to myocardial ischaemia and cerebral stroke (Preiser *et al.* 2002).

Hyperglycaemia is regarded as a physiological parameter. Blood glucose targets are set and are required to be managed to reduce patient mortality and morbidity (Pittas *et al.* 2006). It is therefore important that all critically ill patients have assessment of blood glucose and, if found to be hyperglycaemic, receive appropriate insulin therapy. Prevention of hyperglycaemia with intensive insulin therapy has been shown to decrease morbidity and mortality in critically ill patients in surgical intensive-care units (Van den Burghe *et al.* 2001) and is now widely used, although the mechanisms by which insulin exerts its beneficial effects are uncertain (Preiser *et al.* 2002).

Symptoms and signs

A patient who is critically ill and is hyperglycaemic may not show any clinical signs to lead the practitioner to suspect this. The potential for hyperglycaemia should be considered in the following circumstances:

- any patient who is acutely unwell for whatever reason;
- a patient who is known to have diabetes;
- a patient who is receiving corticosteroid treatment.

Management

Stable patients

If the patient is clinically stable, not dehydrated, not on any diabetic medicine and able to eat but is persistently hyperglycaemic, then monitor blood glucose every 4 hours and consider treating as unstable if hyperglycaemia persists.

Unstable patients

If the patient is clinically unstable the best results are attained in studies using a dynamic scale protocol. The Bath insulin protocol (Laver *et al.* 2004) was developed in response to the evidence that patients with acute critical illness, for example stroke and heart attack, who have hyperglycaemia have better

> **Box 6.4 General principles of the Bath protocol**
>
> - Aim for a target glucose concentration range of 4.5–6.5 mmol/L.
> - Before starting insulin infusion, check the plasma potassium level. If less than 4 mmol/L, seek advice.
> - Before starting insulin infusion, check other infusions for insulin.
> - The standard dilution of insulin is 50 IU in 50 mL of saline solution.
> - Before starting insulin infusion, check if patient received subcutaneous insulin bolus or oral antidiabetic drug in the last 12 hours.
> - When parenteral or enteral nutrition is stopped, stop insulin.
> - The presumption is for a standard glucose intake.
> - In the 2 hours following the start of the insulin infusion, check the glucose and follow the protocol. If not set alternatively, perform the next glucose check in 1 hour.
> - If glycaemia is stable in the two following measurements, the next level could be checked in 4 hours.

outcomes when insulin is used to achieve target blood glucose levels. The general principles for the protocol are given in Box 6.4.

The starting rate for insulin infusion is set out in Table 6.4, and the monitoring protocol is shown in Fig. 6.3.

Table 6.4 Initial insulin infusion for the Bath protocol

Blood glucose (mmol/L)	Starting insulin infusion rate (mL/h)
3–6.1	0
6.2–9.9	1
10–12	2
> 12	4

The protocol should be stopped if blood sugars are stable at between 4 and 7 mmol/L and no insulin has been required for 24 hours. Stop also when the patient is taking food orally. Note that the patient may still need insulin via more usual protocols.

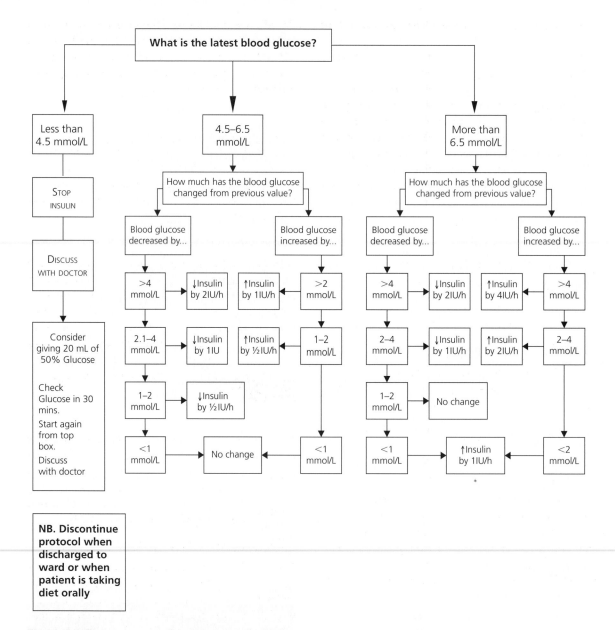

Figure 6.3 Bath protocol, adapted from version v5.4

Surgery

Patients with diabetes have a 50 per cent chance of undergoing surgery at some time during their lives (Page and Hall 1999). Perioperative mortality is up to three times higher among people with DM than among people who do not have DM; this is related to factors such as a greater likelihood of co-morbidities such as coronary heart disease, autonomic neuropathy or renal impairment (Freeman 2005).

Surgery is a form of physical trauma. It results in catabolism, increased metabolic rate, increased fat and protein breakdown, glucose intolerance and starvation. In a patient with diabetes the pre-existing metabolic disturbances are exacerbated by surgery. In addition, either the circumstances that have led to the need for surgery, such as bowel obstruction or trauma, or a need for the patient to be 'nil by mouth', will interfere with the patient's usual medication (Box 6.5).

Correct management of the diabetic patient during surgery reduces morbidity and length of admission as well as resulting in better wound healing and the overall aim to keep the blood glucose within a normal range. This is challenging as surgery and the circumstances surrounding it make normal diabetic management difficult. All hospitals will have protocols in place and these should be adhered to and become familiar.

Blood glucose derangement

Hypoglycaemia

Hypoglycaemia may develop perioperatively due to the residual effects of preoperative long-acting oral hypoglycaemic agents or insulin. It can be exacerbated by preoperative fasting or insufficient glucose administration. Counter-regulatory mechanisms may be defective because of autonomic dysfunction and can lead to irreversible neurological deficits. This can be dangerous in the anaesthetized or neuropathic patient as the warning signs may be absent (Freeman 2005).

Hyperglycaemia

Glucagon, cortisol and adrenaline secretion as part of the neuroendocrine response to trauma, combined with iatrogenic insulin deficiency or glucose over administration may result in hyperglycaemia. This can cause osmotic diuresis, making volume status difficult to determine and risking profound dehydration and organ hypoperfusion. In addition there is increased risk of urinary tract infections and delayed wound healing. Eventually this can result in hyperosmolality with hyperviscocity, thrombogenesis and cerebral oedema.

Underlying complications of surgery

The patient with diabetes may have a number of underlying problems that should be considered because they may have an impact both preoperatively and postoperatively.

Cardiovascular

All these patients should have a cardiovascular examination and an ECG. They must be considered as being at high risk of a myocardial infarction. Patients may suffer a silent MI as cardiac autonomic neuropathy may abolish the heart's response to stress. Most cardiac and antihypertensive drugs should be continued throughout the perioperative period, except aspirin, diuretics and anticoagulants (Freeman 2005).

Renal

Renal dysfunction is a possible complication. Intrinsic renal disease including glomerulosclerosis and renal papillary necrosis enhance the risk of acute renal failure perioperatively, and proteinuria is an early manifestation. These patients also have an increased risk of urinary tract infection (Freeman 2005).

Immune complications and infection risk

These patients are susceptible to infection and have delayed wound healing. Hyperglycaemia facilitates proliferation of bacteria and fungi and depresses the immune system, and proteolysis and decreased amino acid transport retards wound healing. Loss of phagocytic function also increases the risk of postoperative infection. Strict sterile techniques are required and there is a need to assess the risk/benefit ratio for procedures such as catheterization.

Gastrointestinal complications

Some of these patients suffer from autonomic neuropathy which leads to gastroparesis. Diminished gastric motility and delayed stomach emptying may require antiemetic therapy. In advanced autonomic neuropathy, the possibility of excess residual gastric

---

Box 6.5 Factors adversely affecting diabetic control perioperatively

- Diseases underlying the need for surgery (e.g. sepsis, atherosclerosis)
- Hormonal and metabolic responses to trauma
- Starvation accelerating the development of ketosis
- Anaesthetic drugs
- Other drugs (e.g. steroids)
- Nosocomial infection (more common in diabetic patients)
- Anxiety

contents secondary to gastroparesis must be considered because of the risk of aspiration (Watkins *et al.* 2003).

Ophthalmological complications

Clinically significant ocular complications are associated with diabetes, including transient visual disturbances secondary to osmotic changes. Cataracts, glaucoma and retinopathy decrease visual acuity and increase the unpleasantness of the perioperative period (Freeman 2005).

Managing diabetes during surgery

Management of preoperative insulin therapy depends on the baseline blood glucose, the level of diabetic control, the severity of the illness and the proposed surgical procedure. However, the aims for all patients with diabetes are to reduce excess mortality and to prevent an increase in postoperative complications through the achievement of:

● normal wound healing;
● no increase in duration of hospitalization;
● no hypoglycaemia, hyperglycaemia or ketoacidosis.

It should be noted that the following discussion is based on general principles and guidelines. Staff should be aware of their local guidelines and regimes, which should be followed as appropriate.

Improved surgical methods and anaesthesiology together with the implementation of uncomplicated management protocols and well-planned preoperative assessment may have improved the perioperative fate of patients with diabetes in recent times. Heller and Dineen (2002) outlined three alternative strategies for managing these patients: omission of antidiabetic medication and regular monitoring; separate glucose/insulin infusions; or glucose, potassium and insulin (GKI) infusion.

Omission of antidiabetic medication and regular monitoring

This is suitable for all patients undergoing shorter or minor procedures. The strategy is to place the patient first on the morning operating list if possible, and to avoid long-acting glucose-lowering agents such as chlorpropamide, glibenclamide, metformin and ultralente insulin. Blood glucose levels are monitored

hourly and the urine is tested every 8 hours for ketones.

The aim is for a blood glucose of 7–11 mmol/L. If the blood glucose is 17 mmol/L or above, then 6 units of soluble insulin is administered. Once the patient is eating and drinking normally their usual regimen can be restarted.

Separate glucose/insulin infusions

This is suitable for all emergency surgery, for those with type 1 diabetes undergoing moderate or major surgery, or those with type 2 diabetes undergoing major surgery.

The strategy is to avoid long-acting glucose-lowering agents, including chlorpropamide, glibenclamide, metformin and ultralente insulin. The patient should be placed towards the end of the surgical list to ensure a desirable range. A glucose infusion of 500 mL of dextrose 10% with 10 mmol of KCl at a rate of 100 mL/h is started alongside an insulin infusion via a syringe pump of 50 units of soluble insulin in 50 mL saline in a 50 mL syringe. The capillary blood glucose is measured hourly until the operation and a sliding scale is used to adjust the insulin rate (Table 6.5).

Table 6.5 Sliding scale for preoperative insulin infusion

Blood glucose (mmol/L)	Insulin (units/h)
< 4	Stop
4–6.9	1
7–10.9	2
11–16.9	3
≥ 17	4

GKI infusion

This is suitable for moderate or major surgery in type 1 diabetes and major surgery in type 2 diabetes.

The aim is to keep blood glucose within the range 7–11 mmol/L. The strategy is to place the patient first on the morning operating list if possible and to avoid long-acting glucose-lowering agents such as chlorpropamide, glibenclamide, metformin and ultralente insulin. The blood glucose level is monitored hourly. After the patient has started to fast (i.e. become 'nil by mouth'), the serum potassium is checked and a glucose + potassium + insulin regime is commenced:

- A solution of 500 mL glucose 10% with 10 mmol KCl and10 units of actrapid insulin is set to run at 100 mL/h via a volumetric pump.
- The blood glucose is monitored hourly.
- If the blood glucose falls to 4–7 mmol/L in two successive hours, then the solution is changed to 5 IU in 500 mL.
- If the blood glucose rises to 17 mmol/L in two successive hours, then the solution is changed to 20 IU in 500 mL.

The potassium level is checked before commencing the regimen, immediately postoperatively, and at least daily during the infusion. Postoperatively the regimen is continued until the patient can eat and drink normally.

Conclusion

The seriously ill patient with diabetes constitutes a medical emergency requiring immediate medical and nursing care. The speed and accuracy of the initial assessment of the patient and the treatment in the first two to three hours will have an important bearing on the prognosis.

The main goals in patients with diabetes needing hospitalization are to minimize disruption of the metabolic state, prevent an untoward result, and return the patient to a stable glycaemic balance as quickly as possible. These goals are not always easy to achieve. The key to restoring a patient adequately to wellbeing lies in an understanding of the pathophysiological derangement and subsequent attempts at restoring metabolic equilibrium, and in understanding and responding to the patient as a person coping with his or her acute and chronic disease.

The principles underlying the care of such a patient with complications of hyperglycaemia, hypoglycaemia and surgical stress have been outlined. Most seriously ill patients move from a highly dependent situation where those caring for them need to be able to administer a complex treatment regimen, to one of independence enabling the nurse to initiate a review of their overall diabetes management.

Suggested further reading

Baldwin D, Villanueva G, Mcnutt R, Bhatnagar S (2005). Eliminating inpatient sliding-scale insulin: a re-education project with medical house staff, *Diabetes Care* **28**;1008–11.

Jerreat L (2003). *Diabetes for Nurses*, 2nd edn. Oxford: Wiley.

Jerreat L (2009). Treatment of hyperglycaemia in patients with type 2 diabetes, *Nursing Standard* **24**(1); 50–7.

References

American Diabetes Association (2009). Diagnosis and classification of diabetes, *Diabetes Care* **32**(Suppl. 1); s62–7.

Department of Health (DH) (2003) *National Service Framework for Diabetes: Delivery Strategy*. London: The Stationery Office.

Diabetes UK (2010). See www.diabetes.org.uk/.

Dunning T (2003). *Care of People with Diabetes: A Manual of Nursing Practice*, 2nd edn. Oxford: Blackwell.

Freeman A (2005). *Diabetes Perioperative Management*. Available at www.dr-green.co.uk/html/teaching%20 archive.htm#dpm (accessed July 2010).

Heller S, Dineen SF (2002). Surgery in patients with diabetes, *Medicine* **30**(2); 66–7.

Kearney T, Dang C (2007). Diabetic and endocrine emergencies, *Postgraduate Medical Journal* **83**; 79–86.

Krentz AJ (2000). *Churchill's Pocket Book of Diabetes*. Edinburgh: Churchill Livingstone.

Krentz A (ed) (2004). Emergencies in Diabetes: Diagnosis, management and prevention. Chichester: Wiley.

Laver S et al. (2004). Implementing intensive insulin therapy: development and audit of the Bath insulin protocol, *Anaesthesia and Intensive Care* **32**; 311–16.

Lewis R (2000). Diabetic emergencies. 2: Hyperglycaemia, *Accident and Emergency Nursing* **8**(1); 24–30.

Malloch K, Allwinkle J (2006). Endocrine and metabolic disorders. 2: Diabetes mellitus. In: Alexander M, Fawcett J, Runciman P (eds) *Nursing Practice: Hospital and Home*. London. Churchill Livingstone.

Marinac J, Mesa L (2000). Using a severity of illness scoring system to assess intensive care unit admissions for diabetic ketoacidosis, *Critical Care Medicine* **28**; 2238–41.

Mesotten D, van den Berghe ((2003). Clinical potential of insulin therapy in critically ill patients, *Drugs* **63**; 625–36.

Moore T (2004). Diabetic emergencies in adults, *Nursing Standard* **18**(1); 46–52.

Page S, Hall G (1999). *Diabetes: Emergency and Hospital Management*. London: BMJ Books.

Pittas *et al.* (2006). Insulin therapy and in-hospital mortality in critically ill patients: systematc review and meta-analysis of randomized controlled trials, *Journal of Parenteral and Enteral Nutrition* **30**; 164–72.

Preisser JC, Devos P, van den Berghe G (2002). Tight control of glycaemia in critically ill patients, *Current Opinion in Clinical Nutrition and Metabolic Care* **5**; 533–7.

Van den Burghe G *et al.* (2001). Intensive insulin therapy in the critically ill patients, *New England Journal of Medicine* **345**; 1359–67.

Watkins P, Amiel S, Howell S, Turner E (2003). *Diabetes and Its Management*, 6th edn. London: Blackwell.

Williams G, Pickup JC (2004). *Handbook of Diabetes*, 3rd edn. Oxford: Wiley–Blackwell.

World Health Organization (2006). *Definition and Diagnosis of Diabetes Mellitus and Intermediate Hyperglycemia: Report of a WHO/IDF Consultation*. Geneva: WHO Press.

CHAPTER 7

NUTRITION

Mike Macintosh

LEARNING OUTCOMES

On completion of this chapter the reader will:

1 be able to describe the normal process of digestion and metabolism

2 have an understanding of the metabolic response to acute and severe illness

3 have an awareness of the factors contributing to in-hospital malnutrition

4 understand the process of nutritional assessment

5 have an understanding of the approaches to nutritional support.

Introduction

Nutrition is undeniably an important aspect of care of the acutely ill patient. Poor nutrition is associated with delayed healing, longer hospital stay, higher incidence of perioperative complications, and increased mortality (Edington 2000; BAPEN 2003; Age Concern 2006). It is repeatedly reported that patients in hospital are at significant risk of malnutrition, yet for more than 25 years it has also been reported that 'significant protein-calorie malnutrition occurs commonly' in hospitals in both medical and surgical settings (Bistrian *et al.* 1976). Recent evidence suggests that, despite greater awareness and the availability of screening and assessment tools, nutritional assessment and management remains less than ideal (NHS Quality Improvement Scotland 2003; Age Concern 2006), with up to 30 per cent of patients suffering from undernutrition. Older patients are particularly at risk: a recent independent report to the Department of Health cited 6 out of 10 older patients being at risk of malnourishment or their situation becoming worse in hospital (Lishman 2009).

Ensuring adequate nutrition is in one sense quite simple, yet it requires complex organizational systems to be in place to ensure safe and effective management (BAPEN 2007). Part of this is to ensure a basic understanding of nutrition, its assessment and screening, and nutritional support. This chapter introduces these concepts and in particular focuses on assessment and identification of the patient at risk of malnutrition or undernutrition.

Normal digestion, nutrition and metabolism

ACTIVITY ?

Before reading this section, list as many constituents of normal dietary intake as you can.

There are few factors more important to the seriously ill patient than the provision of adequate nutrition. Nutrition is an integral part of health, and public interest in and awareness of nutrition is increasing. Nurses have a major role in promoting and maintaining good nutritional practices in the clinical setting. Knowledge of the physiological processes relevant to nutrition helps provide an understanding of how the body meets its needs. An understanding of what constitutes 'good nutritional status' and 'adequate functioning' of the digestive system are essential for assessing a patient's needs and planning nursing interventions.

Nutrients

Nutrients are chemical substances in food that provide energy, act as building blocks in forming new body components, or assist in the functioning of various body processes (Clancy and McVicar 2009). There are six major classes of nutrients: carbohydrates (CHO), fats (lipids), proteins, minerals, vitamins and water (Box 7.1).

Dietary fibre, both soluble (e.g. gums, mucilages, most pectins) and insoluble (e.g. cellulose, lignin), is an important component of a healthy diet despite the fact that the body is unable to digest it.

- Insoluble fibre holds water and increases stool bulk, reduces colonic intraluminal pressure and binds metals (e.g. zinc), bile acids and cholesterol.

- Soluble fibre slows gastric emptying, provides fermentable material to support colonic bacteria, with the production of gas which aerates the stool and aids defecation.

Both forms of fibre are important in helping to prevent gastrointestinal (GI) disease such as diverticulosis, and may contribute positively to serum lipid and glucose levels related to chronic conditions such as heart disease and diabetes mellitus.

Nutrients present in food are made available to the body cells by the digestive system: the alimentary canal (Fig. 7.1). The transit times for food products vary with the type of nutrient predominant within the meal. For example, high-fat and to a lesser extent protein-rich meals stay in the stomach for a much longer period than high-carbohydrate meals. Meals taken late at night also stay in the stomach for a prolonged period owing to a lowered metabolic rate during sleep. The general rule relating to metabolic rate is: the higher the individual's metabolic rate, the faster the transit time of food through the gastrointestinal tract.

Box 7.1 Nutrients

- **Protein** – a nutrient for growth and repair of muscle tissues, bone, enzymes, hormones, blood cells etc.
- **Carbohydrate** – for energy
- **Fat** – a concentrated source of energy (calories), important for the fat-soluble vitamins A, D, E and K
- **Vitamin A** – for skin and mucosal integrity, regeneration of the visual pigment rhodopsin, it can be converted from carotene and stored in the liver
- **Vitamin B$_1$** (thiamin) – involved in chemical breakdown of carbohydrate foods in the release of energy
- **Vitamin B$_2$** (riboflavin) – involved in cellular aerobic activity, the health of the eyes, the nervous system and during pregnancy
- **Nicotinic acid** – involved in tissue oxidation and fat metabolism (the amino acid tryptophan can be converted to nicotinic acid)
- **Vitamin B$_6$** (pyridoxin) – for a healthy nervous system and the utilization of iron
- **Folic acid** – involved in oxidation reactions and protein synthesis
- **Vitamin B$_{12}$** (cyanocobalamin) – involved in the formation of mature red blood cells and nervous system
- **Vitamin C** (ascorbic acid) – for growth and for the integrity of connective tissue, wound healing, resisting infections and absorption of iron
- **Vitamin D** (cholecalciferol) – essential for absorption and deposition of calcium into bone and can be stored in the liver; it is essential for the absorption of calcium
- **Vitamin E** (tocopherol) – has antioxidant properties
- **Vitamin K** (phytomenadione) – essential for the formation of prothrombin which is involved in blood-clotting
- **Calcium and phosphorus** – for calcification of bone and teeth
- **Iron** – the 'haem' part of haemoglobin, the oxygen-carrying protein in red blood cells

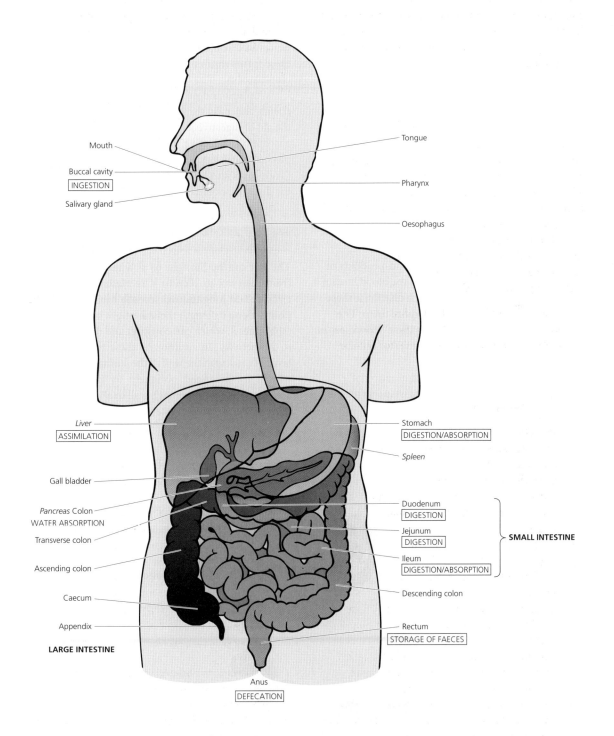

Figure 7.1 The human alimentary canal

Digestive processsses

Digestion comprises five principal physiological processes, all of which may become disrupted during serious illness.

- *Ingestion* (eating) is the process of taking food into the mouth.
- *Movement* is the neuromuscular activity of the gut wall (peristalsis) necessary to move the food through the GI tract in a unidirectional manner from mouth to anus.
- *Digestion* is the physical and chemical breakdown of food involving the muscular movements of segmentation and peristalsis, and the action of various enzymes respectively, to render the food into an absorbable form.
- *Absorption* is the passage of the end-products of digestion from the GI tract into the blood stream and the lymphatic vessels which distribute these metabolites to the cells that require them. The liver assimilates and processes these substances in order to keep blood levels optimal for cellular metabolism.
- *Defecation* (excretion) is the elimination of indigestible and unabsorbed substances from the body.

The *macronutrients* in food are broken down by digestive juices into smaller units: proteins into amino acids, fats into fatty acids and glycerol, and carbohydrates into simple sugars (glucose and galactose). In these forms nutrients pass from the intestine into the bloodstream.

Vitamins and minerals occur in food as *micronutrients* and pass through the intestinal wall without the aid of digestive juices. Figure 7.2 shows the sites of absorption. Effective digestion requires that all five physiological stages be adequately completed (Todorovik and Micklewright 1997). The functions of the digestive organs are given in Table 7.1.

The gut

The gut can be thought of as a muscular tube, and from pharynx to rectum it is made up of layers of circular and longitudinal smooth muscle. At various points along its length there are tight bands of muscle (sphincters), which can constrict and dilate according to gut activity. In addition to these there is an extra layer of muscle in the wall of the stomach, the fibres of which are arranged obliquely to facilitate strong contractions of the stomach wall in all directions. The autonomic nervous system (ANS) innervates the

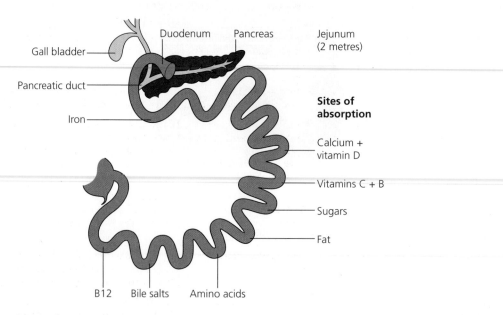

Figure 7.2 Sites of absorption

whole of the gut and generally the parasympathetic branch stimulates peristalsis, whereas the sympathetic branch inhibits it. Hormones such as catecholamines affect motility once the receptors on the smooth muscle in the wall of the GI tract are stimulated. Spasm of this smooth muscle might occur if the tract is over-stimulated by dilation inside the tract, for example by the accumulation of gas or fluid or blockage by foreign body, impacted faeces or

tumour. Such dilation can result in painful stimuli and be experienced as colic.

Regulation

Regulation of food intake involves two centres in the hypothalamic region of the brain: the hunger centre and the satiety centre. The hunger centre is constantly

Table 7.1 Functions of the organs of digestion

Organ	Exocrine secretions	Functions
Mouth and pharynx, teeth, tongue, facial muscles and salivary glands.	Saliva: Salt, water and mucus **Salivary amylase (ptyalin)**	Chewing, mastication, initiation of swallowing reflex. Moistening and lubricating food Carbohydrate (CHO) digesting enzyme.
Oesophagus. Smooth and muscular with mucus glands.	Mucus	Moving the lubricated bolus of food to the stomach by peristaltic waves
Stomach. Thick muscular wall with extra oblique muscle layer, large mucosal folds (rugae), exocrine cells.	Gastric juice: Hydrochloric acid (HCl) **Pepsin** Mucous Intrinsic factor	Storing, mixing and dissolving food. Regulating emptying of liquid food (chyme) into the duodenum. Dissolving food particles, killing microbes, lowering pH. Protein-digesting enzyme. Lubrication and protection of epithelial surface. Necessary for the absorption of vitmin B12 from the diet.
Duodenum. Abundance of villi, vastly increasing luminal surface area, exocrine cells, ducts from gall bladder and pancreas enter here.	Duodenal juice: Bicarbonate **Enterokinase** **Cholecystokinin (CCK)**, **Secretin**	Receives chyme from the stomach, muscular contractions (segmentation) mixes food with alkaline juices, neutralizing the strong acid. Activates the protein-splitting enzymes contained in pancreatic juice. Chemical messenger which stimulates contraction of gall bladder and release of bile into the duodenum. Chemical messenger (hormone) which stimulates release of pancreatic juice into the duodenum.
Pancreas. Exocrine and endocrine producing organ.	Pancreatic juice: Bicarbonate **Amylase** **Lipase** **Trypsinogen** and **chymotrypsinogen**	Secretion of enzymes and bicarbonate to digest nutrients and neutralize stomach acid. CHO digestion Fat digestion. Protein digestion when activated in the presence of enterokinase in duodenum to form **trypsin**.
Gall bladder. Stores bile which is made in the liver.	Bile: Bicarbonate Bile salts Organic waste products	Stored bile is released during a meal and serves to neutralize the acid chyme. Emulsification of fats, facilitating action of pancreatic lipase. Elimination from the body.
Ileum. Villi and microvilli. Exocrine cells, Brunner's glands.	Intestinal juice: **Amylase**, **Trypsin** Salt, water and mucus	Digestion and absorption of most substances, mixing and propulsion of contents. Further digestion of CHO. Further digestion of protein. Lubrication. Action of pancreatic lipase continues.
Colon. Large lumen with no villi.	Mucus (contains bacterial flora)	Storing and concentration of undigested matter by absorption of salt and water. Propulsion of contents. Protection from pathogens. Produces Vitamin K and B complexes.
Rectum		Defecation reflex initiated by distension.

active but may be inhibited by the satiety centre. The centres are stimulated by glucose, amino acids, lipids, body temperature, distension of the gut, and cholecystokinin (CCK), and also by psychological influences.

Energy is required by the body to maintain basal metabolic activities and to sustain an increase in those activities when necessary. The amount of energy required by an individual therefore depends on two factors: the basal metabolic rate (BMR) and the physical activity level (PAL) (Todorovik and Micklewright, 1997). The estimated average requirement for energy can be expressed in kilocalories and/or kilojoules (1 kcal = 4.2 kJ) and is:

$$\text{Energy required} = BMR \times PAL$$

The *caloric value* represents the energy incorporated in chemical bonds that is released during metabolism:

- 1 g of carbohydrate produces 4.1 kcal;
- 1 g of protein produces approximately the same;
- 1 g of fat produces 9.2 kcal.

Metabolism refers to all chemical reactions of the body and has two phases: catabolism and anabolism.

- *Anabolic reactions* consist of a series of synthesis reactions whereby small molecules are built up into larger ones that form the body's structural and functional components. Anabolic reactions require energy whereas catabolism refers to 'breakdown' reactions that release energy.
- *Catabolic reactions* supply the energy required for anabolic reactions and most metabolic reactions are catalysed by enzymes, which are proteins that speed up chemical reactions without themselves being changed.

The *metabolic rate* varies between individuals and tends to slow down with advancing age. PAL values are slightly higher for men than for women, and they also tend to decline with advancing age, resulting in a reduced energy requirement.

Carbohydrate metabolism

During digestion, polysaccharides and disaccharides are converted to monosaccharides which are transported to the liver. *Carbohydrate metabolism is primarily concerned with glucose metabolism.* For more information, see Chapter 6.

The fate of carbohydrates

Some glucose is oxidized by cells to provide energy. It moves into cells by facilitated diffusion, and insulin stimulates glucose movement into the cells. Excess glucose can be stored by the liver and the skeletal muscles as glycogen, or converted to fat.

Glucose catabolism

Glucose oxidation is also called 'cellular respiration'. The complete oxidation of glucose to CO_2 and H_2O involves glycolysis, the Krebs cycle and the electron transport chain.

- Glycolysis, also called 'anaerobic respiration', refers to the breakdown of glucose into two molecules of pyruvic acid. When O_2 is in short supply, pyruvic acid is converted to lactic acid; under aerobic conditions pyruvic acid enters the Krebs cycle. Glycolysis yields two molecules of ATP (energy).
- The Krebs cycle begins when pyruvic acid is converted to acetyl coenzyme A. Then a series of oxidation and reduction reactions take place and the energy originally in the glucose and then the pyruvic acid is transferred to the reduced coenzymes.
- The electron transport chain is a series of oxidation–reduction reactions in which the energy in the coenzymes is liberated and transferred to ATP for storage.

The complete oxidation of glucose can be represented as follows:

$$\text{Glucose} + O_2 \rightarrow 38\,\text{ATP} + CO_2 + H_2O.$$

Glucose anabolism

The conversion of glucose to glycogen for storage in the liver and skeletal muscle is called *glycogenesis*, and is stimulated by insulin. The body can store 500 g of glycogen. The conversion of glycogen back to glucose is called *glycogenolysis*; it occurs between meals and is stimulated by the hormone glucagon. *Gluconeogenesis* is the conversion of fat and protein molecules into glucose.

Lipid metabolism

Lipids are secondary to carbohydrates as a source of energy. During digestion, fats are ultimately broken down into fatty acids and glycerol.

The fate of lipids

Some fats may be oxidized to produce ATP. Some fats are stored in adipose tissue, mostly in the subcutaneous layer. Other lipids are used as structural molecules or to synthesize essential molecules. Examples: phospholipids of cell membranes, lipoproteins that transport cholesterol, thromboplastin for blood clotting, and cholesterol used to synthesize bile salts and steroid hormones.

Lipid catabolism

Fat must be split into fatty acids and glycerol (by enzyme action/chemical digestion in the gut), before it can be catabolized. Glycerol can be converted into glucose by conversion into a substrate in the gluconeogenesis pathway; or similarly, it can enter the pathway in the direction of glycolysis, and yield ATP anaerobically or, in the presence of O_2, enter the Krebs cycle and the electron transport chain (see above) to maximize energy yield aerobically. Fatty acids are catabolized through beta-oxidation, yielding acetyl coenzyme A, which enters the Krebs cycle.

The formation of ketone bodies by the liver is a normal phase of fatty acid catabolism, but an excess of ketones in the body is called ketosis, and may cause acidosis.

Lipid anabolism/lipogenesis

The conversion of glucose or amino acids into lipids is called *lipogenesis* and is stimulated by insulin.

Protein metabolism

During digestion, proteins are broken down into amino acids. Protein anabolism and catabolism must be balanced through daily dietary intake to prevent protein depletion.

The fate of proteins

Amino acids that enter cells are almost immediately synthesized into proteins. Proteins function as enzymes, hormones, structural elements etc. and any excess is stored as fat or glycogen, or used for energy.

Protein catabolism

Before amino acids can be catabolized, they must be converted to substances that can enter the Krebs cycle. Amino acids may also be converted into glucose, fatty acids and ketones.

Protein anabolism

Protein synthesis is directed by DNA and RNA and carried out on the ribosomes of cells. Before protein synthesis can occur, all the essential and non-essential amino acids must be present.

Minerals

Minerals are *inorganic* substances that help to regulate body processes. Minerals known to perform essential functions are calcium, phosphorus, sodium, chlorine, potassium, magnesium, iron, sulphur, iodine, manganese, cobalt, copper, zinc, selenium and chromium.

Vitamins

Vitamins are organic nutrients that maintain growth and normal metabolism, and many function in enzyme systems.

- Fat-soluble vitamins (A, D, E, K) are absorbed with fats.
- Water-soluble vitamins (B, C) are absorbed with water.

Nutrition in acute and severe illness

There are numerous reasons why patients become malnourished following hospitalization, including limited food intake, problems of absorption, alterations to metabolism, altered nutrient and energy requirements, poor nutritional assessment and management, interactions between nutrients and drugs, and the interaction between nutrition and the disease or condition itself, for example, mechanical problems such as dysphagia following a stroke (Feldblum *et al.* 2007). For the severely ill patient the complex metabolic reaction to injury and illness complicates the nutritional picture, so a brief overview of these responses will be given.

Normal response to starvation

It is useful to begin with an overview of the normal response to starvation in the otherwise healthy individual. The normal response is designed to conserve body protein by reducing the rate of depletion and its effect on body weight (Ruderman 1975). Energy requirements are reduced (i.e. basal metabolic rate is reduced) and fat becomes the preferred fuel. Body function is therefore preserved and total starvation can be tolerated for up to 60 days, with compromise of functions such as immune competence around 30 days.

The response is regulated by reduced substrate levels, decreased insulin secretion and increased levels of glucagon in the blood. Ketones are the preferred energy fuel at 14–20 days with some degree of glucose intolerance. Introduction of a sufficient level of substrate (nutritional food) restores metabolic normality.

Derangement during illness

Critical illness such as sepsis and trauma produce a complex phasic response characterized by inflammatory, immune, hormonal and metabolic responses (Singer *et al.* 2004; Hasenboehler *et al.* 2006). These changes negatively impact upon energy production and normal cellular processes, which may lead to multiple organ dysfunction. This metabolic stress response has long been described as having two distinct phases: the ebb phase and the flow phase (Table 7.2).

Table 7.2 Metabolic changes in critical illness (Hasenboehler *et al.* 2006)

Ebb phase (hours)	Flow phase (days to weeks)
Decreased body temperature	Increased body temperature
Decreased oxygen consumption	Increased oxygen consumption
Lactate acidosis	Negative nitrogen balance
Increased stress hormone levels	Increased stress hormone levels
Decreased insulin levels	Normal to increased insulin levels
Hyperglycaemia, insulin resistance	Hyperglycaemia, insulin resistance
Gluconeogenesis	Gluconeogenesis
Increased substrate consumption	Proteinolysis
Hepatic acute-phase response	Lipolysis
Immune activation	Immunosuppression

All diseases associated with an inflammatory response, such as COPD or tissue repair such as trauma or operative surgery, induce a metabolic response. The magnitude of the response is related to the severity of the clinical condition (Gariballa and Forster 2006). The issue of greatest importance, clinically, is the catabolic phase seen during acute illness when the rate of tissue loss and protein depletion can be rapid. The metabolic response to critical disease overrides the normal response to starvation and conservation of body protein and energy is no longer possible. Weight loss and depletion of body protein is accelerated and significant impairment of body function may appear early in the course of the illness. The catabolic nature of the response is related to the disease processes and is unaffected by nutritional intake.

Features of the metabolic response

- *Protein*. Tissue loss occurs mainly in skeletal muscle and is associated with increased urinary excretion of nitrogen, potassium, magnesium, sulphate, phosphate and creatinine. Protein turnover is increased, and the breakdown (catabolism) of protein is increased to a much greater extent, resulting in a net loss of protein from the body. In severe critical illness, the requirements for protein may be increased by 50–80 per cent.
- *Carbohydrate*. There is a state of glucose intolerance with hyperglycaemia, hyperinsulinaemia and insulin intolerance. This is associated with an increase in gluconeogenesis by the liver, principally from tissue protein. Uptake of glucose by the body tissues is reduced due to glucose and insulin intolerance, despite the fact that the tissues are desperate for energy for recovery to take place.
- *Fat*. Lipolysis (fat breakdown) is increased with raised blood levels of free fatty acids and glycerol. By contrast with non-stressed starvation, ketones remain low or absent.
- *Energy*. Resting energy expenditure may increase by 18–30 per cent in multiple fractures, by 30–60 per cent in severe infections, and by 50–100 per cent in severe illness.

The detailed mechanisms that bring about this metabolic response to illness are complex and outside the scope of this chapter; but stimuli such as pain, anoxia, hypercarbia, hypovolaemia and hypotension all operate where there is tissue damage and physiological stress or injury. These all trigger release of ACTH and growth hormone from the hypothalamus, resulting in increased circulating levels of cortisol, glucagon and insulin. Tissue cytokines, released in response to tissue damage and the inflammatory response, are also thought to be involved. This last point is supported by a study finding that the inflammatory marker C-reactive protein (CRP) showed a significant association with measured energy expenditure in hospital patients (Gariballa and Forster 2006).

Clinical implications

- There is loss of body weight at an accelerated rate, which reflects the reduction in lean body mass.
- Muscle function is impaired and experienced as weakness. This has direct implications for respiration and all activities of daily living. A general sense of weakness and illness impairs appetite and the ability to eat.
- The immune function is impaired by traumatic stimuli and by malnutrition, and the cause of death in the critically ill is commonly an infection.
- Mental acuity and performance are impaired, resulting in apathy and depression with loss of morale and the will to recover.

A *severely malnourished person* does not have the nutritional reserves to cope with the increased metabolic demands of severe injury, resulting in organ failure and infection. Organs with rapid cell turnover are the first to fail; for example the GI tract epithelium becomes flattened and the ability to absorb nutrients rapidly declines.

Assessment of nutritional status

ACTIVITY   ?

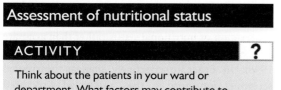

Think about the patients in your ward or department. What factors may contribute to malnutrition in the patients you see?

The nutritional status of a patient is clearly of paramount importance because malnourishment prolongs recovery, increases the need for high-dependency care, increases the risk of serious complications of illness, and at worst leads to death. This is particularly so in the older patient where pre-morbid undernutrition may accelerate these complications.

Assessing those patients at risk of malnutrition may be difficult because of the many factors involved, but the main causes of malnutrition can be identified and listed quite simply as follows:
- impaired intake;
- impaired digestion;
- altered metabolic nutrient requirements;
- excess nutritional loss.

The nurse must be vigilant and observe the patient for signs of poor nutrition. Poor nutrition may have existed before admission or be as a result of the hospitalization and illness. It is important to note, too, that there are many diverse conditions likely to result in nutritional deficiencies (Box 7.2).

Effects of medications

A number of medications, some commonly prescribed, may contribute to malnutrition. Table 7.3 gives a brief list, but nurses should be familiar with the possible impact of drugs used in their own specialities that may have an impact on nutrition.

Table 7.3 Examples of the effects of drugs on nutritional status

Drug	Effect on nutrition
Aspirin and NSAIDs	Blood loss and iron deficiency
Digoxin	Lowered appetite
Purgatives	Potassium loss
Cancer chemotherapy	Anorexia
Diuretics	Potassium loss
Phenformin and metformin	Vitamin B12 malabsorption
Co-trimoxazole	Can antagonize folate

Food can also affect the absorption of certain drugs, but *most* drugs are best taken with or just after meals. This is because it is an easy way to remember to take the drug, and because some are gastric irritants (e.g. aspirin and non-steroidal anti-inflammatory medications such as ibuprofen). Absorption

Box 7.2 Potential causes of inadequate nutritional intake

Mechanical feeding problems

Mechanical feeding problems may be due to poor functioning of oral mucous membranes, teeth, tongue or salivary glands, receding gums, ill-fitting dentures or mouth ulcers.

Physical disability

Physical disabilities include dysphagia due to neuromuscular disorders (e.g. stroke, head injury), Parkinson's disease, achalasia, multiple sclerosis and scleroderma.

Obstruction

Obstruction may result from goitre, acute tonsillitis, cancer neoplasm, chronic oesophagitis or aortic aneurysm.

Psychological causes

These causes may include eating disorders such as bulimia and anorexia nervosa, dementia, clinical depression, general loss of appetite and nausea.

Increased metabolism

Fever, infections or malignancy will cause a metabolic increase, as will hyperthyroidism, surgical stress, trauma and burns.

Increased dietary loss

The patient may have nausea causing vomiting or may have diarrhoea. Decreased transit time through the gut may be caused by pathogenic organisms (e.g. *Salmonella*), gastrointestinal irritation or drug therapy. The patient may have an ileostomy or suffer from malabsorption syndrome.

Defective utilization

This may result from metabolic disease, hepatic insufficiency or renal tubular acidosis.

Defective absorption

This may be caused by pancreatic disease, biliary obstruction, coeliac disease, Crohn's disease or infections such as tuberculosis or *Giardia*. Systemic conditions may reduce absorption, such as scleroderma or diabetes. Certain drugs may be responsible, such as antibiotics or excess laxatives. Surgical procedures such as fistulae formation or aggressive gastric surgery could have this effect.

Defective functions of major organ systems

Conditions such as severe heart disease, chronic obstructive pulmonary disease, liver disease, renal and brain damage may all have a significant effect on nutritional condition and must be taken into consideration.

---

of some drugs is a little delayed, but this is often unimportant and a few are better absorbed when taken with meals (e.g. beta-blockers). A few drugs should be taken half an hour before meals; examples are antibiotics which are labile in acid, such as benzylpenicillin, cloxacillin, erythromycin, tetracycline, rifampicin and isoniazid.

A number of drugs will effect appetite. Appetite may be *decreased* by bulking agents, amphetamines, cardiac glycosides, glucagon, morphine, indomethacin, cyclophosphamide, cytotoxic therapies, and salbutamol. Appetite may be *increased* by chlorpromazine, androgens, anabolic steroids, corticosteroids, insulin, lithium, amitriptyline, benzodiazepines and metoclopramide. *Malabsorption* for one or more nutrients may be induced by neomycin, chlortetracycline, cyclophosphamide, methotrexate and methyldopa.

Healthcare practitioners need to be aware of all these complicating factors when making the initial assessment, during continual reassessment, and at the evaluation of their interventions.

Assessment principles

Nursing assessment has tended to rely on general observation of nutritional status rather than accurate and systematic screening and early referral (Reilly 1996). In order to effectively manage nutritional screening for those at risk, a detailed structured assessment should be a routine aspect of in-hospital care. General factors to consider in patient assessment include the following:

- height and weight, for the body mass index (BMI) calculation and for obvious signs of weight loss;

- direct observation/measurement of muscle bulk, subcutaneous fat, dehydration and grip strength;
- observation of general signs of malnourishment, such as delayed wound healing, repeated infections, loose or fragile skin;
- a biochemical profile to determine deficiencies and abnormalities;
- the impact of the disease and treatment on swallowing and digestion (drugs taken, investigations done and therapy);
- whether the patient has particularly high needs for some or all nutrients;
- whether there is excessive loss of nutrients;
- a dietary history investigating the patient's 'normal diet', recent changes and weight loss;
- fluid balance.

Body mass index is a commonly used measurement for estimating or predicting malnourishment. BMI is weight divided by the height squared (w/h^2), and the optimum range is 20–25. While the BMI is not a perfect guide it is a widely used standard measure and provides a good basis for assessment.

Alongside a general observation of potential risk, it is recommended that an *holistic assessment* be carried out routinely. NHS Quality Improvement Scotland (2003) have published standards for nursing assessment which state that an holistic assessment should be recorded within one day of admission and should include:

- height and weight;
- eating and drinking likes/dislikes;
- food allergies and need for a therapeutic diet;
- cultural/ethnic/religious requirements;
- social/environmental mealtime requirements;
- physical difficulties with eating and drinking;
- the need for equipment to help with eating and drinking.

More specifically there are a number of screening and assessment tools currently recommended for in-hospital use. They include: the Subjective Global Assessment (SGA) questionnaire (Detsky *et al.* 1987); the Malnutrition Universal Screening Tool (MUST) (Elia 2003); and the Nutritional Risk Screening tool 2002 (NRS-2002) (Kondrup *et al.* 2003). These three tools have been subjected to rigorous review. A recent evaluation reported that they are appropriate for assessing nutritional status and risk in hospitalized patients (Kylea *et al.* 2005).

Using the MUST

The tool currently being promoted within the National Health Service is MUST. It has been developed by the British Association for Parenteral and Enteral Nutrition (BAPEN). The tool is given on p. 220. It can also be downloaded from the BAPEN website at www.bapen.org.uk with comprehensive screening guidelines.

This screening tool is a five-step aid for use in adults to identify those who are either malnourished or at risk of malnutrition. The five steps are as follows.

1. Calculate BMI (from weight and height) and score it using the MUST chart. If it is not possible to measure the patient's height it can be estimated from the ulna length. If the weight is not known and patient cannot be weighed, the BMI is estimated from the upper arm circumference.
2. Using the MUST tables, any unplanned weight loss is scored.
3. The presence of acute illness is scored.
4. The scores are added to gain an *overall risk category*: low risk, medium risk or high risk.
5. The final step is to follow management guidelines. For the low-risk patient this is to repeat the screening weekly. Medium risk requires observation of dietary intake for three days, then reassess; if there is no improvement and/or there is clinical concern, then local hospital policy for assisted nutrition should be followed. High risk requires treatment and referral to a dietician.

CASE STUDY 7.1

Mr Jennings is a 78-year-old man who lives alone. He has been admitted to a surgical ward from the A&E department having been diagnosed with an 'acute abdomen'. He has been unwell for several days with abdominal pain and nausea. He will be going for a laperotomy in the next few hours. He is a slight-looking gentleman and his height and weight give a BMI of 19.

- Is Mr Jennings at risk of undernutrition? If so, why?
- How do you think he would score on the MUST?

The MUST is fairly simple to administer and has a high degree of sensitivity, which means it has a high probability of detecting those at risk. Current UK clinical guidelines support the use of MUST. However, it is acknowledged that there are other tools available, and MUST is described here to illustrate the value of using a structured assessment of risk.

Providing nutritional support

Malnutrition can detrimentally affect every system of the body. The evidence suggests that effective nutritional support can reduce mortality, complications after illness, length of hospital stay and readmission rates, and have a positive impact on economics and quality of life (Stratton *et al.* 2003). There are a number of options in providing nutritional support (Fig. 7.3).

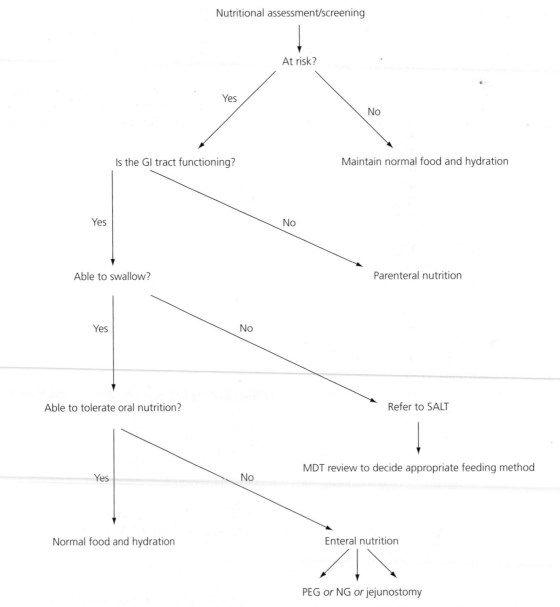

Figure 7.3 Nutritional assessment/screening: MDT, multidisciplinary team; SALT, speech and language therapist; NG, nasogastric; PEG, percutaneous endoscopic gastrostomy

In the last 30 years, modern management has enabled patients to survive acute episodes of critical disease where impaired nutritional status would have had a serious impact on survival.

Goals for nutritional support

The goals are straightforward:

- to achieve nutritional balance, i.e. prevent further depletion;
- to restore depleted tissue, i.e. regain the negative protein balance and return to normal function.

The options are summarized in Fig. 7.4 and listed below:

- a *normal diet* with or without the addition of frequent small appetising snacks between meals;
- *sip feeding* with a balanced composition similar to

a normal diet and/or fortified liquid foods, or special liquid feeds composed of amino acids, glucose and lipid which may be required for particular conditions (e.g. to reduce intestinal inflammation in patients with Crohn's disease);

- *enteral tube feeding* – the administration of specially formulated liquid nutrients through a tube directly into the gut either by nasogastric, nasoduodenal or nasojejunal routes (suitable for short-term measures), or by percutaneous endoscopic gastrostomy (PEG) and jejunostomy (for long-term measures);
- *parenteral tube feeding* – the introduction of digested nutrients directly into a vein, so bypassing the intestine.

In order to choose the most appropriate method, the answer to this fundamental question is required: *Is the enteral system/gut functional?* If it is functional,

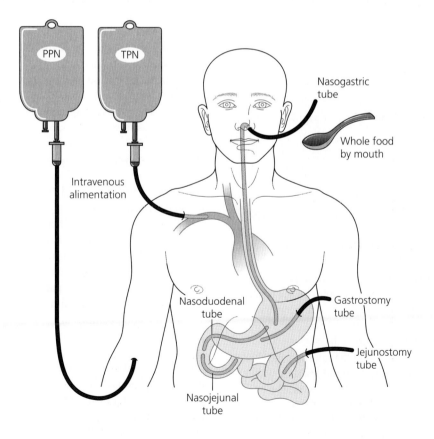

Figure 7.4 Alternative ways of feeding a patient

then enteral feeding is the optimal course of action to promote and maintain a healthy functioning GI tract.

Enteral feeding

Enteral feeding is indicated in patients with increased nutritional needs and whose GI tract is functioning (Finlay 1997), but who might have compromised oral access to the GI tract, an inability or unwillingness to eat, and where there is a danger of aspiration.

Box 7.3 Procedure for nasogastric (NG) tube insertion (NPSA 2005; Baillie 2009)

1. Obtain informed consent and maintain communication with the patient throughout.
2. Assist the patient to sit up, well-supported by pillows.
3. If unconscious, the patient should be on his/her side.
4. Clean the nostrils, or get the patient to blow his/her nose. Assess the patency.
5. Estimate the required length of tube by measuring the distance from the tip of the nose to the ear lobe and to the xiphisternum.
6. Check that the patient can swallow.
7. Lubricate the tip of the tube with sterile water.
8. Insert the tube into the nostril, passing along the floor of the nasopharynx to the oropharynx. If any obstruction is felt, withdraw the tube and try again in a slightly different direction.
9. As the tube passes the oropharynx, ask the patient to swallow.
10. Gently advance the tube as the patient swallows, to the estimated point on the tube.
11. If the patient shows any sign of respiratory distress – coughing, gasping, cyanosis – withdraw the tube immediately.
12. Confirm the position of the tube by gently passing a small amount of fluid (about 0.5–1 mL) and testing with pH indicator strips. The pH should be 5.5 or below.
13. If there is any doubt about the position of the tube it should be checked with a chest X-ray.
14. Secure the tube in place.

Administering enteral nutrition

Insertion of nasoenteric tubes may be generally carried out by qualified and experienced nurses (Box 7.3). Doctors are responsible for the insertion of fine-bore feeding tubes in patients who have maxillofacial disorders or following surgery, laryngectomy, and any disorder of the oesophagus.

A patient who requires prolonged enteral nutrition will have a percutaneous endoscopic gastrostomy (PEG) tube inserted by staff trained in the technique. PEG is a procedure performed under local anaesthetic whereby the tube is placed endoscopically. Some tubes are kept in place by means of a retention balloon while others are sutured. Drug therapy in solution can be administered via the tube.

The functioning and safety of the method of feeding must be monitored constantly. An awareness of the potential complications of enteral feeding is important, as shown in Box 7.4 (Palmer and MacFie 1997). Enteral tubes have become commonplace, but it must be recognized that they are not without risks: the National Patient Safety Agency (2005) have highlighted a number of deaths and complications from NG tube misplacement. The crucial point is to check the tube position using approved methods (pH indicator strips or chest X-ray) and not to administer anything down the tube if there is the slightest doubt about the position.

Composition of an enteral diet

An average patient will need 2000–3000 kcal (35 kcal/kg per day) and 10–15 g of nitrogen, corresponding to 60–90 g of protein (1.5 g/kg per day) in 2–3 L of fluid. The proportion of energy provided by fat should be about 30–40 per cent. The mixture should contain essential minerals, trace elements, vitamins and essential fatty acids. Some patients may need extra micronutrients and macronutrients.

Specific compositions are available for particular patient needs. In the acute seriously ill patient suffering from trauma or sepsis, up to 50 per cent additional protein may offset the adverse impact of the hypermetabolic response in the first 24–48 hours (Jivnani *et al.* 2010), although caution must be exercised if the patient is at risk of refeeding syndrome (described later). NCCAC (2006) guidelines recommend starting feeds with only 50 per cent of the target energy and protein needs and building up over 24–48 hours.

Box 7.4 Avoiding or resolving the complications of enteral feeding

Tube blockage

Flush the tube with water when the feed is interrupted or stopped. Maintain a continuous flow using a correct combination of tube and nutrient solution, and replace the tube regularly.

Misplacement or displacement

Insert the correct type/length of tube with the patient in an upright position. Check tube position by aspiration and pH/X-ray, and secure firmly.

Aspiration

Elevate the head of the bed during continuous feeding. Check the position of the tube before each feed. Avoid large-bore tubes. Use nasojejunal feeding if the patient is supine, unconscious or when the cardiac sphincter is incompetent.

Discomfort

Secure the tube firmly to avoid mucosal erosion. Encourage nose breathing. Ensure hydration and oral hygiene. Lubricate lips and inspect nostrils daily.

Contamination

Practise good personal hygiene when handling feeds and equipment. Avoid non-sterile feeds. Change giving sets regularly. Practise aseptic care of a PEG tube site, and change bags every 24 hours.

Nausea and vomiting

Avoid high-lipid or hyperosmolar feeds. Use low-lactose or lactose-free formulas and dilute when necessary. Avoid rapid infusion rates, and increase concentration and rate slowly.

Diarrhoea

Dilute the feed or change to lactose-free and isotonic formula if appropriate. Monitor antibiotic therapy and hydration, and consider IV fluids for better absorption. Check the feed for contamination.

Constipation

Monitor hydration and use fibre-containing feed.

Parenteral nutrition

Parenteral nutrition is indicated in patients with increased nutritional needs and whose GI tract is not functioning, and who may have fistulae, multiple trauma/burns, inflammatory bowel disease with complications, multiple organ failure, pancreatitis, prolonged paralytic ileus, peritoneal sepsis or short bowel syndrome.

Administering parenteral nutrition

Central venous catheters are inserted by experienced medical staff and managed by suitably qualified medical and nursing personnel. The potential complications of parenteral nutrition are listed in Box 7.5.

The subclavian vein is the preferred site (see Fig. 1.4b on page 8). In patients with poor venous access or in whom a central line is contraindicated, a peripherally inserted central catheter (PICC) may be used, although ideally only for a limited period.

The infusion enters the vein at a point where it will be rapidly diluted by high-volume flow past the catheter tip.

Nutrients used in parenteral feeding

The feed is tailored to a patient's individual requirements. A stable patient with intestinal failure usually requires about 10.5 MJ (2500 kcal) of energy and 12 g of nitrogen as crystalline amino acids in 2500 mL of fluid. Energy is provided using glucose and lipid emulsion (usually soya bean oil). Lipid usually provides about 30 per cent of the calories infused. Amino acid provision includes all the essential amino acids and a wide range of the non-essential ones. Mixed into the bag with the above are the normal daily requirement of electrolytes, trace elements and vitamins. For patients with sepsis and increased metabolic requirements, the feed needs to be modified with additional amounts of vitamin B complex, trace elements and electrolytes. Nutrients are administered to the patient from a 3 L bag.

Box 7.5 Avoiding or resolving the complications of parenteral feeding

Catheterization insertion

Dangers include air embolism, arterial puncture, chylothorax, haemothorax, pneumothorax, nerve injury and arrhythmias. Correctly insert the central line, confirm its position and document and firmly secure it. Tilt the patient into a 200 head-down position prior to venepuncture. Use silicone catheters in preference to plastic in order to minimize damage to the lining of the vein. Withdraw the catheter slightly as the catheter tip can be too close to the sinoatrial node (pacemaker). The catheter tip should lie in the superior vena cava (see Fig. 1.4).

Indwelling catheter issues

Dangers include sepsis and septicaemia. Insert the catheter under full sterile conditions, cover the entry site with a sterile adhesive dressing, and change this when necessary in accordance with strict aseptic technique. Ensure infusion solutions are sterile, and change infusions and giving sets only by experienced nurses wearing sterile gloves. Monitor the patient for pyrexia. Inspect the catheter site, swab and culture blood and catheter tip for micro-organisms and sensitivity.

Catheter blockage

Dangers include air embolism and blood clot. Maintain an adequate infusion rate using a volumetric infusion pump. Check clamps, taps and devices. Change empty fluid containers promptly. Ensure there are locking connections to prevent accidental disconnections.

Metabolic disturbances

Dangers include hyperglycaemia, hypoglycaemia, urea and electrolyte imbalances, hyperosmolar diuresis, nutritional deficiences, overhydration and circulatory overload. Ensure the feed solution meets the specific needs of the patient and control the rate of infusion. Disturbances may be due to the nutrient proportions in the feed: too much glucose can cause dehydration, respiratory distress due to CO_2 build-up, and coma. Energy can be provided in the form of more lipid and proportionally less glucose. Feed composition is very important and comprises pre-digested macronutrients: glucose, lipid emulsions, L-amino acids and micronutrients (electrolytes, trace elements, vitamins and water).

All feeds are specially prepared by the pharmacist according to medical prescription and dietetic recommendations based on individual patient needs, extent of trauma, preoperative repletion, postoperative management etc. A regular rate of infusion is ensured by using a constant-volume infusion pump, which incorporates alarms to warn of air in the infusion system and changes in flow rate.

Dietary interventions or therapeutic diets are considered for acute renal failure, cancer, cirrhosis of the liver, Crohn's disease, coeliac disease, constipation, diabetes mellitus, diverticulitis, gastrectomy, hyperlipidaemia, liver transplantation, malabsorption syndrome and obesity.

Refeeding syndrome

Refeeding syndrome is a life-threatening complication of rapid feeding following a period of starvation. It is mediated by metabolic and hormonal changes after refeeding by enteral or parenteral routes. It may lead to severe metabolic derangement and can be fatal.

The syndrome is characterized by hypophosphataemia, hypokalaemia, hypomagnesaemia, and fluid balance abnormalities. On refeeding following starvation, the increased blood glucose levels increase insulin and decrease glucagon secretion, which results in an anabolic state with the synthesis of glycogen, fat and protein. This requires minerals such as phosphate and magnesium which are soon used up. Insulin stimulates the absorption of potassium into the cells and water moves into the intracellular space. This results in decreased serum levels of phosphate, potassium and magnesium and fluid overload. There is also retention of sodium which compounds the volume overload (Mehenna et al. 2008).

Clinically the patient may show signs of weakness, confusion, fits or coma. The initial signs are those of cardiac failure, such as tachycardia and increasing breathlessness. If these are seen the feeding should be temporarily stopped and the patient urgently assessed.

NICE guidelines have listed those considered to be at risk of refeeding problems (Box 7.6). For those considered at risk, feeding should be started slowly and at reduced level of nutritional support of 10 kcal/kg per day, increasing slowly over 4–7 days and providing supplements of thiamine, vitamin B complex, potassium, phosphate and magnesium (NCCAC 2006).

Conclusion

In-hospital malnutrition remains common particularly in the elderly, although there is far greater awareness of the importance of structured assessment to identify those at risk and structured screening tools widely available. Acutely ill patients pose particular challenges for the healthcare team, especially those who are seriously ill from trauma, infection or other severe illness. The reader is encouraged to refer to the many clinical guidelines and recommendations now available to support the practitioner in the assessment and management of nutrition in hospital.

Suggested further reading

Garrow JS, James WPT (eds) (1993). *Human Nutrition and Dietetics*, 9th edn. London: Churchill Livingstone.

Box 7.6 Criteria for determining people at high risk of developing refeeding syndrome (NCCAC 2006)

Patient has *one or more* of the following:
- BMI less than 16 kg/m^2
- unintentional weight loss greater than 15% within the last 3–6 months
- little or no nutritional intake for more than 10 days
- low levels of potassium, phosphate or magnesium prior to feeding;

OR

patient has *two or more* of the following:
- BMI less than 18.5 kg/m^2
- unintentional weight loss greater than 10% within the last 3–6 months
- little or no nutritional intake for more than 5 days
- a history of alcohol abuse or drug use, including insulin, chemotherapy, antacids or diuretics.

Hinchliffe S, Norman S, Schober J (1994). *Nursing Practice and Health Care*. London: Arnold.

Jivnani S, Iyer S, Umakumar K, Gore M (2010). Impact of enteral nutrition on nitrogen balance in patients with trauma, *Journal of Emergencies, Trauma and Shock* 3(2); 109–14.

References

Age Concern England (2006). Hungry to be Heard campaign; see www.ageconcern.org.uk/AgeConcern/hungry2bheard.asp (accessed July 2010).

Baillie (2009) *Developing Practical Adult Nursing Skills*, 3rd edn. London: Hodder Arnold.

BAPEN (2003) *Malnutrition Universal Screening Tool: MUST*. Redditch: British Association for Parenteral and Enteral Nutrition.

BAPEN (2007). *Organisation of Food and Nutritional Support in Hospitals*. Redditch: British Association for Parenteral and Enteral Nutrition.

Bistrian BR, Blackburn G, Vitale J, Cochran D, Naylor J (1976). Prevalence of malnutrition in general medical patients, *Journal of the American Medical Association* 235; 1567–70.

Clancy J, McVicar AJ (2009). *Physiology and Anatomy: A Homeostatic Approach*, 3rd edn. London: Hodder Arnold.

Detsky AS, McLaughin JR, Baker JP et al. (1987). What is subjective global assessment of nutritional status? *Journal of Parenteral and Enteral Nutrition* 11; 8–13.

Edington J, Boorman J, Durrant ER et al. (2000). Prevalence of malnutrition on admission to four hospitals in England, *Clinical Nutrition* 19(3); 191–5.

Elia M (2003). *Screening for Malnutrition: A Multidisciplinary Responsibility. Development and Use of the Malnutrition Universal Screening Tool (MUST) for Adults*. Redditch: BAPEN.

Feldblum I, German L, Castel H et al. (2007). Characteristics of undernourished older medical patients and the identification of predictors for undernutrition status, *Nutrition Journal* 6; 37.

Finlay T (1997). Making sense of parenteral nutrition in adult patients, *Nursing Times* **93**(2); 35–6.

Gariballa SE, Forster S (2006). Effects of acute phase response on nutritional status and clinical outcome of hospitalised patients, *Nutrition* **22**; 750–7.

Hasenboehler E, Williams A, Leinhase I *et al.* (2006). Metabolic changes after polytrauma: an imperative for early nutritional support, *World Journal of Emergency Surgery* **1**; 29.

Kondrup J, Allison SP, Elia M, Vellas B, Plauth M. (2003). ESPEN guidelines for nutrition screening 2002. *Clinical Nutrition* **22**; 415–21.

Kylea U, Kossovskyb M, Karsegarda V, and Pichard C (2005). Comparison of tools for nutritional assessment and screening at hospital admission: a population study, *Clinical Nutrition* **25**; 409–17.

Lishman G (2009). *Nutrition Action Plan Delivery Board End-of-Year Report.* London: Department of Health.

Mehenna H, Moledina J, Travis J (2008). Refeeding syndrome: what it is and how to prevent and treat it, *British Medical Journal* **336**; 1495.

National Collaborating Centre for Acute Care (2006). Nutrition Support in Adults: Oral Nutrition Support, Enteral Tube Feeding, and Parenteral Nutrition. London: NCCAC.

National Patient Safety Agency (2005). *Patient Safety Alert: Reducing Harm from Misplaced NG Tubes.* London: NPSA/Department of Health.

NHS Quality Improvement Scotland (2003). *Food, Fluid and Nutritional Care in Hospitals: Clinical Standards.* Edinburgh: NHS Quality Improvement Scotland.

Palmer D, MacFie J (1997). Alternative intake, *Nursing Times* **93**(Suppl.); 49.

Reilly H (1996). Nutritional assessment, *British Journal of Nursing* **5**(1); 18–24.

Ruderman NB (1975). Muscle amino acid metabolism and gluconeogenesis, *Annual Review of Medicine* **26**; 248.

Singer M, De Santis V, Vitale D, Jeffcoate W (2004). Multiorgan failure is an adaptive, endocrine-mediated, metabolic response to overwhelming systemic inflammation, *Lancet* **364**; 545–8.

Stratton RJ, Green CJ, Elia M (2003). *Disease-related Malnutrition: An Evidence-based Approach to Treatment.* Oxford: CAB International.

Todorovik VE, Micklewright A (eds) (1997). *A Pocket Guide to Clinical Nutrition.* London: British Dietetic Association.

LEARNING OUTCOMES

On completion of this chapter the reader will:

1 be able to describe the physiological phases of the pain process

2 have a good understanding of the assessment of pain in the acute setting

3 be able to describe the main approaches to pain management in the acute setting.

Introduction

This chapter discusses the physiology of pain and highlights some of the factors that will influence the effectiveness of the assessment and management of acute pain. The chapter focuses largely on pain assessment and briefly discusses pain relief strategies.

Overview

Pain is probably the most common symptom experienced by patients in hospital and one of the principal clinical features that lead to admission. Patient surveys show that more than two-thirds of patients experience pain while in hospital (Garrett and Boyd 2008), and pain is the most common presenting complaint in patients admitted to A&E departments (Todd *et al.* 2007). It has been said that effective pain management is a fundamental human right (Macintyre *et al.* 2010) and the relief of pain and suffering is arguably the raison d'être of nursing and healthcare. It is clearly a core aspect of care and one that patients would expect to be high on the list of priorities in the acute care setting.

While there have been significant improvements in pain management over time, there remains evidence that pain may go under-assessed and under-managed (Dolin *et al.* 2002; Strohbuecker *et al.* 2005). This is particularly so in vulnerable groups, and a recent review of surgical care in the elderly reported that postoperative pain management was poor in up to 20 per cent of cases (NCEPOD 2010). However, there is now much clearer understanding of the knowledge and systems that need to be in place to ensure effective acute pain management with clear guidelines and models of practice (RCoA and The Pain Society 2003; Macintyre *et al.* 2010).

It is clear that there are costs and consequences arising from poor acute pain management. Poor outcomes associated with ineffective pain management include extended hospital stay, more postoperative complications, lower patient and nurse satisfaction, and greater incidence of subsequent chronic pain (Macintyre and Ready 2002). It should be noted here that acute pain stimulates the immune response to injury including the production of inflammatory cytokines, increased levels of catecholamines and decreases in insulin sensitivity; if severe and prolonged this injury response becomes counter-productive (Chapman *et al.* 2008).

In the acute care setting pain has been described as the 'fifth vital sign' and it is important that health professionals caring for acutely ill patients have a good understanding of pain assessment and management.

Good pain management requires an understanding of the phenomenon of pain. The sensation of pain is an important defence mechanism essential for survival. The essential nature of the pain experience is made obvious in conditions where pain is not felt, as in rare cases of congenital analgesia or the more common cases of analgesia caused by lesions of the nerve pathways. Patients may sustain extensive tissue damage without being aware of any noxious stimuli which can lead to serious and life-threatening complications.

Definitions of pain

Definitions of pain are many and varied and often reflect an underpinning approach or philosophy. A widely cited definition is that of the International Association for the Study of Pain from 1974 (Merskey and Bogduk 1994):

Pain is defined as an unpleasant sensory and emotional experience associated with actual or potential tissue damage or described in terms of such damage.

This definition has stood the test of time, but it has been criticized for focusing explicitly on tissue damage.

Within nursing the classic definition proposed by McCaffery (1968) continues to be used:

Pain is whatever the experiencing person says it is, existing whenever he says it does.

This is less of a definition and more of a statement of intent or approach. The patient is viewed as the best judge of his or her own pain, and the health professional takes a compassionate approach, seeing the patient at the centre of pain management.

Pain is a subjective experience that is unique to each individual. The experience of pain is influenced not only by the neurological processes but also by a complex mix of physiological, psychological, social and cultural factors. According to Macintyre *et al.* (2010):

Pain is an individual, multifactorial experience influenced by culture, previous pain events, beliefs, mood and ability to cope.

Acute pain can be defined as pain of recent onset and probably of limited duration. It usually has an identifiable temporal and causal relationship to injury or disease. In other words, acute pain usually follows tissue damage. This damage activates receptors which leads to the transmission of this information to the brain and which is perceived as pain. The process by which the damage or potential damage is transmitted to the brain is called *nociception*. However, this seemingly simple process of receptor stimulation, transmission and perception is complex and influenced by many factors. Here a brief and simplified description is given; for a fuller account there are numerous textbooks devoted to the subject of pain.

The physiology of pain

The receptors that are stimulated in response to injury, or 'noxious stimuli', are called *nociceptors*. Nociceptors are free nerve endings and are found in all tissues and organs of the body except for the brain. They have a defined area of tissue from which they receive information resulting from tissue damage. This is the first stage in the sensation or perception of pain.

The pain process comprises four major phases (Fig. 8.1):

- *transduction* – the detection of a noxious stimulus by peripheral nerve receptors;
- *transmission* – the relaying of information from the peripheral nerve system to the central nervous system;
- *perception* – perceiving a stimulus as painful;
- *modulation* – alteration of information by other nerve activity in the nervous system.

Transduction

Nociceptors are usually divided in two main types (Table 8.1):

- fast-conducting mechanoreceptors (A-delta) which respond to stimuli such as strong pressure, sudden heat, or a sudden sharp stimulus, and produce a 'sharp' pain;

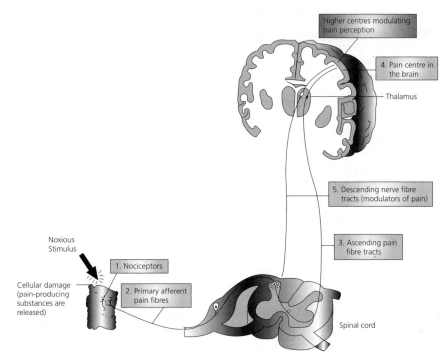

Figure 8.1 Four phases of the pain process

- the relatively slower conducting polymodal or C-type receptors which respond directly to tissue damage and to the chemical mediators that are released on injury, and produce a dull, longer-lasting pain or 'ache'.

Sources of stimuli that may result in nociception include:

- *mechanical* – from external traumatic injury (crushing or wounding), or from internal pressure such as from a tumour;

- *chemical* – such as the release of mediators during ischaemia or from infection;
- *thermal* – such as thermal trauma from a burn.

Such sources lead to the stimulation of nociceptors by the release of algesic or pain-producing substances. These chemical mediators act by either directly stimulating nociceptors or by potentiating the effects of the directly acting substances. Chemicals released include prostaglandins, bradykinin, potassium ions, substance P and histamine.

Table 8.1 Characteristics and functions of C and A-delta fibres

	C fibres	A-delta fibres
Characteristics	Primary afferent fibres Small diameter Unmyelinated Slow conducting	Primary afferent fibres Large diameter Myelinated Fast conducting
Receptor type	Polymodal (respond to more than one type of noxious stimuli): mechanical, thermal, chemical	High-threshold mechanoreceptors respond to mechanical stimuli over a certain intensity
Pain quality	Diffuse Dull Burning Aching Referred to as 'slow' or second' pain	Well-localized Sharp Stinging Pricking Referred to as 'fast' or 'first' pain

The initial sensation of pain resulting from injury is called *primary hyperalgesia*. Following this initial sensation there is wider sensitization of the nociceptors to stimuli, which leads to an area wider than that of the original site of injury becoming painful. This is called *secondary hyperalgesia*.

Transmission

The pain-producing power of the chemical mediators is proportional to their local concentration. When nociceptor stimulation reaches a particular threshold, depolarization of the nociceptor membrane occurs, this through the changing concentrations of sodium and potassium, and a pain impulse, or action potential, is sent along the nerve. The greater the number of impulses that are transmitted, the more severe the pain sensation.

Sensory impulses for pain are conducted to the central nervous system (CNS) along the spinal and cranial nerves. The spinal cord is composed of both grey and white matter; the grey matter forms the H-shaped area of the spinal cord that is surrounded by white matter (Fig. 8.2). The region of grey matter located to the back of the spinal cord is known as the posterior or dorsal horn. The dorsal horn is where C fibres and A-delta fibres enter the spinal cord, where they synapse with nociceptive dorsal horn neurones (NDHN). The synapse between the A-delta fibres and C fibres and the NDHN is crossed by releasing neurotransmitters including ATP, nitrous oxide, substance P, and bradykinin. The NDHN fibres then cross the cord and travel up the spinothalamic tract and the spinoreticular tract to the brainstem and thalamus.

When there has been deep tissue damage then 'afferent barrage' may occur. Because of a continuous barrage of nerve activity inputting the spinal cord interneurones, a pain message continues to be sent up the spinothalamic tract even when the stimulus has been removed. This may account for phantom limb pain.

Some patients develop chronic pain where the original injury may have healed. This may be related to changes in the neurones in the dorsal horn which become hypersensitive. Also, damaged nerves may grow new alternative synapses with neighbouring neurones ('crosstalk'). In effect, wires get crossed and signals go astray. Sensory stimuli such as touching, brushing or stroking can find their way down alternative pathways and end up generating pain sensations to the brain.

Perception

The perception of pain is where the neurological activity becomes a conscious experience. The pain signals from the A-delta and C fibres are relayed via the brainstem and the thalamus to areas of the cortex, especially the somatosensory area, as well as the limbic system which is associated with memory and emotion. The cortex can identify the area from which the message is sent, which will result in actions such as looking at the area that is injured. The area within the brainstem known as the reticular formation is responsible for the autonomic response. This includes the withdrawal reflex, for example the reflex removal of the hand from a hot surface, and the general autonomic response resulting in an increase in heart rate and blood pressure, changes in local blood flow, piloerection and sweating.

Modulation

Modulation refers to changing or inhibiting the transmission of pain signals. This may occur through descending pain pathways. As nociceptive afferents enter the spinal cord they form synapses with other nerve endings. Some of these nerve endings are from the neurones whose cell bodies are in the brain and whose axons form a descending pathway. These

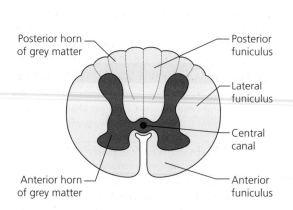

Posterior horn of grey matter — Posterior funiculus — Lateral funiculus — Central canal — Anterior horn of grey matter — Anterior funiculus

Figure 8.2 Simplified cross-section of the spinal cord

descending pathways function to modulate activity in the nociceptive pathway. One pathway begins in the reticular formation. From there, there is a projection to the dorsal horn of the spinal cord via the descending tract. Therefore the transmission of the pain message can synapse with the descending pathway sending a message down to the dorsal horn. This causes the release of enkephalin which is found in the interneurones. This inhibits the excitory neurotransmitters and prevents the pain message crossing through the dorsal horn.

Natural neural mechanisms exist to modulate pain transmission and perception. When we perceive pain our natural opiates – endorphins and enkephalins – are released in the brain to decrease the perception. Enkephalins function as inhibitory neurotransmitters and are found in the substantia gelatinosa – the 'spinal gate' – thereby inhibiting the transmission of pain, and in the limbic system (which explains the emotional effects of natural and synthetic opioids). Endorphins bind to various opiate receptors in the brain and appear to function as endogenously produced analgesia, but their exact role remains unknown.

This endogenous pain modulation partly explains variations in the perception of pain as individuals produce different amounts of inhibitory neurotransmitters.

The gate control theory of pain

In 1965, Melzack and Wall proposed their gate control theory. There have been other theories – for example the specificity theory and the pattern theory – but the gate control theory is the most established.

The gate control theory focuses on specific nerve cells, termed substantia gelatinosa, which are found in the dorsal horn. It is here that the passage of impulses from A-delta and C fibres are regulated (gate cells are nerve cells of the substantia gelatinosa). Gate control focuses on the concept that if impulses along the slow C fibres or the A-delta fibres outnumber impulses from fast A-beta (touch) fibres, the gate opens and pain impulses are transmitted and perceived. Stimulation of more A-beta touch fibres, until they outnumber the C fibre or the A-delta fibre impulses, will close the gate, inhibiting the transmission and therefore perception of pain. This is referred to as the 'counter-irritant theory'.

This theory helps to explain why a massage, or rubbing a painful area, can lesson the intensity of pain.

Referred pain

A feature of visceral pain is that it is often perceived as coming from a site that is different from its true point of origin. Referred pain occurs because the area to which the pain is referred and the visceral organ involved receive their innervation from the same segment of the spinal cord (they share a *dermatone*). For example, afferent fibres from the heart, the skin over the heart and the left upper extremity enter spinal cord segments T1 to T4, so pain is typically felt in the skin over the heart and along the left arm.

Factors influencing the assessment of pain

Everyone perceives pain at the same stimulus intensity that is at the same threshold. For example, heat is perceived as painful at 44–46°C, because that is when tissue damage begins. However, *pain tolerance* varies widely and is influenced greatly by cultural and psychological factors. Note that the term 'pain threshold' is sometimes used inappropriately when the term 'pain tolerance' should be used.

Pain has two components: the original sensation or perception and the reaction to the sensation. The reaction to the sensation is called *pain behaviour* and includes facial expressions, mood change, engaging in particular activity such as rubbing the injury or restlessness, and the use of language to express the sensation of pain. The assessment of pain takes into account both the sensation and the reaction.

The assessment of pain must take into account the wide range of factors that will influence the perception, interpretation and expression of pain by the individual. A recent review of the evidence for acute pain (Macintyre 2010) has pointed to such factors as:

- preoperative anxiety predicting postoperative pain;
- a tendency towards anxiety (trait anxiety) being associated with increased pain perception;
- the meaning of the pain (such as the threat that is posed by the cause of the pain) influencing its perception;

- previous pain experiences influencing perception through expectations of both the intensity of the pain and of the response of health professionals;
- cultural factors, such as norms of pain behaviour which may vary significantly between different groups.

An individual's coping response is associated with pain behaviour, and a number of studies have reported pain catastrophizing, or catastrophic thinking, being influential in the pain behaviour (Vancleef and Peters 2006).

There are barriers within the health profession that may interfere with effective pain assessment and its management. These have been reported as problems of inadequate knowledge, attitudes and beliefs about pain (Hall-Lord and Larsson 2006). Perhaps the most important is the suggestion that a health professional, particularly a nurse, may distrust a patient's self-reporting of pain and have preconceived ideas of, for example, how much pain the patient should be experiencing for a particular trigger (Watt-Watson *et al.* 2001). Such barriers make it essential that an *objective* assessment be made, with the patient providing the information for the assessment. In other words, the patient should assess his or her own pain and the health professional should record this assessment.

Practical pain assessment

Pain should be assessed during deep breathing, during coughing and during other movements, not just at rest. Regular patient assessments of their pain and nausea, combined with nursing assessments of respiratory rate, level of sedation, heart rate and blood pressure, should be taken in acute pain, using standard observation charts.

History and observation

Assessment begins with identifying the cause of the pain. In some instances this will be obvious, as with postoperative wound pain or pain associated with traumatic injury such as a fracture. In other cases, even in severe acute pain, the cause can be difficult to identify. For example, chest pain which could be associated with anything from a heart attack to indigestion to an aortic aneurysm. In such cases a

good history must be taken which considers a range of clinical features. Having a guide to help remember the key aspects is useful, and a commonly used mnemonic for taking a pain history is SOCRATES (Box 8.1).

There are also non-verbal accompaniments to pain. Examples are immobilization of the part of the body involved, purposeless movements, protective movements, rubbing and rhythmic movements, facial expressions (clenched teeth, wrinkled forehead, biting of lower lip) and behavioural changes.

There are usually physiological changes. Pain usually activates the sympathetic nervous system, so that adrenalin is released which increases the pulse, respiration rate and blood pressure; perspiration,

---

Box 8.1 Taking a history in acute pain

SOCRATES

- *Site*. Can the patient point to where the pain is? If in more than one place, where is it most severe? Remember that pain may be referred.
- *Onset*. How did the pain start? Was it a sudden onset or gradual? What was the patient doing when the pain started – for example, asleep, running, eating?
- *Character*. What words can be used to describe the pain – for example, sharp, throbbing, aching, burning? Somatic pain is often described as sharp or stinging and is generally well localized. Visceral pain is often dull, may be described as colic, and have local tenderness.
- *Radiation*. Does the pain radiate anywhere? Examples are chest pain radiating to the arm in myocardial ischaemia, and abdominal pain radiating to the shoulder tip.
- *Associations*. Any other signs or symptoms associated with the pain – for example, nausea or vomiting, diarrhoea, blurred vision!
- *Time course*. Does the pain follow any pattern? Is it worse at a particular time of day?
- *Exacerbating or relieving factors*. Does anything change the pain? Is it changed by position, for example sitting forward or lying back? Is it worse or better after eating?
- *Severity*. How bad is the pain, for example by using a numerical rating scale?

pallor, dilated pupils, nausea, and muscle tension are other signs. However, it should also be recognized that some visceral pain of severe intensity can stimulate a response in the parasympathetic system which can lower the pulse and blood pressure; for example pain in the distal colon, bladder and rectum.

Tools for pain assessment

Tools are used to minimize bias, increase an awareness of the nature of the pain being experienced by the patient, and assess the effectiveness of pain-relieving interventions. The oft-used quote 'pain cannot be said to have been relieved unless pain or pain relief has been directly measured' (Huskisson 1974) makes the point nicely. Using a scoring tool with the patient may also give the patient some sense of control and involvement with the assessment process.

The available tools include uni-dimensional scales such as simple descriptive rating scales, graphic rating scales, numerical rating scales, pain thermometers, visual analogue scales, and faces rating scales; examples of these are shown in Fig. 8.3. The value of a simple uni-dimensional scale is that it is quick and simple to use, which makes it useful in the acute setting. The choice of tool will often be decided locally and it is probably sensible that whatever tool is used is

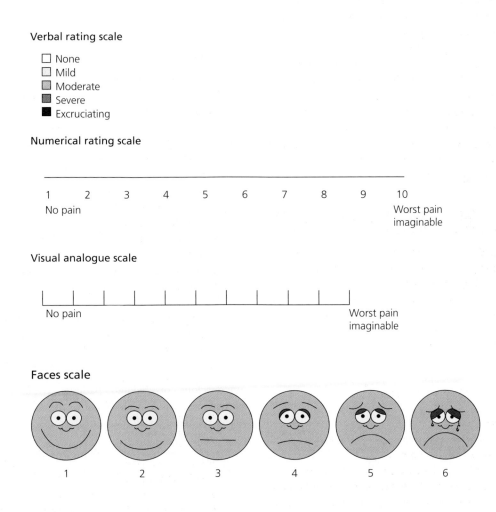

Figure 8.3 Pain assessment tools

consistently used within that particular area so that continuity and experience can develop. There may be specific circumstances that dictate which of these scales can be used; for example it may not be appropriate to use a visual analogue scale with a visually impaired patient.

The FAS (functional activity scale) score assesses whether the patient can perform a particular activity given his or her current level of pain and pain control (Scott and McDonald 2008). For example, in postoperative situations it may be important for the patient to be able to take a deep breath or to cough, or to be able to begin to mobilize. The patient is asked to perform the activity – cough, try to sit forward – and the assessment is made (Fig. 8.4). The FAS score will assist in determining whether further pain relief may be needed to allow the activity to be performed.

Some tools have been developed that are multidimensional and use a combination approach, with the McGill pain questionnaire the most commonly cited of these. Tools such as the McGill questionnaire are designed to include both qualitative and quantitative data and are particularly useful in the assessment and management of chronic pain.

There are limitations in assessment tools. Simple pain scales focus exclusively on the intensity of the pain and fail to take account of its context (Brown 2009), whereas multidimensional tools may be time-consuming. The full McGill questionnaire may take up to 30 minutes to administer and require good verbal skills and a degree of concentration by the patient. A short-form version of the McGill questionnaire, the SF-MPQ (Fig. 8.5), is quicker and easier to use and may be appropriate in the acute setting where pain control is proving difficult or pain is chronic or ongoing.

Pain relief tools can be used in conjunction with pain assessment tools. The simplest approach is to use a similar approach to that used with the pain intensity scales in Fig. 8. 3. For example, if the visual analogue scale is used to rate the pain then similarly a visual scale can be used, from 'No pain relief' to 'Complete pain relief'. If a verbal rating scale is used then, again, a similar approach can be used, so that pain relief is 'Complete', 'Good', 'Moderate', 'Slight' or 'None'.

Regular assessments

The purpose of pain assessment is to aid understanding of the underlying cause of the pain, to provide information on which to base pain relief interventions, and to allow for evaluation of the effectiveness of interventions. Whatever assessment strategy or tool is used, the approach to assessment is based on a shared philosophy of compassion and belief in the patient's experience (Roach 2002; Moskow 1987). Pain assessment should be carried out with appropriate frequency and must always be repeated following a pain-relieving intervention. There is good evidence that regular pain assessment leads to better acute pain management (Macintyre et al. 2010).

Pain assessment in the 'non-verbal' patient

In the acute setting there will be situations where self-reporting of pain is not possible, examples being cognitive impairment such as dementia, and the unconscious or sedated patient. These patients provide a significant challenge to the health professional in the provision of effective assessment and management of pain.

Approaches to assessment in these groups has been the subject of specific clinical guidelines (Herr et al. 2006) which suggest that, in all situations, assessment should be based on a 'hierarchy of assessment techniques' (McCaffery and Pasero 1999) which includes the following.

A — no limitation: the patient is able to undertake the activity without limitation due to pain

B — mild limitation: the patient is able to undertake the activity but experiences moderate to severe pain

C — significant limitation: the patient is unable to complete the activity due to pain, or pain treatment-related side effects

Figure 8.4 FAS: functional activity score

Self-report

Always attempt to gain a self-report of pain from the patient. This may be simply a 'yes' or 'no' response, or even a non-verbal response such as blinking or squeezing a hand.

Look for potential causes of pain

If there is evidence of painful injury or other painful pathology it should be assumed that pain is present. Similarly when carrying out painful procedures, for example venepuncture or wound care, assume that it will produce pain and treat accordingly.

SHORT-FORM McGILL PAIN QUESTIONNAIRE

	NONE (0)	MILD (1)	MODERATE (2)	SEVERE (3)
THROBBING	_____	_____	_____	_____
SHOOTING	_____	_____	_____	_____
STABBING	_____	_____	_____	_____
SHARP	_____	_____	_____	_____
CRAMPING	_____	_____	_____	_____
GNAWING	_____	_____	_____	_____
HOT–BURNING	_____	_____	_____	_____
ACHING	_____	_____	_____	_____
HEAVY	_____	_____	_____	_____
TENDER	_____	_____	_____	_____
SPLITTING	_____	_____	_____	_____
TIRING–EXHAUSTING	_____	_____	_____	_____
SICKENING	_____	_____	_____	_____
FEARFUL	_____	_____	_____	_____
PUNISHING–CRUEL	_____	_____	_____	_____

NO PAIN |——————————————————————————————| WORST POSSIBLE PAIN

PPI

0 NO PAIN	_____
1 MILD	_____
2 DISCOMFORTING	_____
3 DISTRESSING	_____
4 HORRIBLE	_____
5 EXCRUCIATING	_____

Figure 8.5 Short form of the McGill pain questionnaire (SF-MPQ). Reproduced from Melzack 1987, with permission. Descriptors 1–11 represent the sensory dimension of pain experience and 12–15 represent the affective dimension. The present pain intensity (PPI) of the standard long form and the visual analogue are included to provide overall intensity scores.

Observe patient behaviours

Where self-report is not possible pain may be assessed by observing behaviours that may indicate pain. Such behaviours may include groaning, facial expressions such as wincing or frowning, movements such as rigidity or restlessness. While such behaviours are not completely reliable they are still an appropriate part of pain assessment.

A number of tools have been developed for assessing patient behaviours. For example, in advanced dementia there is the PAINAD scale (Warden 2003), and for critically ill sedated patients there is the BPS (Payen *et al.* 2001). PAINAD uses indicators such as breathing, vocalizations, facial expressions and consolability; the BPS uses facial expressions, upper limb movements and compliance with ventilation.

Surrogate reporting of pain and behaviour changes

Relatives and carers can be a valuable source of information. Subtle changes in behaviour may be identified by those who know the patient best. Relatives and usual care givers should be encouraged where possible to be involved in pain assessment and in assessing the effectiveness of pain relief.

Analgesic trial

When pain is suspected but there is uncertainty, an analgesic trial may be appropriate. Analgesia is given, the type and amount based on the pathology and the perceived intensity, and the patient is reassessed using the above methods.

Pain assessment in older people

Assessing pain in older people is challenging for a number of reasons. However, given the increasing age of the acute hospital population, and evidence that pain is under-recognized and under-treated in older people (Ferrell 1995; Helme and Gibson 2001), it is essential that health professionals working in acute care make every effort to ensure that pain management in this group is given particular attention.

Explanations for this relatively poor pain management begin with difficulties in assessment. Older people may be more reluctant than younger people to report pain (Yong 2001); may be less confident that their pain may be relieved (Yates *et al.* 1995); are more likely to have complicating co-morbidities;

and are more likely to have cognitive and communication difficulties. In the acute setting where the patient may have a serious or life-threatening injury or pathology (e.g. hip fracture or acute coronary syndrome), this creates a significant challenge to both diagnosis of the underlying problem and pain management.

Specific guidelines have been published by the British Pain Society and the British Geriatrics Society which give practical guidance and an assessment algorithm (BPS/BGS 2007). The guidelines largely follow the principles of assessment suggested for the 'non-verbal' patient set out above and focus on the importance of not relying on self-reporting, using observations of facial expressions and behaviour, and including pain assessment as a routine part of general patient assessment. The use of simple tools such as those described above is recommended along with pain maps where the patient is asked to point to the part of the body that has pain.

When considering the use of systemic medications for pain relief (see later) there are a number of complicating factors that should be taken into account in the older person. These include (Banicek 2010):

- greater sensitivity to NSAIDs;
- altered distribution and drug half-life due to changes in body composition;
- reduced first-pass metabolism which for some agents may indicate that a lower dose should be used;
- reduction in renal function with age which will influence clearance of some drugs;
- the greater risk of interactions given the higher likelihood of polypharmacy in the older person.

CASE STUDY 8.1

Mrs Brown is an 82-year-old woman who has been brought into the emergency department following a fall. A wrist fracture is suspected and she is awaiting X-ray examination.

- What approach should be taken to Mrs Brown with regard to pain assessment?

CASE STUDY 8.2

Mr Peters is a 68-year-old man who had abdominal surgery one day ago. He is to be seen today on the ward by the physiotherapist.

- What consideration should be made with regard to management of his pain today?

Pain relief

Pain relief strategies should be in place and should be able to respond effectively to both predictable pain, such as postoperative pain, and unexpected pain such as the patient with a traumatic injury or undifferentiated medical diagnosis. It is also important to plan for interventions that are known to be painful. The six most common procedures producing pain in acute patients are (Puntillo *et al.* 2001):

- turning;
- wound drain removal;
- tracheal suctioning;
- femoral catheter removal;
- placement of central lines;
- changing of wound dressings.

While there are a number of pain relief methods, the mainstay of acute pain control is systemic analgesia administration. The World Health Organization (WHO) summarizes the principles of pain management with systemic analgesia as follows.

- Use the oral or another non-invasive route of administration whenever possible.
- Individualize analgesia.
- Other than for patients presenting with very severe or excruciating pain, the sequence of analgesic therapy should follow the 'analgesic ladder'. When the combination of non-narcotic and weak narcotic analgesics no longer controls the pain, the patient should be started on potent narcotic analgesics.
- Dose by the clock. Less analgesia is required to prevent the recurrence of pain than to treat it after it recurs.
- Use adjuvants.

The 'analgesic ladder' referred to in the above principles was developed by the WHO in 1990 primarily for treating cancer pain. For acute pain management, the World Federation of Societies of Anaesthesiologists analgesic ladder was developed, in particular for postoperative pain.

The ladder represents a stepwise approach to pain management, starting at the lowest step with mild analgesia and escalating the strength if not effective. In the acute setting, however, postoperative pain, trauma pain or medical pain from heart attack, where pain may be expected to be severe, may need controlling with strong intravenous or intramuscular analgesics at the top of the ladder. As the pain comes under control then the next rung comes into play and finally the lowest rung.

It is beyond the scope of this chapter to review the full range of analgesic medication that could be used. Rather the main groups will be described and examples given. For a full discussion of effects, indications, adverse effects and drug interactions you should refer to the latest edition of *British National Formulary*. Analgesics are generally classified as opioid or non-opioid.

Non-opioid analgesics

This group is effective for mild to moderate pain. It includes paracetemol and the non-steroidal anti-inflammatory drugs (NSAIDs) such as diclofenac and ibuprofen, and the COX-2 inhibitors such as celcoxib. While the NSAIDs are the best of the oral analgesic drugs, paracetamol alone or with another drug such as codeine is also effective (McQuay *et al.* 1997). Adding paracetamol to an opioid can reduce the amount of opioid needed, which increases safety. The mechanism of action of paracetamol in pain relief is unclear but it has an advantage over the NSAIDs in that there are fewer adverse effects at appropriate doses.

NSAIDs work by interfering with prostaglandin production (prostaglandins promote inflammation and are key substances in pain transduction). Adverse effects of NSAIDs include gastrointestinal bleeding, water retention and platelet dysfunction. These effects should be considered when administering NSAIDs in the acute setting where the patient may be presenting with acute heart failure or gastrointestinal symptoms.

Opioid analgesics

Opioid (narcotic) analgesics include both opium derivatives such as morphine and synthetic agents that mimic the action of natural narcotics, such as pethidine. Opioids work by mimicking the effect of natural endorphins. Opioids can be further divided into weak and strong types.

Weak opioids

Codeine and tramadol are weak opioid agents and are used alone or in combination with non-narcotics such as paracetamol to treat mild or moderate pain.

Strong opioids

Examples include morphine, diamorphine, pethidine and fentanyl. Most opioids can cause respiratory depression, sedation, pruritis, nausea and vomiting, and constipation. Pethidine is a synthetic opioid but shorter acting. Strong opioids are the first-line treatment for severe pain. Fears among health professionals of respiratory depression are usually unfounded unless the drugs are used inappropriately (Pasero and McCaffery 1994), but it is important to monitor patients carefully following administration of strong opioid analgesia and it may be necessary to use a sedation scoring tool. The key is to titrate the dose against pain relief while avoiding the unwanted side-effects of compromised respiration.

If the patient is still in pain following initial administration it is usually safe to give a second smaller dose. The time between the first and second dose depends on the route of administration: 5 minutes after intravenous, 60 minutes after subcutaneous or intramuscular, 90 minutes after oral morphine. If this is still ineffective then the route of administration could be changed, for example from intramuscular to intravenous.

It should be noted that slow- or delayed-release analgesia is inappropriate in acute pain as it makes rapid titration difficult or even dangerous and unpredictable; this is particularly so in the case of strong opioid analgesia (Macintyre et al. 2010). Similarly, compound preparations are probably less appropriate than single-drug preparations as there is more control over the latter.

It has been suggested that health professionals,

particularly nurses, sometimes under-administer opioid analgesia because of fears of addiction. Such fears are without merit; addiction resulting from opioids being administered for pain relief is extremely rare (Porter and Hicks 1980).

Patient-controlled analgesia (PCA)

PCA is now a common method of administration. The patient chooses when to have analgesia, which therefore leads to patient control and empowerment. The aim with PCA is to keep plasma levels of opioid steady and avoid peaks and troughs. The patient needs to be physically and mentally able and patient education is vital. PCA is most commonly used in postoperative pain management where patients can be prepared for it preoperatively. Some equipment allows the use of a background infusion that can be 'topped up' by the patient.

Adjuvant drugs

Adjuvant drugs are drugs that have a primary indication other than pain relief but which can be used in combination with analgesics in particular circumstances.

- *Steroids.* Corticosteroids such as prednisolone enhance or produce analgesia by preventing the release of prostaglandins and commonly stimulate appetite and elevate mood. This anti-inflammatory action may relieve pressure on compressed structures and therefore can be effective for pain caused by compression of nerves, spinal cord and intracranial metastases.
- *Antidepressants.* These may assist by elevating mood, increasing sedation, and may potentiate narcotics. Some agents will stimulate descending pathways in the spinal cord to release endogenous opiates.
- *Anxiolytics.* Anti-anxiety drugs such as diazepam may be indicated in the management of acute anxiety associated with pain. Diazepam also acts as a muscle relaxant.
- *Local anaesthetics.* These can be administered by wound infiltration, nerve or nerve plexus blocks, and epidural infiltration.

Route of administration

By mouth

This is the most acceptable route and should be the route of choice if available. However, the nature of the drug may prevent the oral route, and in certain situations (e.g. in the immediate postoperative phase) it may be contraindicated due to reduced gut motility.

Per rectum

Paracetamol and NSAIDs can be administered like this, but the route is clearly less acceptable to patients.

Intravenously

The intravenous (IV) route clearly has important advantages in severe acute pain and when the oral route is unavailable. It is fast-acting, easy to titrate, but may require very careful observation if administering narcotic analgesia.

Intramuscularly

The intramuscular (IM) route is usually used for as-required medication where the oral route is unavailable or inappropriate. The pharmokinetics are less predictable with the intramuscular route.

Epidural

This involves the injection of drugs into an epidural space. Usually a mixture of opioids (diamorphine and fentanyl which diffuse into the dura into the cerebrospinal fluid) and local anaesthetic (bupivacaine) is used in a continuous infusion. Careful monitoring of the patient is important as serious complications, while not common, may still occur. Usual observations are 2-hourly for the first 24 hours and thereafter 4-hourly and should include 4-hourly measurement of motor or sensory function. Problems to be observed include displacement of the catheter, hypotension as a result of sympathetic blockade, migration of the epidural catheter, epidural haematoma, epidural abscess, headache, and local anaesthetic toxicity.

Summary of acute pain management

Guidelines for managing acute pain are based on understanding the principles discussed so far. It is essential to select the most appropriate drug and determine its optimal dose and route of administration for each patient on the basis of:

- the intensity and duration of the pain;
- the physical and mental state of the patient;
- the pharmacology and side-effects of the drug;
- the optimal route.

A stepped approach to analgesia should be used, combining analgesics where appropriate. If the pain is not severe, paracetamol should be used first with other analgesics added to paracetamol in a stepped fashion according to the severity of the pain and patient response. Combining analgesics from different groups can have an additive affect. For example, adding paracetamol to diclofenac for moderate pain or adding paracetamol and diclofenac to morphine for severe pain which may reduce the amount of morphine needed and is therefore safer.

Where pain can be predicted, analgesia should be used early, either before pain begins as in postoperative situations, or to prevent mild pain becoming moderate or severe.

In severe pain or where pain is expected to be severe (e.g. postoperatively), the ladder is *descending* – starting with a strong opioid, via either bolus injections or continuous infusion via PCA or epidural infusion. This may be with or without local or regional analgesia. The next step down is a weak opioid, with or without NSAIDs, this followed on the next step by non-opioid analgesia.

Pain services

It is beyond the scope of this chapter to discuss the organization of pain services, but it is worth highlighting the growth in pain management as a specialty over the past two decades. Rigorous evaluation of the impact of pain services is made difficult because there is no clear consensus on the structure and organization of such services, but a recent review of the evidence suggests the following possible outcomes from acute pain teams: better pain relief, fewer adverse reactions, and lower postoperative morbidity and mortality (Macintyre *et al.* 2010). Recommendations are that specialist multidisciplinary pain teams should be in place at all acute hospitals to provide specialist advice, education, support and practice, and that more effective acute pain management may result from these organizational interventions than from the analgesic interventions.

Conclusion

Pain management is an essential part of acute care. Poor pain management is associated with adverse outcomes including lengthened stay in hospital. Pain assessment is at the heart of good pain management and should be seen as important as the pulse rate or blood pressure and treated as the 'fifth vital sign'. Pain relief should be approached using a stepped process following well-established guidelines but always tailored to the individual, recognizing that no two people experience pain in the same way or respond the same to pain relief.

References

Banicek J (2010). How to ensure acute pain in older people is appropriately assessed and managed, *Nursing Times* **106**(29); 14–17.

British Pain Society and British Geriatrics Society (BPS/BGS, 2007). *The Assessment of Pain in Older People*. London: BPS.

Brown D (2009) Principles of acute pain assessment. In Cox F (ed.) *Perioperative Pain Management*. Oxford: Wiley–Blackwell.

Chapman CR, Tuckett RP, Song CW (2008). Pain and stress in a systems perspective: reciprocal neural, endocrine, and immune interactions, *Journal of Pain* **9**(2); 122–45.

Dolin SJ, Cashman JN, Bland JM (2002). Effectiveness of acute postoperative pain management: evidence from published data, *British Journal of Anaesthesia* **89**; 409–23.

Ferrell BA (1995). Pain evaluation and management in the nursing home, *Annals of Internal Medicine* **123**; 681–7.

Garrett E, Boyd J (2008). *Key Findings Report for the 2007 Inpatient Survey* (Co-ordination centre for the NHS hospital patient survey programme). Oxford: Picker Institute Europe.

Hall-Lord ML, Larsson BW (2006). Registered nurses' and student nurses' assessment of pain and distress related to specific patient and nurse characteristics, *Nurse Education Today* **26**; 377–87.

Helme RD, Gibson SJ (2001). The epidemiology of pain in elderly people, *Clinics in Geriatric Medicine* **17**; 417–31.

Herr K, Coyne J, Key T *et al.* (2006). Pain assessment in the nonverbal patient: position statement with clinical practice recommendations, *Pain Management Nursing* **7**(2); 44–52.

Huskisson EC (1974). Measurement of pain, *Lancet* **2**; 1127–31.

Macintyre PE, Ready LB (2002) *Acute Pain Management: A Practical Guide*, 2nd edn. London: WB Saunders.

Macintyre PE, Schug SA, Scott DA *et al.* (APM SE Working Group of the Australian and New Zealand College of Anaesthetists and Faculty of Pain Medicine, 2010). *Acute Pain Management: Scientific Evidence*, 3rd edn). Melbourne: ANZCA and FPM.

McCaffery M (1968). Nursing Practice Theories related to cognition, bodily pain, and man-environment interactions. Los Angeles: VCLA Students Store.

McCaffery M, Pasero C (1999). Assessment: underlying complexities, misconceptions, and practical tools. In McCaffery C, Pasero C (eds) *Pain: A Clinical Manual*, 2nd edn. St Louis: Mosby.

McQuay HL, Moore A, Justins D (1997).Treating acute pain in hospital, *British Medical Journal* **314**: 1531–35.

Melzack R (1987). The short-form McGill Pain Questionnaire. *Pain* **30**(2); 191–7

Melzack R, Wall P (1965). Pain mechanisms: a new theory, *Science* **150**; 971–9.

Merskey H, Bogduk N (1994). *Classification of Chronic Pain* (IASP Task Force on Taxonomy). Seattle: IASP Press.

Moskow SB (1987). *Human Hand and Other Ailments*. Boston: Little Brown.

NCEPOD (2010). *An Age Old Problem: A Review of the Care Received by Elderly Patients Undergoing Surgery* (report by the National Confidential Enquiry into Patient Outcome and Death). NCEPOD.

Pasero C, McCaffery M (1994). Preventing and managing opioid induced respiratory depression, *American Journal of Nursing* **94**(4); 25–31.

Payen J, Bru O, Bosson J *et al.* (2001). Assessing pain in critically ill sedated patients by using a behavioural pain scale, *Critical Care Medicine* **29**; 2258–63.

Porter J, Hicks J (1980). Addiction rate in patients treated with narcotics, *New England Journal of Medicine* **302**; 123.

Puntillo KA, White C, Morris AB *et al.* (2001). Patients' perceptions and responses to procedural pain: results from Thunder Project II, *American Journal of Critical Care* **10**(4); 238–51.

RCoA and The Pain Society (2003). *Pain Management Services: Good Practice.* Available at www.rcoa.ac.uk/docs/painservices.pdf.

Roach SM (2002). *Caring, the Human Mode of Being: A Blueprint for the Health Professions*, 2nd edn. Ottawa: Canadian Hospital Association Press.

Scott DA, McDonald WM (2008) Assessment, measurement and history. In: Macintyre PE, Rowbotham D, Walker S (eds) *Clinical Pain Management: Acute Pain*, 2nd edn. London: Hodder Arnold.

Strohbuecker B, Mayer H, Evers G, Sabatowski R (2005). Pain prevalence in hospitalized patients in a German university teaching hospital, *Journal of Pain and Symptom Management* **29**; 498–506.

Todd KH, Ducharme J, Choiniere M *et al.* (2007). Pain in the emergency department: results of the pain and emergency medicine initiative (PEMI) multicenter study. *Journal of Pain* **8**; 460–6.

Vancleef LM, Peters ML (2006). Pain catastrophizing, but not injury/illness sensitivity or anxiety sensitivity, enhances attentional interference by pain, *Journal of Pain* **7**(1); 23–30.

Watt-Watson JB, Stevens B, Garfinkel P, Streiner D, Gallop R (2001). Relationship between nurses' knowledge and pain management outcomes for their postoperative cardiac patients, *Journal of Advanced Nursing* **36**: 535–45.

Warden V, Hurley A, Volicer L (2003). Development and psychometric evaluation of the pain assessment in advanced dementia (PAINAD) scale, *American Medical Directors Association* **4**; 9–15.

World Health Organization (1990). *Cancer Pain Relief and Palliative Care.* Geneva: WHO.

Yates P, Dewar A, Fentiman B (1995). Pain: the views of elderly people living in long-term residential care settings, *Journal of Advanced Nursing* **21**; 667–74.

Yong H-H, Gibson SJ, de L Horne DJ, Helme RD (2001). Development of a pain attitudes questionnaire to assess stoicism and cautiousness for possible age differences, *Journal of Gerontology* **56B**; P279–84.

CHAPTER 9

THE PATIENT AND FAMILY: SUPPORT AND DECISION-MAKING

Nicola Morton and Sue Snelson

LEARNING OUTCOMES

On completion of this chapter the reader will:

1 have an increased understanding of the ethical issues that arise when caring for seriously ill patients

2 have gained an insight into some of the psychological issues that can affect patients with a serious illness

3 recognize the importance of the healthcare professional's role in issues relating to consent and confidentiality

4 appreciate the importance of involving the patient and the family in ethical decision-making

5 have an awareness of the ethical dilemmas that can arise during end-of-life care.

Introduction

This chapter will explore some of the ethical dilemmas that healthcare professionals who care for seriously ill patients may have to face. Concepts of consent and confidentiality will be addressed. We will explore the psychological assessment and support needed by seriously ill patients and their families. Perhaps the most difficult topic for health professionals is end-of-life care. This will be addressed with discussion surrounding euthanasia, advanced directives, do-not-resuscitate (DNR) orders, withdrawal of treatment and family-witnessed resuscitation. Case studies will be used to illustrate specific issues and to promote reflective clinical practice.

Ethical practice

'Ethics' is a general term used to describe ways of examining and understanding moral life (Beauchamp and Childress 2009). Initially it is important to understand ethical terms, principles and theories. This chapter will endeavour to explore how the healthcare professional can both fulfil moral obligations and uphold the professional obligation of duty of care. Many healthcare workers use models to aid clinical decision-making, and this can be a useful approach to the ethical decision-making process too. Perhaps the most widely known model is that produced by Beauchamp and Childress (1989), who provide a framework that is simple to remember when in the stressful environment of caring for seriously ill patients (Box 9.1).

The model has four principles. These have been criticized on the basis of their ritualistic approach and lack of definitive courses of action, but they are useful starting points for any discussion. As with all tools to aid decision-making, they should evolve and be open to revision where necessary.

Healthcare workers are bound by a professional code to act in the best interests of their patients, but it

Box 9.1 The Beauchamp and Childress (1989) framework

- **Beneficence** – the obligation to act for the benefit of others
- **Non-maleficence** – the obligation not to inflict harm on others
- **Respect for autonomy** – the obligation to respect the decision-making ability of autonomous individuals
- **Justice** – obligations of fairness in the distribution of benefits and risks

is not always easy to determine the best way to achieve this. Moral decision-making can be extremely difficult. This can be complicated further when the potential intervention initially causes harm to the patient despite the final outcome being positive. This is called the principle of 'double effect'.

This may be regarded as 'the end justifies the means' ethics and considers the addition of consequences to actions. An example of this theory is 'consequentialism' which considers that the value of an action is solely derived from its consequences, the concept of 'the greatest good for the greatest number'. Similarly, 'utilitarianism' considers that the action achieves 'the most happiness for the most people', a doctrine appearing in the work of John Stuart Mill (1806–1873) who based his work on that of Jeremy Bentham (1748–1832).

In contrast, the concept of 'natural law' ethics appeals to the belief that the correct course of action is always self-evident. Deontology is based on the work of Emmanuel Kant (1724–1804) and suggests that one's own concept of duty promotes equality, so the action is always intrinsically good. While consequentialism and utilitarianism aim to provide a good ending, deontology seeks to follow self-evident paths where the object of the intervention is an end in itself. This may seem complicated, but ask yourself the question 'Who benefits?' With the first two theories it is necessary that people other than the patient benefit from the intervention too, while with deontology others may benefit but not necessarily.

The NMC Code of Professional Conduct places expectations upon nurses to serve the best interests of the patient and society while upholding trust and confidence. However, certain interventions that benefit a specific patient may not benefit society at large, thereby causing potential conflict. Nevertheless, the general tone of the Code suggests that the needs of the individual patient are paramount. Whatever decisions are made relating to the care of a patient, particularly those that have a high moral investment, there must be clear demonstration and clarity as to why and how those decisions were reached. In this chapter we will explore ways in which this moral reasoning can bring about good and enhance patient care.

Consent

Healthcare professionals have a responsibility to participate in discussions relating to the patient's ability to consent. There are three overriding responsibilities:

- to make the care of people our primary concern and ensure consent is obtained before any intervention is undertaken;
- to ensure that the obtaining of consent is rigorous and transparent and demonstrates a high level of professional accountability;
- to accurately document all discussions and decisions relating to the obtaining of consent.

If a patient is touched without consent, or other lawful justification, then the person has the right of action in a civil court to sue for trespass to the person – battery (where the person is actually touched) or assault (where he fears he may be). To be valid, consent must be given voluntarily by a mentally competent adult without any duress or fraud.

Every adult must be presumed to have the mental capacity to consent or to refuse treatment unless he or she is:

- unable to take in or retain information provided about the treatment;
- unable to understand the information provided;
- unable to weigh up the information as part of the decision-making process.

Another individual cannot consent for an adult who has the competence to give consent personally. However, you may find yourself in an emergency situation where the patient is temporarily unable to consent. The patient may be unconscious and may need to receive treatment to preserve life. The law allows care to be delivered in these situations, without the patient's consent, provided it is in the person's best interests.

Jean is making a decision that could put her life at risk. Legally, a competent adult can refuse treatment even if that decision may result in death. Although Jean's condition is life-threatening she is competent to give consent. What should be done? The NMC Code of Professional Conduct states that nurses should always act in the best interests of a patient, so it is essential to determine what those are for Jean. Using the principles of Beauchamp and Childress discussed earlier may help in the decision-making process. Think back to those four principles:

- beneficence
- non-maleficence
- respect for autonomy
- justice.

ACTIVITY ?

- What course of treatment will be of the greatest benefit to Jean?
- What would cause her the most harm?
- Does she have the knowledge and ability to make these decisions?

Respect for *autonomy* focuses on the right of the individual to take control over his or her own life. It could be argued that Jean's overwhelming fear is reducing her ability to make a sensible decision. So what is the role of the nurse in this situation?

Consent must be obtained with *effective communication*. When a person is told about possible treatment and care it is important that the information be given in a sensitive and understandable way.

The patient should have time to ask questions. The nurse should try to address Jean's fears by discussing with her the advantages and disadvantages of surgery.

If we look at the principle of *beneficence*, the team needs to act in such a way that promotes the most good for Jean. Would Jean's best interests be served by not having surgery? It may be possible that allaying the fears that Jean has through effective communication and the delivery of information we can allow her to make a decision which will have a positive outcome for her. However, if Jean continues to refuse surgery and her condition deteriorates as a result of not accepting surgery, the healthcare professionals could be seen to be negligent in their duty of care towards her. So, clear documentation is essential, outlining that the risks and benefits have been fully explained to Jean in a manner she could understand. It would be sensible to ensure that another healthcare professional is present when these issues are discussed and all conversations and reason for actions taken documented fully.

ACTIVITY ?

- What information do you think should be given to Jean to enable her to make an informed decision?
- Who do you think should give this information, and why?
- What is the role of the nurse in this process?

It is essential that enough information be provided to Jean. This may include specific details of the surgery, postoperative recovery, and risks and benefits of the surgery. Usually the person undertaking the intervention obtains consent, in this instance the surgeon. In a situation such as this the nurse should be present to offer support and reassurance to Jean and to members of her family. It is important to establish the level of Jean's understanding of her condition and aim the discussion at this level. Ensure that the discussion takes place in an environment conducive to the situation and not inhibiting to the patient. Think about this. How would you feel in this situation? Would you be scared? How would you want to be supported? Think about the old adage, 'Treat others as you yourself would wish to be treated.'

Types of consent

Consent in writing is by far the best form of evidence available to the healthcare professional. Written consent should always be obtained if the intervention is lengthy, complex or considered to be risky. It stands as a record that a discussion has taken place and that the patient is happy to proceed with the intervention.

However, what should a nurse do if he or she feels that the patient has not been fully informed yet has signed a consent form?

CASE STUDY 9.2

Emily, aged 21, has been admitted to hospital for the removal of a benign ovarian cyst. She has never been in hospital before and is very anxious about the surgery. The doctor obtaining the consent explains the procedure but the staff nurse is aware that he does not mention the possibility of the removal of the ovary if the cyst is too entwined. Emily signs the consent without appearing to take in much of the discussion.

- What should the staff nurse do?

There is a legal and an ethical duty to patients. If the nurse feels that a patient does not understand information given by the doctor, then the doctor should be asked to return to the patient and discuss it further. Any additional procedures carried out other than those expressly consented to should happen only if there is a life-threatening emergency. In the case of Emily, the removal of an ovary could result in a successful action for negligence as the relevant information was not made available to her, preventing her from making an informed choice.

Verbal consent is valid but more controversial. Less risky treatments are often given with verbal consent, such as the administration of injections, venepuncture and cannulation. Many day-to-day nursing duties involve verbal consent.

Implied consent is not supported in law. There must always be evidence that a patient accepts the treatment on offer. It can be argued that if a patient holds up his sleeve thinking a nurse wishes to take his blood pressure then consent is achieved. However, if that nurse was actually going to give him an injection then an allegation of trespass may be successful. It is safer to clearly state your intention prior to any intervention at all, thus avoiding any misunderstanding.

Capacity

If all steps have been taken to assist the patient through the decision-making process but a final decision has not been reached, an assessment of capacity may be needed. The Mental Capacity Act 2005 sets out the criteria for ascertaining decision-making capacity. Section 1(2) of the legislation uses the so-called 'five-principle' approach, and Section 2 outlines what constitutes 'lack of capacity' (Box 9.2).

Box 9.2 Some principles from the Mental Capacity Act 2005

Five principles of capacity

- A person must be assumed to have capacity unless it is established that he lacks capacity.
- A person is not to be treated as unable to make a decision unless all practicable steps to help him to do so have been taken, without success.
- A person is not to be treated as unable to make a decision merely because he makes an unwise decision.
- An action done, or decision made, under this Act for or on behalf of a person who lacks capacity must be done, or made, in his best interests.
- Before the action is done, or the decision is made, regard must be given to whether the purpose for which it is needed can be as effectively achieved in a way that is less restrictive of the person's rights and freedom of action.

Incapacity

- A person lacks capacity in relation to a matter if at the material time he is unable to make a decision for himself in relation to the matter because of an impairment of, or a disturbance in, the functioning of the mind or brain.
- It does not matter whether the impairment is permanent or temporary. Examples of impairment/disturbance may be dementia or a significant learning disability.

The Act suggests that a patient is unable to make a decision if he or she is unable to:

- understand relevant information;
- retain that information;
- use or weight that information in order to make an informed decision;
- communicate his or her decision.

CASE STUDY 9.3

John has Alzheimer's disease. He has alternating periods of lucidity and confusion. The doctor wants John to consent to a colonoscopy to investigate rectal bleeding.

- Can John give informed consent?
- Can you apply the principles of the Mental Capacity Act?

For John, the healthcare workers would need to assess the position using the criteria set out by the Act. Fluctuating capacity will not mean that John is unable to make all treatment decisions himself. The Act sets out a clear test for assessing capacity, which should guide the staff dealing with this situation. The Act also offers statutory protection from liability where a person is performing an action in connection with the care or treatment of someone who lacks capacity. This means that giving medical treatment in these circumstances can be done lawfully provided there is proof that it is in the patient's best interests.

The European Court of Human Rights has said that the rights of people who cannot make decisions and who need to have their liberty removed in hospitals and care homes must be strengthened. This group of people need more care and protection than others to ensure they suffer no harm. The Deprivation of Liberty Safeguards associated with the Mental Capacity Act 2005 aim to protect such people who cannot make decisions regarding their care or treatment and who need to be cared for in a restrictive way. The law says that the Safeguards must be used if people need to have their liberty taken away in order to receive care/treatment that is in their best interests and protects them from harm.

Confidentiality

Confidentiality is a fundamental part of professional practice that protects human rights. The NMC Code of Professional Conduct states:

- you must respect people's right to confidentiality;
- you must ensure people are informed about how and why information is shared by those who will be providing their care;
- you must disclose information if you believe someone may be at risk of harm, in line with the law of the country in which you are practising.

So, what is confidentiality? When information is disclosed from one person to another it is reasonable to expect that the information will be held in confidence. This duty of confidence arises from:

- common law – the decisions of the Courts;
- statute law – which is passed by Parliament.

Concern about the way in which information was being managed by the National Health Service prompted the Caldicott Report (DH 1997). Included in the report was the need to raise awareness of confidentiality requirements, and it recommended the establishment of Caldicott Guardians throughout the NHS. A Guardian is expected to liaise with others involved with patient information, such as IT security and data protection officers. Guardians are responsible for ensuring that Trusts are upholding national guidance/policy and law regarding the protection and use of patient-identifiable information. A key recommendation of the Caldicott committee was that every use of such information should be regularly justified and tested against the six principles developed in the report (Box 9.3).

Since the appearance of the report, developments in information management have added further dimension to the Caldicott Guardian role. These include:

- the Data Protection Act 1998;
- the Freedom of Information Act 2000;
- the NHS Code on Confidentiality 2003;
- the Mental Capacity Act 2005;
- the Cayton review of NHS Information Governance 2006.

Box 9.3 Six principles arising from the Caldicott Report

- Justify the purpose(s) for using confidential information.
- Use the information only when absolutely necessary.
- Use the minimum information that is required in the circumstances.
- Access should be on a strict need-to-know basis.
- Everyone must understand his or her responsibilities in this regard.
- Understand and comply with the law.

ACTIVITY ?

In light of the six principles in Box 9.3, consider Jean's case (Case study 9.1 on page 193). Make a list of all the people you think will be involved in her care. Who do you think should have access to information relating to her care and treatment, and why?

How can we ensure that those involved in the care of Jean have access to relevant information? Disclosure means the giving of information. It is only lawful and ethical if the individual has given consent, and such consent should be freely and fully given. Consent to disclosure may be:

- explicit or implied;
- required by law;
- capable of justification by reason of public interest.

Explicit and implied consent are discussed in the previous section. Public interest describes a situation where an individual's right to confidentiality can be overruled by wider social interest, such as in cases of rape or child abuse. Even so, disclosures should be limited to relevant details only. There are six possible exceptions to maintaining confidentiality (Dimond 2005):

- if the patient gives consent to disclosure;
- if it can be demonstrated that it is in the best interests of the patient;
- if a court has ordered the release of information;
- if there is a statutory duty to release the information;
- if disclosure is in the public interest;
- if requested to do so legitimately as part of a police investigation.

How does your Code of Conduct guide you in these situations? Could you use the ethical principles discussed earlier to guide your judgement?

ACTIVITY ?

A doctor is standing at the nurses' station discussing in depth Jean's diagnosis with a medical student. The ward is very busy and, as it is visiting time, relatives are constantly approaching the station enquiring about their loved ones. Is this a breach of confidentiality?

A risk of breach of confidentiality may arise from individual behaviour or be a result of organizational systems and procedures. Nurses have a professional duty to ensure the protection of people in their care. Any failure to take action could amount to misconduct on their part. The information concerning Jean is relevant only to her and her healthcare team. It is unacceptable to discuss her diagnosis in such an open environment, and it would be appropriate to suggest that the conversation take place at a more private location. It may also be appropriate to ask Jean if she is happy for her case to be discussed with a student.

One of the most common situations regarding access to information is via the telephone. It is very common to receive an enquiry about the condition of a patient via the telephone, so record-keeping is essential to avoid inadvertent breaches of confidentiality. Many hospitals have a password system whereby designated family members can access information with the full consent of the patient. However, how should the nurse act in an emergency situation when not able to gain consent to divulge information owing to the patient's condition?

Think again about the ethical principles of beneficence and non-maleficence outlined in Box 9.1. Nurses have a professional responsibility to demonstrate that they have acted in someone's best interests when providing care in an emergency. This extends to the care given to the loved ones also, and may mean that information is given without the explicit consent of the patient but in his or her and the family's best interests. However, in some situations patients do not want information about their diagnosis, prognosis or treatment discussed with loved ones, and this must be respected.

Caring for highly dependent, seriously ill patients can be challenging with regard to confidentiality. Many disciplines may need access to medical notes, observation charts and prescription sheets, including doctors, nurses, clinical nurse specialists, pharmacists and physiotherapists. So, in order to interact with Jean in an ethical manner, the nurse must always remember to minimize harm and promote autonomy.

Psychological assessment and support

Research into health outcomes following critical illness was traditionally focused on morbidity and mortality, but in recent years there has been a move to measure quality of life as a secondary outcome in studies. Understanding the relationship between supportive behaviour and the psychological adjustment of critically ill patients and family members is important for nursing care provision. Emotional distress, anger, sense of loss, depression and anxiety are all problems reported by this group of patients. Critically ill patients have feelings of hopelessness, inability to cope and isolation from family members. Failure to recognize the psychological dimension can affect adversely the rehabilitation of critically ill patients.

Sense of coherence

Nursing researchers have used Antonovsky's model (Antonovsky 1987; Fok *et al.* 2005). 'Sense of coherence' (SOC) is the central concept of his model and is built around three components:

- comprehensibility;
- manageability;
- meaningfulness.

Sense of coherence is defined as:

A global orientation that expresses the extent to which one has pervasive, enduring and thorough dynamic feelings of confidence (1) that the stimuli deriving from one's internal and external

environments in the course of living are structured, predictable and explicable (comprehensibility); (2) the resources are available to one to meet the demands posed by these stimuli (manageability); and (3) these demands are challenges, worthy of investment and engagement (meaningfulness).

(Antonovsky 1987)

A strong SOC is required to cope successfully with the stressors of living and maintenance of health.

Antonovsky asserts that life experiences from childhood are sources of SOC and the degree of success depends on the individual's capacity, knowledge and skill in managing the stressors, which leads to strengthening of the SOC.

Coping has been identified as an important factor in explaining the differences in patients' reactions when facing episodes of critical illness. Although SOC does not refer to a specific type of coping strategy, it encompasses factors that are a basis for successful coping. Therefore it can be suggested that individuals with a strong SOC have greater ability to cope effectively and reduce tension. In others with a weaker SOC this tension can lead to stress and declining health. Strengthening a patient's SOC is an important nursing intervention to enhance the internal and external resources of seriously ill patients.

To enhance a patient's internal resources, nursing staff can encourage self-reliance and autonomy, giving hope and control and promoting an experience of wholeness. To enhance external resources we can provide understandable healthcare information, encourage open channels of communication, address the needs of the patients' support networks and utilize these support systems effectively. Nurses should support and encourage patients to take control of their lives as their condition allows. It may be something very small such as brushing the teeth. Within the dimensions of a strong SOC, seriously ill patients who are able to understand their illness and its impact on their life may show better ability to cope.

Coping with illness

Coping can be described as the process of managing difficult circumstances, expending effort to solve personal and interpersonal problems, and seeking to master, minimize, reduce or tolerate stress or conflict.

Wieten and Lloyd (2006) suggest that in coping with stressful situations we tend to use one of three main coping strategies:

- appraisal-focused;
- problem-focused;
- emotion-focused.

Appraisal-focused strategies are used when a person tries to modify the way he or she thinks in order to make a difficult situation appear easier. Examples are denial or distancing oneself from the problem, or changing beliefs and values, such as by seeing humour in the situation.

Problem-focused strategies aim to deal with the cause of the problem. This may be done by finding out about the particular condition and altering one's life to accommodate the disease. Finally, emotion-focused strategies involve releasing emotions, managing hostile feelings or using relaxation aids.

A mixture of these strategies is possible, and over time they may change. The literature suggests that a problem-focused strategy is the most effective and will support a better adjustment to the situation.

An alternative distinction that is often discussed in the literature is between active and avoidant coping strategies. *Active strategies* are either behavioural or psychological responses designed to change the nature of the problem or how the individual perceives it. *Avoidant strategies* lead people into alternative activities (e.g. alcohol) or mental states (e.g. withdrawal) that prevent them from addressing stressful events. Generally speaking, active strategies will have a more positive impact on the individual.

All humans are likely to experience a crisis at some time. The experience and the way we react to it is as individual as everything else about us. The changing nature of the crisis response can be confusing both to the individual and to others.

Psychologically we are equipped to deal with various aspects of crisis and our reactions can vary considerably. Some of the appropriate reactions to a crisis are:

- fear;
- stress;
- anger;
- guilt/shock/disbelief.

CASE STUDY 9.4

Consider again Jean's case (Case study 9.1 on page 193). Jean consented to theatre and had an emergency laparotomy. She went to the intensive care unit where she spent 11 days. She was treated for sepsis due to faecal peritonitis, was ventilated and required multi-organ support. Jean was transferred back to the surgical ward. Do you think Jean can employ coping strategies to assist with her personal crisis?

Just as in the grieving process, the crisis response has definite phases. Jean may not go through each phase and may not go through them in a fixed order, but it is highly likely that she will experience the process set out below.

- *Shock.* She has never been this ill before. She is scared and disbelieving that she is so unwell.
- *Denial.* 'This can't be happening to me.'
- *Overwhelming thoughts or emotions.* These can be anxiety, depression, fear or anger.
- *Acceptance.* She develops an awareness of events and is ready to work through the problems and how they may impact on her life.
- *Conclusion.* Jean is left with a desire to see things to their conclusion, be that a successful discharge home or a peaceful and dignified death.

This is not the time for criticism and judgement. This is a time to listen to the patient and offer comfort, support and empathy.

Practical nursing support

Advances in intensive care mean that many patients survive a critical illness who would previously have died. This in turn means that ward-based staff care for more patients requiring both physical and psychological support. Anxiety, stress and post-traumatic stress disorder have been well documented in this group of patients. These psychological consequences can have a marked impact on recovery. Let us consider a few elements of intensive care treatment and what feelings they may engender.

ACTIVITY   ?

Think about these aspects of critical care and how they may have affected Jean:

- invasive treatments such as ventilation;
- lack of privacy;
- reduction in mobility;
- altered sleep pattern;
- flashbacks.

Jean may be frightened, anxious or scared about her future. Knowing that she will be confined to bed she might feel helpless. She might feel isolated now that she is back on the ward, which could affect her emotional state.

The Hospital Anxiety and Depression Scale

Emotional outcome following critical illness has been assessed mainly using standardized questionnaires with demonstrated reliability and validity. The Hospital Anxiety and Depression Scale (Zigmond and Snaith 1982) is a self-report questionnaire with increasing scores indicating whether a patient is more likely to have an anxiety or depressive disorder. Scores of 11 and above suggest the probable presence of the condition. It is easy for the patient to complete and can be done as part of the assessment following discharge from ICU. It is not exclusive to critically ill patients and may be useful in a variety of other patient groups.

ACTIVITY   ?

Obtain a copy of the Hospital Anxiety and Depression Scale and think about how it could be used in caring for seriously ill patients.

Post-traumatic stress disorder

Post-traumatic stress disorder (PTSD) has been widely documented as a reaction following a period of critical illness. It has been suggested that up to 27 per cent of ICU patients may develop a post-traumatic reaction (Cuthbertson *et al.* 2004). Many of the symptoms can be mistaken as normal in the initial days following critical illness, as it is common to have poor sleep and nightmares. Normal reactions are separated from those seen in PTSD by their severity and duration. The diagnosis is not made until one month after the illness and the symptoms should be present for one month.

Patients with PTSD may re-experience their trauma by having intrusive thoughts, often in the form of flashbacks and nightmares. These are often described as being persecutory in nature, reliving a previous event or fighting for survival. The lack of memory for actual events means that patients process these delusions as real and this results in longer term psychological problems. The Impact of Events Scale (Horowitz *et al.* 1979) is another self-report questionnaire that can easily be completed by the patient. If PTSD is suspected, specialist psychiatric help is required.

Communication and empathy

Good communication is essential to the nursing role, both as an advocate for the patient and when caring for the patient directly. In today's healthcare there is a danger of overlooking the importance of talking to patients. The nursing Code of Conduct tells us to treat people kindly and considerately, listening to the people in our care and supporting them to improve and maintain their health (NMC 2008). We can make so much progress with patients if we take the time to listen to their concerns and try to empathize.

It may be that a nurse can answer many of the questions asked by a patient, such as 'Am I getting better?' or 'Can I start to walk soon?' The patient may be experiencing flashbacks to events while having intensive care, or have a lack of understanding regarding a specific aspect of his or her care. With the advent of Critical Care Outreach teams, specialist intensive care nurses now review patients following discharge from ICU and those suffering critical illness on the wards. They are expert in critical care nursing and can be used as an effective resource for both the patient and the staff. There has also been much research into the benefit of patient diaries to try to help them gain understanding about their experiences. They can be compiled by nurses or relatives and can orientate the patient to the timescales involved. They may act as a de-briefing tool and can be read at the convenience of the patient. However, caution is advised: avoidance of reminders is important in PTSD.

Family involvement

It has been suggested that the patient's family is a very important influencing factor. Family members' anxiety can affect the patient's recovery owing to their inability to understand the significance of events, which therefore impairs their decision-making. A family with a high level of uncertainty about the illness, treatment and outcome for their loved one have a reduced ability to apply coping mechanisms, which can negatively impact on patient outcome. The family may struggle to come to terms with reduced monitoring and reduction in nurses on the ward. Their loved one may have lack of recall and understanding about his or her condition, which can be distressing for the family. So how can nurses help the family?

Moulter (1979) developed the Critical Care Family Needs Inventory (CCFNI) to formally assess their needs. The inventory has five domains (Box 9.4).

Box 9.4 Domains of the Critical Care Family Needs Inventory (CCFNI; Moulter 1979)

- **Support** (resources and support systems)
- **Comfort** (family members' personal comfort)
- **Information** (consistent, realistic and timely)
- **Proximity** (personal contact and being physically and emotionally close to the patient)
- **Assurance** (feeling hope for the desired outcome)

Items from the proximity and assurance domains have been cited as the most important, with 'having hope' as the most important need. Additionally, how healthcare professionals deliver information has been ranked highly, emphasizing the importance of effective communication. Relatives want their questions to be answered honestly and to be kept updated on their loved one's condition. Information must be given in understandable terms, avoiding medical terminology while considering the issues around consent. Family satisfaction is an important measurement of quality of care.

Effective interventions are imperative to support relatives through a potentially long and slow recovery period. Relatives may use a range of coping mechanisms that can vary according to demographic and cultural factors. Many relatives focus on the immediate – suppressing anxiety despite feelings of uncertainty and turmoil. Support mechanisms may be vital but sometimes not available within the family network. Nurses are often required to fulfil this role and this should be seen as a positive and worthwhile aspect of the job. Instilling hope can have an empowering effect on the family's ability to cope. This can sometimes be difficult when the patient's prognosis is poor, but with effective communication such a situation can be made easier for the relatives to accept and thus cope with.

End-of-life issues

Dealing with end-of-life issues can be very difficult for healthcare professionals because they generally perceive their role as getting patients back to good health and see any death as a failure. Sometimes death is inevitable despite our best efforts.

Advances in medicine and technology have led to patients having more complex therapies and interventions to keep them alive for longer, sometimes to the point when the situation becomes futile. This arises regularly in critical care environments and is becoming more commonplace in general wards where healthcare professionals are now caring for more highly dependent patients. Consequently working in these areas involves participating in difficult decisions.

According to Oberle and Hughes (2008), misunderstandings can result from differing perceptions of ethical problems, highlighting the importance of appreciating the perspectives of others when difficult decisions have to be made. Therefore it is essential that healthcare professionals involve the patient and his or her family wherever possible when end-of-life issues are discussed.

The Department of Health (DH 2008) has issued an end-of-life care strategy to enable patients and their families to make care choices. However, many patients become seriously ill with an acute unexpected illness and may not have had the need or opportunity to consider these issues and their feelings may not be known.

Euthanasia and assisted suicide

The principle of respect for autonomy acknowledges the right of the patient to have control over his or her own life, including decisions about the end of that life.

The word 'euthanasia' originated in Greece and means 'a good death'. This could be interpreted as a timely, dignified and peaceful death in preference to suffering a long and painful terminal illness. Hendrick (2004) suggests that voluntary euthanasia is easy to justify on the grounds of autonomy as it is based on a patient's free and informed choice. However, when discussing the issue of autonomy there are further considerations that should be taken into account, such as whether the patient has the mental competence to make such a decision. In addition it is more difficult to justify involuntary euthanasia where ending someone's life is brought about without their informed consent supposedly in their best interests.

ACTIVITY   ?

Look back to Box 9.2 for the five-principles approach to determining a patient's decision-making capacity set out in the Mental Capacity Act 2005.

After the introduction of the Suicide Act 1961, committing suicide was no longer a criminal offence. Until then, anyone who attempted suicide and failed could have faced criminal prosecution. However, it is still against the law to deliberately end someone's life or to assist him or her in suicide. The Act clearly states:

A person who aids, abets, counsels or procures the suicide of another or an attempt by another to commit suicide shall be liable on conviction or indictment to imprisonment for a term not exceeding fourteen years.

Dimond (2009) noted the case of a husband who suffocated his wife who was suffering from multiple sclerosis. He admitted aiding and abetting his wife's suicide and was given a 12-month suspended sentence.

Nurses have to uphold the NMC Code of Professional Conduct, whatever ethical dilemmas they are facing. The code clearly states:

You must adhere to the laws of the country in which you are practising.

The media have reported on a number of cases where terminally or chronically ill people have travelled to European countries such as the Netherlands and Belgium where the law permits euthanasia. There has also been a particular focus on the Dignitas clinic in Zurich where physician-assisted suicide is permitted in certain circumstances.

CASE STUDY 9.5

Dimond (2009) noted the case of Debbie Purdy, a woman with multiple sclerosis who wanted her husband to be able to take her abroad to commit suicide if her condition became unbearably painful. She went to the High Court to seek clarification of the law with regard to assisted suicide in an effort to ensure that he would not be prosecuted for aiding and abetting her suicide.

The High Court said that, while it had great sympathy for Ms Purdy and others in similar situations, the law was clear on assisted suicide and for it to be permitted required Parliament to change the law. She was given leave to appeal, which was heard in February 2009. The High Court's earlier decision was confirmed, but the appeal judges identified that there were broad circumstances in which aiding and abetting suicide would not be prosecuted.

Following this case, the House of Lords instructed the Director of Public Prosecutions to clarify the factors taken into account when deciding whether to prosecute relatives who assist a suicide, while a review was undertaken of the arguments for and against prosecution.

It is important to differentiate between active euthanasia and passive euthanasia.

- Active euthanasia occurs when a death is brought about by an action such as administering a lethal injection, and is unlawful.
- Passive euthanasia occurs when a patient is allowed to die by *omitting to act*, such as withholding or withdrawing life-saving treatment, which is lawful.

The landmark case that established this legal principle was that of *Airedale Trust* v *Bland* (1993). Permission was given to discontinue artificial nutrition to Tony Bland who was in a permanent vegetative state (PVS) as a result of the injuries he sustained during the Hillsborough football disaster. He could not see, hear, taste, smell, speak nor communicate, so the doctors caring for him believed it would be of no benefit to the patient to continue futile treatment. In this instance the withdrawal of artificial nutrition and hydration was seen as an act of omission rather than commission.

The issue of euthanasia has been widely debated for many years with compelling arguments both for and against. In 2005, a House of Lords Select Committee took evidence from expert witnesses and visited countries in Europe where assisted suicide is practised. In 2008, the National Council for Palliative Care opposed a bill by Lord Joffe which sought to legalize 'assisted dying'. It was considered in the House of Lords but was defeated on its second reading in 2006. The Royal College of Nursing (2009) changed its position from one of opposition to assisted suicide to one of neutrality, where it neither supports nor opposes people's right to take their own life.

CASE STUDY 9.6

One argument that supporters of euthanasia raise is that of a patient's right to die with dignity. In 2002, Diane Pretty, who had motor neurone disease and was paralysed from the neck down, applied to the European Court of Human Rights for a ruling that would allow her husband to assist her to commit suicide without facing prosecution (after losing her case in the House of Lords). She based her application on Article 2 of the European Convention on Human Rights, which she argued protects the right to life and the right to choose the manner of death. She had a poor life expectancy and wanted a dignified pain-free death. The court ruled against her application, finding that her human rights had not been violated. They did not find that Article 2 created the right to die, and that the need to protect vulnerable citizens justified the prohibition of assisted suicide. Diane Pretty reportedly died shortly afterwards.

The term 'death with dignity' is commonly used in nursing but what does it mean? According to the Royal College of Nursing:

Dignity is concerned with how people feel, think and behave in relation to the worth or value of themselves and others. To treat someone with dignity is to treat them as being of worth in a way that is respectful of them as valued individuals.

CASE STUDY 9.7

Mary, a 77-year-old woman, has chronic obstructive airways disease (COPD) and has had increasingly frequent admissions to hospital with acute exacerbations of the disease. She is brought into the A&E department in acute respiratory failure, very distressed, stating that she wants to die. Mary asks for help to end her life.

Patients like Mary may feel that they are deprived of their dignity if they have to spend their final days attached to tubes, infusions and other devices rather than having a peaceful death.

Hendrick (2004) identified how the courts have recognized that Article 3 of the Human Rights Act 1998 – which covers the prohibition on torture as well as cruel and inhuman treatment – encompasses the right to die with dignity. However, a key argument against euthanasia is the doctrine of the sanctity of life, which argues that all human life has a worth and that it is wrong to end a person's life directly or indirectly no matter what the quality of life. Opponents of euthanasia also argue that, if it were made legal, the laws could be abused and people would be killed who did not really want to die. Hendrick (2004) wrote about the 'slippery slope' whereby, once we start to kill people who have requested it, we will find ourselves sliding down a slope that leads to unwanted killings, such as the terminally or chronically ill who have become a burden to their families or society. Wright (2004) wrote that patients who are chronically ill or dying often state that they do not want to be a burden and he suggests that nurses should challenge the assumption that dependency is bad.

Nurses in the United Kingdom have a responsibility to act in the patient's best interests. If we consider the concept of non-maleficence (Box 9.1), which is the obligation not to inflict harm intentionally, it is difficult to justify assisting someone to commit suicide as it is hard to see how death can be a benefit to the patient. However, in certain circumstances where the patient's quality of life is very poor then it might be argued that prolonging his or her life may not be of benefit to the patient.

How can we assess someone's quality of life, and who should determine what it is? Johnstone (1999) suggested that most people use the term 'quality of life' in one of three ways (Box 9.5).

Box 9.5 Three ways to describe quality of life (Johnstone 1999)

- **Descriptively**. This involves identifying certain traits or features a person might have, such as the patient is 'in pain' or 'is totally dependent on others'.
- **Evaluatively**. Here some value is attached to a particular trait or characteristic, such as the pain suffered by the patient is 'bad' or regaining independence is 'good'.
- **Prescriptively**. A prescriptive statement involves a moral judgement. Examples are: 'a life of such pain is not worth living' or 'being so dependent it is not in the patient's best interests to go on living'.

Healthcare professionals and a patient's family may perceive a patient's quality of life differently from how the patient sees it. Paterson (2003) describes how patients wish to be in control of their death and emphasizes that to some a 'good death' is as important as a 'good life'. Therefore it would be good practice to ensure that everyone is involved in making a judgement in end-of-life discussions where quality of life is an issue.

If a patient is mentally competent (see Box 9.2), he or she has the right to give or refuse consent to treatment even if the latter will result in death. The person does not have the right to request that any healthcare professional actively causes their death. However, if Mary (Case study 9.7) made such a request, consideration should be given as to why she wants to die.

According to Jeffrey (2006), the majority of requests for euthanasia or assisted suicide arise from poor symptom control, depression, poor social and family support as well as a loss of autonomy. The request may be a 'cry for help' rather than a desire to die.

Poor pain control is a significant issue in end-of-life care. Sutherland (2000) states:

There is abundant evidence to indicate that healthcare professionals consistently underestimate patients' pain and thus under-treat pain.

It could be argued that if a patient receives effective pain and symptom control as well as support to cope with other problems he or she is experiencing, the person may feel more able to go on with life and not want to die prematurely. This could be achieved by involving the palliative care team in the care of the patient. The World Health Organization in 2009 defined palliative care as:

An approach that improves the quality of life of the patient and family facing the problems associated with life-threatening illness through the prevention and relief of suffering by means of early identification, impeccable assessment and treatment of pain and other problems.

One issue that can arise when providing adequate pain relief is that large doses of a strong analgesic (e.g. an opiate) may cause shortening of life. This is known as the doctrine of 'double effect', which argues that there is a moral distinction between acting with the deliberate intention of causing someone's death and undertaking an act where death is a foreseen but indirect, unintended consequence. Pattinson (2006) noted a case where a general practitioner was acquitted from a murder charge following the administration of large doses of opiates to an elderly, incurably ill patient, where the judge stated to the jury:

A doctor is entitled to do all that is proper and necessary to relieve pain and suffering, even if the measures that he takes may incidentally shorten human life.

However, in the case of *Regina* v *Cox* (1993), Dr Cox, a consultant, administered an injection of potassium chloride with the intent to kill a patient who had uncontrollable pain from severe arthritis. The patient had asked to die and the doctor may have believed he was acting compassionately, but this was seen as active euthanasia and as such illegal. Sutherland (2000) argued that, if the doctor had administered a drug with analgesic properties, leading to her death, it would have been considered a legal act. Because he used potassium chloride, which has no analgesic effects and is known to cause cardiac arrest when it is given as a large bolus dose, he would not have been able to use the double effect in his defence. If any healthcare professional had undertaken the same course of action they would have been accountable both legally and professionally.

In conclusion, a nurse is personally accountable for any actions or omissions in his or her practice and must always be able to justify decisions made. While active euthanasia remains against the law, there can be no justification for practising it.

Advance directives

Appropriate circumstances

Although a person cannot expect a healthcare professional to assist with suicide, as a mentally competent adult he or she can refuse treatment for any reason – even if that decision is likely to lead to death. For example, Mary (Case study 9.7) could refuse artificial ventilation having been told that she will die without it.

Nevertheless, some patients do lack the mental capacity to make informed decisions about their treatment in certain circumstances, for example if they are confused, unconscious or have severe brain damage (see Box 9.2). In these situations healthcare professionals have a legal and ethical obligation to act in the best interests of the patient – as in the case *Airedale Trust* v *Bland* (1993) discussed on page 202. However, the House of Lords stipulated that if there had been an advance directive outlining his wishes if he were mentally incapacitated these should be taken into account in the assessment of best interests. This case was important in establishing the validity of advanced directives.

An advance directive – or 'living will' as they are sometimes called – is a statement made by a competent adult about the way he or she wishes to be treated if in the future he or she becomes no longer able to make decisions or communicate wishes. Hendrick (2004) suggests that advance directives can be considered as a type of informed consent for the future.

Advance directives can also be seen as promoting patients' autonomy by allowing them some control over their treatment at the end of life. Cardozo (2005) argues that many people fear that if they become seriously ill they will be given treatment when there is little or no chance of recovery, or treatment that leaves them in a condition with which they could not cope.

It might seem obvious that healthcare professionals should encourage patients to make their wishes known not only to their family but also to those responsible for caring for them when they are ill. Unfortunately, discussing end-of-life issues can be difficult because many people do not like to address their own mortality. In contrast, for some people – particularly those who have an incurable or chronic illness – this may not be the case. They may have very definite views about how they wish to be treated if they become seriously ill and unable to make their wishes known.

An advance directive does not give someone the right to refuse basic care that is essential to keep them comfortable, such as washing, pain relief, oral food and drinks. However, the person can refuse to have artificial nutrition and hydration.

A patient cannot use an advance directive to *demand* that he or she be given a particular treatment if the healthcare team considers it to be inappropriate or not in the patient's best interests.

Validity

Certain conditions have to be met for an advance directive to be valid (Box 9.6). Note that an advance decision to refuse treatment does not have to be made in writing, so if a patient states to a healthcare professional that he does not want to have a particular treatment in certain circumstances in the future this would be valid if the conditions in Box 9.6 were met.

However, the Mental Capacity Act 2005 rules that, where advance decisions relate to life-sustaining treatment, they must be in writing, signed and witnessed, and must specify clearly that the decision applies even if life is at risk. For example, if a patient with chronic respiratory disease states that she does not want to be invasively ventilated if brought into hospital with severe respiratory failure in the future, it is essential that the healthcare professional documents her wishes in the medical notes. This would then be seen as a valid advance directive and should be

Box 9.6 Conditions for an advance directive to be valid

- It has to be made by a competent adult aged 18 or over.
- It has to be entered into voluntarily and not be unduly influenced by anyone else.
- The individual has to be sufficiently informed about the nature of the treatment he or she is refusing and the potential consequences of doing so.
- There must be evidence that the directive was witnessed.
- The directive is applicable to the specific circumstances that arise.

respected if this situation occurs and the patient is admitted to hospital seriously ill and unable to make her wishes known.

If there are any doubts about the validity of an advance directive it could cause an ethical dilemma for the healthcare team concerned. According to the British Medical Association (2001):

> Where there are good grounds for genuine doubt about the validity of an advance refusal, there should be a presumption in favour of life and emergency treatment should be provided. Treatment may, however, be withdrawn at a later stage should the validity or existence of a valid advance directive become clear.

In cases where an advance directive is valid and applicable to the treatment in question, the person's relatives do not have the right to challenge the decision to withhold treatment. Relatives cannot give or withhold consent on behalf of another adult. However, under the Mental Capacity Act 2005, a patient can create a 'lasting power of attorney' which allows the person to choose who should make decisions about treatment if he or she is not able to do so.

If a healthcare professional ignores a valid directive and treats the patient against expressed wishes, that professional could be found guilty of trespass to the person (battery) or of assault. Healthcare professionals therefore have a duty in law to respect an advance refusal of treatment if it applies to the specific situation stated.

One issue of concern with advance directives is the possibility that a particular patient may have changed his mind by the time he is unable to make his own decisions. The Mental Capacity Act advocates that anyone who has made an advance directive should regularly review and update it if necessary. Healthcare professionals should encourage patients to do this and ensure that their medical records reflect any updated wishes.

Withdrawal of treatment

Caring for seriously ill patients involves ethical dilemmas for healthcare teams in deciding to withhold or withdraw treatment when it is deemed to be no longer of benefit to the patient. This includes withholding lifesaving measures in the event of a cardiopulmonary arrest. A 'do not attempt resuscitation' (DNR) order clarifies the resuscitation status of the patient for all those involved. DNR decisions should be reviewed regularly, and in particular whenever there are any changes in the patient's condition.

According to the NHS Executive (2000), cardiopulmonary resuscitation (CPR) should be withheld *only* in the following situations:

- when a mentally competent patient has refused treatment;
- when a valid advance directive (living will) has been made by the patient;
- when effective CPR is unlikely to be successful;
- where successful CPR is likely to be followed by a length and quality of life that would not be in the best interests of the patient to sustain.

Situations can arise shortly after a person is admitted to hospital with cardiopulmonary arrest where the full medical history and the person's express wishes are not known. In such cases all reasonable efforts should be made to resuscitate the person. Then, if further information becomes available about the person's clinical condition indicating that CPR would not be successful, it would be deemed inappropriate and the resuscitation attempt stopped (Resuscitation Council 2007).

CASE STUDY 9.8

Caroline, a 68-year-old woman, has had breast cancer with lymph node involvement. She has had a mastectomy, chemotherapy and radiotherapy. Her mobility is very limited due to severe osteoarthritis. Her daughter states that she is becoming frailer and more dependent on others for her care.

Caroline is admitted to hospital with increasing shortness of breath and chest pain. She is also hypotensive and tachycardic. The healthcare team stabilize her with high-flow oxygen, intravenous fluids and pain relief. A chest X-ray reveals a suspicious shadow.

Caroline has not made an advance directive and her wishes are not known should her condition deteriorate further or if she has a cardiopulmonary arrest.

- Should the healthcare team consider a DNR order for Caroline?

Discussing DNR decisions with patients is not easy, but in cases such as Caroline's it would be very important to establish what her wishes were in relation to this sensitive issue. It would be better to do this in advance of a crisis occurring to avoid unnecessary interventions and distress to those involved. In order to promote autonomy, Caroline should be involved in any discussions regarding resuscitation and other end-of-life care. Involving her family would also be good practice provided that Caroline agreed to their presence, as they may be able to offer her support and add further information to aid the decision-making.

We should also consider the principles of beneficence, non-maleficence and justice to ensure that any decisions are made in Caroline's best interests (see Box 9.1). It would be important to ensure that she and her family understood all the implications of CPR as the public may have unrealistic perceptions of a resuscitation attempt from television dramas where interventions are often brief and have a successful outcome. The reality of CPR is often very different, with poor survival rates even when the cardiac arrest occurs in hospital. The chances of surviving CPR and being discharged home from hospital are at best 15–20 per cent (Resuscitation Council 2007).

Even when CPR is successful in restarting the heart initially, it can be harmful in its outcome. It can,

for example, result in hypoxic brain damage and admission to intensive care, with all the associated invasive monitoring and procedures, only for the patient to die hours or days later.

Therefore it is essential to weigh up the potential benefits against the possible harm from CPR. The Gold Standards Framework (2008) suggests that cancer, organ failure, general frailty, dementia and severe stroke are not associated with successful CPR. Therefore, if we balance Caroline's illness as well as her increased frailty and dependence on others against the chances of surviving a resuscitation attempt without undue harm, it would be justifiable to agree to a DNR order. Such a decision would allow Caroline the benefit of dying peacefully if her heart stopped, rather than the indignity of a futile resuscitation attempt.

Situations can arise where a patient may still request CPR to be attempted even if there is only a very small chance of success and despite being informed of the risks involved. The Resuscitation Council (2007) recommend that the patient's decision should be respected and no DNR order made, while adding that in the event of a cardiac or respiratory arrest the decision should be reviewed.

One concern that patients and their families may have with a DNR decision is that this would also imply no 'active' treatment. Healthcare professionals should strive to reassure them that they will continue to receive all other appropriate treatment and care even if a DNR order is in place. However there may be a limitation of treatment offered. For example, it may be deemed in Caroline's best interests not to have further surgery if the harms outweigh the benefits. Similarly, a patient with end-stage respiratory disease and severe acute respiratory failure may be given non-invasive ventilation in a respiratory ward but a decision be made not to progress to invasive ventilation in ICU.

If, despite all appropriate treatment, the patient's condition continues to deteriorate, a decision may be made to withdraw all life-sustaining treatment and allow the patient to die. In such situations the Liverpool Care Pathway (LCP) could be utilized to ensure the patient receives appropriate evidence-based multidisciplinary care in the last days of life (Marie Curie Palliative Care Institute 2005). All healthcare professionals should endeavour to provide high-quality individualized end-of-life care. They would be failing in their duty of care if patients were offered anything less.

Family-witnessed resuscitation

When a patient has a cardiopulmonary arrest in hospital the family tend to be escorted away from their loved one into a waiting room while life-saving measures are attempted. A pioneering nine-year study was undertaken by the Foote Hospital in Michigan, USA, after staff were forced to question this policy following two incidents in 1982 where family members demanded to be present during resuscitation, as a result of which a guideline for family presence during resuscitation was developed (Hanson and Strawser 1992). Despite more recent professional recommendations supportive of family presence during CPR, the practice is often discouraged and many hospitals do not have guidance for staff to help them deal with such a situation.

Nevertheless, family-witnessed resuscitation appears now to be more widely accepted in A&E departments and is also being introduced into other critical care environments. It is common practice when the patient is a child. Therefore, can healthcare practitioners justify excluding relatives in the same situations in other areas of the hospital?

CASE STUDY 9.9

Paul, a 42-year-old man, is admitted to hospital with chest pain, accompanied by his wife Lynne. He is generally fit and well. He has recently returned from a holiday in Thailand and on examination is found to have a swollen and painful right calf. He is suspected to have had a pulmonary embolism.

Shortly after admission Paul becomes acutely short of breath and very distressed. He collapses and is unresponsive. The nurse who is present quickly identifies that he has had a cardiac arrest. When the staff nurse asks Lynne to wait in the visitors' room she refuses to leave her husband.

- Should Lynne be allowed to stay?
- What would be the most ethical approach for the team to take in Paul's case?

Allowing relatives to be present during resuscitation attempts can be seen as a more family-centred approach to care. Eichhorn et al. (1996) suggested that moves towards this approach are the result of the moral and ethical imperative for preserving the wholeness, dignity and integrity of the family unit from birth to death. How can healthcare professionals practice holistic care if family members are made to leave the room while resuscitation takes place?

The Human Rights Act 1998 grants individuals the right to have their family life respected, so it might give relatives the right to be present with their loved one as they die, if this is interpreted as a 'family life' event.

There appears to be evidence that relatives not only want the choice to witness the resuscitation of their loved one but that they also benefit from being present. Wieliczka (2007) was present while her mother was being resuscitated. She described how having the opportunity to stay gave her the satisfaction of knowing that her mother was well cared for and the chance to say goodbye, stating that she would have felt cheated if she had not been given the choice to be present. Ardley (2003) gave an account of how a senior nursing sister was physically but gently restrained from entering the room where her daughter was being resuscitated and afterwards regretted not forcing her way in, because she was left with feelings of anger that she had left her daughter alone to die among total strangers.

If Paul's wife Lynne were allowed to stay in the room it might help her to understand the seriousness of the situation and enable her to see that the healthcare team were doing everything possible to help Paul. That said, concerns have been raised about the psychological effects of witnessing a resuscitation attempt on a relative. This can be a traumatic experience for anyone, particularly if it involves their loved one. Exposure to medical documentaries and television dramas may mean that relatives are more aware of what to expect, but the reality may seem very different in comparison. It is inevitable that family members will become upset and distressed, whether they are present or not, but this should not be a reason to prevent them from witnessing what could be the final moments of their relative's life.

Questions have been raised as to who benefits from relatives being present during a resuscitation attempt, the patient or the family. Could we be respecting the wishes of the living without knowing those of the dying patient? In emergency situations it is virtually impossible to establish what the patient's wishes are, but it seems reasonable to assume that someone close to dying would normally want a loved one close by.

McMahon-Parkes *et al.* (2009) believe that resuscitation survivors have a unique and potentially valuable perspective on family-witnessed resuscitation. Their study found that, compared with patients without the experience of resuscitation, resuscitated patients were more likely to want a family member nearby, believed that loved ones benefited from the experience, and wished to be present themselves if a relative required resuscitation.

It is to be expected that not all relatives would want to be present during resuscitation. However, it is possible that if relatives are offered the choice they may feel obliged to stay even if they don't want to. It is crucial that family members not be pressurized into witnessing resuscitation, but they can be made aware that it may help them through the grieving process if they choose to stay. A member of staff should remain throughout the process to provide information about what is happening.

Ultimate responsibility for all decisions, including family presence at resuscitation, remains with the healthcare professional leading the resuscitation attempt, although ideally it should be a team approach.

There are reasons why healthcare professionals might prefer not to have the family present. A key concern might be that they will complain or consider legal action if they believe that too little has been done, or if they feel that mistakes have been made. Complaints and litigation often arise from lack of information, mistrust or misunderstanding of the situation, which highlights the importance of having someone specifically to support the family during and after the resuscitation attempt.

A further issue is that the resuscitation attempt may be prolonged because staff find it difficult to make a decision to stop with the relatives present, or the relatives want the resuscitation to continue even though it has been deemed futile by the team. The decision to end a resuscitation attempt will need to be dealt with in a sensitive manner, and ideally the team should involve the family members in this. The reasons for stopping should be fully explained so that they understand the futility of continuing.

Other negative perceptions of having the family present are that the team will not function as well as they might do otherwise, and that it will make the situation more stressful for the staff.

In order to support staff involved in witnessed resuscitation, debriefing following a cardiac arrest where the family have been present may be helpful.

This would enable them to reflect on the situation as a team, identify what they did well, as well as what issues arose and identify what they might do differently should they be involved in a similar situation in the future.

Change is inevitable in healthcare as research and evidence in practice encourage us to take an innovative approach to meeting the needs of patients and their families. Therefore healthcare professionals should be open-minded with regard to family-witnessed resuscitation as they may then develop more confidence in participating in the process and recognize the benefits once they have had the opportunity to participate in such a situation.

Conclusion

It is apparent that, in order to ensure an ethical approach to healthcare, we need to understand the beliefs, values and wishes of the patients. Healthcare professionals must also adhere to the relevant laws and be guided by professional recommendations when difficult ethical decisions have to be made. It is important that the patient and his or her family be involved in the decision-making process wherever possible. Difficult dilemmas can arise when the patient's wishes conflict with what is considered to be in his or her best interests or those of society. The use of an appropriate ethical decision-making model can provide the healthcare team with a framework to assist in considering the options available and to provide a rationale for whatever course of action is chosen. Whatever decision is reached, the basis on which it was made should be clearly documented and communicated to other members of the multidisciplinary team.

Ethical decision-making can be particularly difficult when end-of-life issues are involved. Healthcare professionals should endeavour to handle these situations sensitively to minimize the risk of distressing the patient and his or her family.

Suggested further reading

Crown Prosecution Service. DPP Publishes Interim Policy on Department of Health (DH) (2000). *Comprehensive Critical Care: Review of Adult Critical Care Services*. London: NHS Executive.

Department of Health (2005). *Mental Capacity Act.* London: The Stationery Office.

Department of Health (2006). *The Caldicott Guardian Manual.* London: The Stationery Office.

Department of Health (2008). What are the Mental Capacity Act 2005 Deprivation of Liberty Safeguards? See www.dh.dov.uk/publications.

Fulbrook S (1998). Legal implications of relatives witnessing resuscitation, *British Journal of Theatre Nursing* 7(10); 33–35.

McHale J (2009). Capacity to consent: health care law and adult patients, *British Journal of Nursing* 18; 639–641.

Nursing and Midwifery Council (2008). *Code of Professional Conduct.* London.

Nursing and Midwifery Council (2008). *Consent.* London.

Nursing and Midwifery Council (2009). *Advice Sheet: Confidentiality.* London.

Paul F, Rattray J (2007). Short- and long-term impact of critical illness on relatives: literature review, *Journal of Advanced Nursing* 62; 276–92.

Rattray J, Hull A (2008). Emotional outcome after intensive care: literature review, *Journal of Advanced Nursing* 64; 2–13.

Resuscitation Council UK (1996). *Should Relatives be Allowed to Witness Resuscitation?* London: Resuscitation Council.

Salovey P, Rothman A, Detweiler J, Steward W (2000). Emotional states and physical health, *American Psychologist* 55; 110–21.

Sully P, Dallas J (2005). *Essential Communication Skills for Nursing.* London: Elsevier Mosby.

References

Airedale NHS Trust *v* Bland (1993). A.C.789; ALL ER 821.

Antonovsky A (1987). *Stress and Coping.* San Franscisco: Jossey-Bass.

Ardley C (2003). Should relatives be allowed in the resuscitation room? *Intensive and Critical Care Nursing* 19; 1–10.

Beauchamp T, Childress J (1989). *Principles of Biomedical Ethics*, 3rd edn. Oxford: Oxford University Press.

Beauchamp T, Childress J (2009). *Principles of Biomedical Ethics*, 6th edn. New York: Oxford University Press.

British Medical Association (2001). *Withholding and Withdrawing Life Prolonging Treatment: Guidance for Decision-making*, 2nd edn. London: BMA.

Cardozo M (2005). What is a good death? Issues to examine in critical care, *British Journal of Nursing* 14; 1056–60.

Cuthbertson B, Hull A, Strachan A, Scott J (2004). Post-traumatic stress disorder after critical illness requiring general intensive care, *Intensive Care Medicine* 30; 450–5.

Department of Health (DH) (1997). *The Caldicott Report.* London: The Stationery Office.

Department of Health (2008). *End of Life Care Strategy: Promoting High Quality Care for all Adults at the End of Life.* London: The Stationery Office.

Dimond B (2005). *Legal Aspects of Nursing.* London: Pearson Education.

Dimond B (2009). Assisted suicide and euthanasia: unravelling the law, *British Journal of Neuroscience Nursing* 5(3); 125–7.

Eichhorn DJ, Meyers TA, Mitchell TG, Guzzetta CE (1996). Opening the doors: family presence during resuscitation, *Journal of Cardiovascular Nursing* 10(4); 59–70.

Fok SK, Chair SY, Lopez V (2005). Sense of coherence, coping and quality of life following a critical illness, *Journal of Advanced Nursing* 49; 173–81.

Gold Standards Framework (2008). *Prognostic Indicator Guidance.* See www.goldstandardsframework.nhs.uk/.

Hanson C, Strawser D (1992). Family presence during cardiopulmonary resuscitation: Foote Hospital emergency department's nine-year perspective, *Journal of Emergency Nursing* 18(2); 104–6.

Hendrick J (2004). *Law and Ethics: Foundations in Healthcare*, Cheltenham: Nelson Thornes.

Horowitz M, Wilner N, Alvarez W (1979). Impact of Event Scale: a measure of subjective stress, *Psychosomatic Medicine* 41; 209–18.

Jeffrey D (2006). *Patient Centred Ethics and Communication at the End of Life.* Oxford: Radcliffe Publishing.

Johnstone M J (1999). *Bioethics: A Nursing Perspective*, 3rd edn. Marrickville, NSW: Saunders.

Marie Curie Palliative Care Institute (2005). Liverpool Care Pathway: Care of the Dying, version 11. Liverpool.

McMahon-Parkes K, Moule P, Benger J, Albarron J (2009). The views and preferences of resuscitated and non-resuscitated patients towards family witnessed resuscitation: a qualitative study, *International Journal of Nursing Studies* 46; 220–9.

Moulter NC (1979). Needs of relatives of critically ill patients: a descriptive study, *Heart and Lung* **8**; 332–9.

National Council for Palliative Care (2008). *Euthanasia and Assisted Dying*. Available at www.ncpc.org.uk/ethics/assisted_dying.html (accessed December 2010).

NHS Executive (2000). *Resuscitation Policy*. HSC 2000/028. London: NHS Executive.

Oberle K, Hughes D (2008). Doctors' and nurses' perceptions of ethical problems in end-of-life decisions, *Journal of Advanced Nursing* **33**; 707–15.

Paterson I (2003). The ethics of assisted suicide, *Nursing Times* **99**(7); 30–1.

Pattinson S (2006). *Medical Law and Ethics*. London: Sweet & Maxwell.

Resuscitation Council UK and the Royal College of Nursing (2007). *Decisions Relating to Cardiopulmonary Resuscitation: Joint Statement*. London: BMA, RC(UK), RCN.

Sutherland P (2000). Ethical issues. In: Bassett C, Makin L (eds) *Caring for the Seriously Ill Patient*. London: Hodder Arnold.

Wieten W, Lloyd MA (2006). *Psychology Applied to Modern Life*. California: Thompson Wadsworth.

Wieliczka ML (2007). My experience of being present during resuscitation, *Critical Care Nurse* **27**; 17.

Wright S (2004). Speak up for life, *Nursing Standard* **19**; 1.

Zigmond AS, Snaith RP (1982). The Hospital Anxiety and Depression Scale, *Acta Psychiatrica Scandinavica* **67**; 361–70.

LEARNING OUTCOMES

On completion of this chapter the reader will:

1　have an awareness of the impact of suboptimal care on the acutely ill patient

2　have an understanding of the involvement of teams in the management of the acutely ill patient and those at risk of clinical deterioration

3　appreciate the impact of track-and-trigger scoring systems on the care and management of the acutely ill patient

4　understand the impact of systematic patient assessment and effective communication on patient outcome.

Introduction

Over the past ten to fifteen years the care and management of patients in acute hospitals have come under increasing scrutiny. In particular there has been a growing awareness of the need to develop well-organized systems to guarantee the safe and effective management of the acutely ill and deteriorating patient. This chapter will outline some of the commonly used systems that are now in place in most acute care settings, including systems for assessing and identifying acutely ill patients and those at risk of deterioration, systems for communicating clinical concerns within the healthcare team, and systems for responding swiftly with appropriate care and management. The chapter will start with a brief review of the background that has led to the current position.

Background

Early-warning scoring tools and critical-care outreach teams are just two examples of developments that have evolved rapidly in the past ten years. The key drivers for systems such as these come from the simple but troubling revelation that some patients die unnecessarily in acute hospitals. For example, the National Patient Safety Agency (NPSA 2007) reported on data collected in 2005 that demonstrated 1804 serious incidents resulting in death. Of these incidents, 576 were interpreted as potentially avoidable and related to patient safety issues. Of these deaths, 425 occurred in acute/general hospitals, with 71 relating to a range of diagnostic errors, 64 relating to unrecognized patient deterioration or recognized deterioration that was not acted upon, and 43 involving problems with resuscitation after cardiac arrest – including delays in starting resuscitation because staff did not recognize the acute situation, failure to call the resuscitation team, and failure in attempting themselves to resuscitate the patient.

The failings identified in this report followed previous concerns that harm was being done to patients in acute care due to lack of appropriate assessment and management from such sources as the National Confidential Enquiry into Patient Outcome and Death (NCEPOD 2005) and the Department of Health (DH), and mirrored similar observations from the USA. Conclusions were drawn that suggested that many patients were dying as a result of poor organization of care; that the clinical evidence is there to guide appropriate interventions but patients were being denied the best possible chance of survival owing to a range of structural and system-based failures such as those listed in Box 10.1.

Box 10.1 Causes of patient deterioration (NPSA 2007)

- Deterioration is not recognized.
- Deterioration is not appreciated or not acted on sufficiently quickly.
- Communication and documentation are sometimes poor.
- Experience is sometimes lacking.
- Provision of critical-care expertise (including admission to critical-care areas) can be delayed.

The NPSA (2007) suggested that some of these problems may be overcome through the sharing of ideas and information. It was recommended that every acute hospital trust develop a multidisciplinary deterioration recognition group with the sole purpose of optimizing patient safety through the improvement and development of local healthcare systems and processes that enable early recognition and management of the patient at risk of deterioration.

Patient safety reporting is a relatively new development nationally and internationally, but systems such as the National Reporting and Learning System in England and Wales should enable the identification of hazards and help to evaluate why patients are being harmed rather than helped by their healthcare organizations.

Every year 13 million people on average are admitted to acute hospitals in England and Wales. Inevitably some of these people will die as a result of their illness. However, there remain a number of patients whose death was not inevitable.

Patients admitted to hospital believe they are entering a place of safety where they, their families and carers have a right to believe that they will receive the best possible care. They feel confident that should their condition deteriorate they are in the best place for prompt and effective treatment. That deterioration leading to catastrophic events such as cardiac arrest sometimes goes undetected is clearly avoidable.

Indeed, many patients give physiological signals that help to detect clinical deterioration hours or even days before deterioration becomes catastrophic. For example, Hillman *et al.* (2001) noted that 60–84% of patients suffering a cardiorespiratory arrest with subsequent intensive care admission or death had identifiable deterioration of vital signs as much as 48 hours prior to the event.

There is a clear need for strategies that enable healthcare practitioners to systematically assess patients for signs of clinical deterioration, summon the correct help in a timely manner, and communicate effectively to ensure the correct level of care is provided to the patient at the correct time. Such strategies can be seen in the use of clinical scoring and assessment tools, in the development of critical-care outreach, and in the use of structured communication processes.

Critical-care outreach teams

The origins of critical-care outreach lie in the development of the Medical Emergency Team (MET), alternatively known as a Rapid Response Team. These were introduced in 1990 following grave concerns of suboptimal care in Australia. The teams, which consisted of a group of physicians, anaesthetists and senior nurses similar to those found on the original cardiac arrest team, were designed to improve the early identification and management of vital sign abnormalities in acutely deteriorating ward patients. The intention of the MET was to quickly assess and manage patient deterioration before the patient's condition became increasingly critical.

The concerns in Australia were soon mirrored by the United Kingdom. In 2000, the Department of Health recommended the establishment of Critical Care Outreach Services with three main purposes:

- to reduce intensive care unit (ICU) admissions consistent with earlier intervention and treatment of seriously ill ward patients;
- to enable patient discharge from critical-care areas to general wards;
- to share critical-care skills and knowledge with ward-based staff (DH 2000).

Outreach care is a systems approach for recognizing and managing patients at risk of deterioration through a collaborative style, rather than providing a service through an external group. The most common model of critical-care outreach teams (CCOTs) consists of expert critical-care nurses with a clear function to empower ward-based staff by providing them with the skills, knowledge and support they need to deliver the correct form of care in a timely manner. The aims are summarized in Box 10.2.

Box 10.2 Aims of critical-care outreach teams (NCEPOD 2005)

- Avert admissions to critical care.
- Facilitate timely admission to critical care and discharge back to the ward.
- Share critical-care skills and expertise through an educational partnership.
- Promote continuity of care.
- Ensure audit and evaluation of outreach services.

Referral to the CCOT is mainly undertaken by ward staff when a patient triggers a response on the track-and-trigger scoring system. The CCOT also provides support and training on other occasions, including the provision of taught programmes and telephone advice.

While the purpose of CCOTs has been clearly defined by the Department of Health, acute Trusts have been given the freedom to develop the service in a way deemed appropriate for their individual needs. Clearly this has enabled the development of a service more attuned to individual Trust requirements, but equally it has created a problem for generalizable evaluation of a consistent model and attempts at demonstrating definite positive outcomes have been disappointing (Gao et al. 2007a), although individual single-centre studies have shown some positive impact (Esmonde et al. 2006). More studies are therefore needed to evaluate the efficacy of this development.

Further information and links to critical-care outreach resources can be found by going to the website of the National Critical Care Outreach Forum (NORF) at www.norf.org.uk.

Track-and-trigger systems

Alongside CCOTs has been the implementation of a 'scoring system' on to the wards for tracking clinical deterioration in patients and triggering expert referral. To date three main types of scoring system exist, although many Trusts have adapted these to meet their individual needs. The main system categories are:

- single-parameter systems (although their use is confined to Australia);
- multiple-parameter systems;
- aggregated scoring systems.

In 2007, the National Institute for Health and Clinical Excellence (NICE) recommended the introduction of either the multiple-parameter system or the aggregated scoring system into acute Trusts within the UK. The multiple-parameter system, first piloted in England in 1997, requires that more than one abnormal criterion be met for system activation (Fig. 10.1). To date this particular version of track-and-trigger is used in few Trusts within England.

The more commonly used tool in acute hospitals in the UK is the aggregated scoring system (Fig. 10.2). This system, first developed by Morgan et al. (1997), can now be found in at least 95 acute hospitals in England. It works by assigning an increasing number of points to deranged physiological parameters in patients at risk of deterioration. When scores reach a predefined threshold level, the patient's medical team or CCOT are alerted.

NICE (2007) suggested that, within each scoring system, be it multiple-parameter or aggregated scoring, the following physiological parameters be included as a minimum: heart rate; respiratory rate; systolic blood pressure; level of consciousness; oxygen saturation; temperature. NICE also recommends a graded trigger response to the acutely ill patient, with the patient described as falling within a low scoring group (as defined by the track-and-trigger score), a medium scoring group or a high scoring group – with different actions determined by grouping (Box 10.3).

Despite the introduction of systematic track-and-trigger scoring systems, reports of missed deterioration in patients, untimely management of deterioration and inappropriate treatment continue. This is supported in a recent systemic review of physiological track-and-trigger warning systems where results showed that the commonly used warning

Any 3 or more of the following			
Physiological parameters	Trigger 1 value	Trigger 2 value	Trigger 3 value
Heart rate	<55 per min	≥110 per min	
AVPU	Not fully alert and responsive		
O$_2$ saturation	<90%		
Respiratory rate	<10 per min	≥25 per min	≤35 per min
Urine output	<100 mL over past 4 hours		
Systolic BP	<90 mmHg		
Other			
OR:	Patient not fully alert and orientated AND respiratory rate ≥35/min OR heart rate ≥140/min		
Response	Call outreach team		

Figure 10.1 A multiple-parameter system

Parameter	A	B	C	D	E	F	G
Score	3	2	1	0	1	2	3
AVPU				Alert	Voice	Pain	Unresponsive
Heart rate (per min)		< 40	41–50	51–100	101–110	111–129	≤ 130
Respiratory rate (per min)	< 9			9–14	15–20	21–29	≥ 30
Systolic BP (mmHg)	< 70	71–80	81–100	101–199		> 200	
Temperature (°C)		< 35		35–38.4		≥ 38.5	

Score	Response
5 or more	Alert appropriate medical staff and CCOT

Figure 10.2 MEWS: an aggregate scoring system

Box 10.3 Graded response strategy for the patient at risk of deterioration (NICE)

Low scoring group

These patients (who are triggering but at the lower end of the trigger value) need the frequency with which their observations are recorded to be increased. It is also necessary to alert the nurse in charge that this action is needed for this patient.

Medium scoring group

These patients require an urgent call to the primary medical team. A call to the CCOT or their equivalent (e.g. Hospital at Night Team) must be made at the same time.

High scoring group

These patients require an emergency call to the critical-care team that have the skills and competencies needed for advanced airway and resuscitation management. An immediate response from the critical-care team must be provided.

systems had little reliability, validity and utility (Gao et al. 2007b). The review suggests that they be used only as adjuncts to clinical judgement as many at-risk patients will be missed if ward staff rely only on such objective criteria. The authors are currently involved in research that seeks to more fully understand the reasons for failure to rescue deteriorating patients.

The 'chain of response'

In addition to the recommendation that Trusts introduce a track-and-trigger scoring system on to their wards with a graded trigger response, NICE (2007) also proposed the development and attainment of relevant competencies for health-care staff. The suggested areas of proficiency included competence in monitoring, measuring and interpreting vital signs in the acutely ill patient based on the role of staff in the described 'chain of response' approach to care (Fig. 10.3).

The 'chain of response' reflects a team approach to care where levels of intervention escalate as the acute patient becomes more ill. As with many team-based processes, individual staff have roles within the team. These are described as non-clinical staff, recorder, recognizer, primary responder, secondary responder and, where appropriate, tertiary responder (critical care) – recognizing that one person may undertake more than one role in the chain. In addition, the identified competencies (NICE 2007) are consistent with the knowledge, skills and attitudes expected of the primary, secondary and tertiary responders (Box 10.4).

Box 10.4 Roles in the 'chain of response' (NICE)

- **Non-clinical staff** (may include the patient or visitor).
- **Recorder**. This person takes designated measurements, records information and records observations.
- **Recognizer**. This person monitors the condition of the patient and interprets measurements, observations and information. He or she adjusts the frequency and level of monitoring/observation as appropriate.
- **Primary responder**. This person interprets the measurements, observations and information and commences a clinical management plan.
- **Secondary responder**. This person is called to attend to the patient if he or she fails to respond to the primary intervention or continues to trigger a response on the EWS/Multiple Parameter Scoring Tool. The secondary responder assesses the effect of the primary intervention, forms a diagnosis, reassesses the management plan and alters this as needed. The person will initiate a secondary response and recognize when the patient's condition requires referral to critical care.
- **Tertiary responder**. This person has the skills and knowledge consistent with critical care: advanced airway management, resuscitation management, clinical examination and interpretation skills.

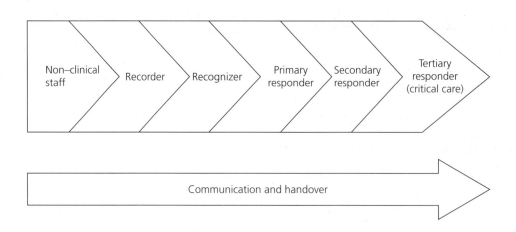

Figure 10.3 The 'chain of response'

The following case studies require you to explore your actions as primary responder.

ABCDE systematic assessment strategy

The Resuscitation Council UK (2006) recommends that staff follow the ABCDE (airway, breathing, circulation, disability, exposure) approach for assessing acutely ill patients. This approach helps to ensure prompt identification and initial management of the deteriorating patient and has been applied to courses such as ALERT and provides the basic structure of many advanced life-support programmes. Based on simplicity, the approach provides a systematic framework for completing the initial assessment of the acutely ill patient that every member of staff will remember with ease. This reduces the likelihood of mistakes or misunderstandings, and ensures that the whole team works together.

In addition, the ABCDE assessment framework is consistent with the analysis of events that precede critical care, such as cardiac arrest. Several studies have demonstrated significant alterations in airway, breathing and circulation prior to catastrophic patient deterioration (Franklin and Mathew 1994; Hillman *et al.* 2001; Resuscitation Council 2000). In 2004, Kause and co-workers reported significant physiological deterioration in up to 60 per cent of patients prior to cardiac arrest, death and unanticipated admission to intensive care. For some of these patients abnormal physiological data was noted up to 24 hours preceding the critical event.

The ABCDE assessment process

A = Airway

Important aspects to note when assessing the airway include airway patency/obstruction (partial or complete) and degree of airway protection. Observe for signs of obstruction, including abnormal retraction of interspaces during inspiration and 'tracheal tug'. There is more information in Chapter 2.

If partial airway obstruction is evident, high-concentration oxygen must be administered using a mask with a reservoir bag and immediate assistance called for.

If your airway assessment suggests complete airway obstruction and no air movement can be felt, administer an airway manoeuvre immediately – head lift, chin lift or jaw thrust – and summon help.

B = Breathing

Once assessment of the patient's airway has been safely undertaken, you can then assess the breathing. Alterations in respiratory rate and levels of oxygen saturation are noted in several studies as early indicators of patient deterioration, both indicating the person's attempt to increase oxygen delivery to the cells (Hillman *et al.* 2001; Cuthbertson *et al.* 2007; Duckitt *et al.* 2007). Each of these physiological parameters is easy to assess in practice. More detailed observation and assessment include skills of auscultation, palpation and percussion, which are examined in Chapter 2.

Unless it is contraindicated, administer high-flow oxygen using a mask with a reservoir bag.

C = Circulation

Once treatment of an altered airway and/or breathing has been initiated, assessment of the patient's circulation can begin. This includes initial observation for: distress; clammy/cold peripheries; capillary refill time less than 2 seconds; peripheral pulses; altered heart rate; evidence of bleeding/fluid loss (remember that bleeding may not be external so check for signs of internal haemorrhage/fluid loss); signs of cardiac failure; reduced level of consciousness; oliguria; pulse

pressure less than 35–45 mmHg. Chapter 1 has m... information.

Immediate treatment will depend on the cause of the cardiovascular failure (e.g. blood loss, arrhythmia or pump failure) and therefore may range from volume replacement to inotropic support (see Chapter 1).

D = Disability

Disability addresses the responsiveness of the patient and his or her level of consciousness. This is undertaken quite simply using the AVPU approach:

A How **A**lert is the person?
V Can the patient respond **V**erbally?
P Does the patient respond to **P**ainful stimuli?
U How **U**nresponsive or responsive is the patient?

Assessment of disability must also address levels of hypoxia, hypercapnia and cerebral hypoperfusion since these are the most common causes of unconsciousness in the seriously ill. If a patient has altered levels of consciousness it is important to also check blood glucose to rule out a hypoglycaemic incident.

The patient's drug administration record must also be examined to exclude an adverse reaction to recent drug treatment.

Pupillary response to light must be undertaken, noting especially pupil size, equality of pupils and their reaction to light.

If time allows, a Glasgow Coma Score should be performed. This will provide a more in-depth record of the patient's consciousness level. See Chapter 4 for more information.

E = Exposure/examination

Exposure of the patient is sometimes necessary to examine for injury or bleeding, or for the insertion of an intravenous cannula. If treatment and further assessment requires the patient's clothing to be loosened and/or removed, do consider the risk of hypothermia. Equally respect the patient's dignity and privacy. During exposure observe for rashes and/or hives that may indicate infection, sepsis or anaphylaxis, and look for wounds and scars from previous injury/surgery.

Effective communication: SBAR

Studies repeatedly cite deficient communication between healthcare professionals as a central cause of inadequate patient care (NPSA 2007; NICE 2007). In many instances poor communication has been a key feature reported in serious untoward incidents.

One reason stated for inadequate communication is that less-experienced staff often find it a challenge to make recommendations for patient care to more senior staff. Having a structure within which to present patient care recommendations may be one

---

Box 10.5 The SBAR scheme

Prior to placing the call, gather the patient's medical and nursing notes, medication chart, fluid balance chart and observation records.

S = *Situation*

- State your name and that of the ward.
- Give the name of the patient you are calling about and the reason for your call.
- Describe your concern.

B = *Background*

- Explain why the patient was admitted.
- Explain significant medical history.
- State the admitting diagnosis, the date the patient was admitted and any procedures undertaken, medications, allergies, laboratory results and any results from other investigations/tests.

A = *Assessment*

- State vital signs, including track-and-trigger scores.
- Give a clinical impression and state your concerns (i.e. consider the reasons for the patient's deterioration prior to making the call and present these to the doctor).

R = *Recommendation*

- State what action you would like to happen (e.g. that the doctor visit the patient).
- Make a specific time frame within which you would like this action to happen.
- Make suggestions for further action.
- Clarify expectations again.

---

way to improve the situation. This is supported by Andrews and Waterman (2005) who claim the definitive way for a nurse to convince a doctor of the need to review a patient is by presenting quantifiable evidence.

SBAR (situation, background, assessment, recommendation) is a tool that can be used to frame verbal communication, especially those relating to critical issues. It helps healthcare practitioners to provide clarification of information through a series of steps, thus contributing to patient safety. Patient handover and communication has been shown to improve when using standardized tools such as SBAR (Clark *et al.* 2008). The tool comprises four sections each with its own standardized prompt questions (Box 10.5).

CASE STUDY 10.3

Mrs Hussein is a 79-year-old woman in Bay 5 of Harlow Ward. She was admitted yesterday with an exacerbation of COPD. Her oxygen saturation has fallen to 86 per cent on 3 litres of oxygen via nasal cannulae, and her respiration has increased to 26 breaths/min. Her heart rate has increased to 110/min and her systolic blood pressure is 120 mmHg. She seems to be slightly confused.

- List the information you would gather prior to making a call to the doctor.
- Use the SBAR tool for communication to present the conversation that you would like to take place with regard to Mrs Hussein.

While SBAR is the tool most widely used and recommended, there are numerous reports of adaptations of SBAR and of tools of a similar nature, such as I-Pass BATON. Recently there has been interest in the development of patient and/or relative triggering referral to outreach teams, which has led to the development of tools to make this feasible.

Conclusion

Unrecognized patient deterioration, untimely actions and poor communication have led to the development of a number of well-organized systems to guarantee the safe and effective management of the acutely ill and deteriorating patient. These include the development of critical-care outreach teams (CCOTs), track-and-trigger scoring systems, patient assessment frameworks and communication frameworks. These systems of care are mechanisms for supporting decisions that optimize the safety of acutely ill patients, and as adjuncts to clinical judgement they are pivotal.

Healthcare staff and organizations can make a real impact on the safety of patients by identifying a clinically deteriorating patient and acting early.

References

Andrews T, Waterman H (2005). Packaging: a grounded theory of how to report physiological deterioration effectively, *Journal of Advanced Nursing* **52**; 473–81.

Clark E, Squire S, Heyme A, Mickle ME, Petrie E (2009). The PACT Project: improving communication at handover, *Medical Journal of Australia* **190**(11 Suppl.); S125–7.

Cuthbertson BH, Boroujerdi M *et al.* (2007). Can physiological variables and early warning scoring systems allow early recognition of the deteriorating surgical patient? *Critical Care Medicine* **35**; 402–9.

Department of Health (DH, 2000). *Comprehensive Critical Care*. London: DH.

Duckitt RW, Buxton-Thomas R, Walker J *et al.* (2007). Worthing physiological scoring system: derivation and validation of a physiological early-warning system for medical admissions. An observational, population-based single-centre study, *British Journal of Anaesthesia* **98**; 769–74.

Esmonde L, McDonnell A, Ball C *et al.* (2006). Investigating the effectiveness of critical care outreach services: a systematic review, *Intensive Care Medicine* **32**; 1713–21.

Franklin C, Mathew J (1994). Developing strategies to prevent in-hospital cardiac arrest: analysing responses of physicians and nurses in the hours before the event, *Critical Care Medicine* **22**; 244–7.

Gao H, Harrison DA, Parry GJ *et al.* (2007a). The impact of the introduction of critical care outreach services in England: a multicentre interrupted time-series analysis, *Critical Care* **11**; R113.

Gao H, McDonnell A, Harrison DA *et al.* (2007b). Systematic review of physiological track and trigger tools: systems of identifying at risk patients on the ward, *Intensive Care Medicine* **33**; 667–79.

Hillman K, Parr M, Flabouris A, Bishop G, Stewart A (2001). Redefining in-hospital resuscitation: the concept of the medical emergency team, *Resuscitation* **48**; 105–10.

Kause J, Smith G *et al.* (2004). A comparison of antecedents to cardiac arrests, deaths and emergency intensive care admissions in Australia, New Zealand and the United Kingdom in the ACADEMIA study, *Resuscitation* **62**; 275–82.

Morgan RJM, Williams F, Wright MM (1997). An early-warning scoring system for detecting critical illness, *Clinical Intensive Care* **8**; 100.

NCEPOD (2005). *An Acute Problem? National Confidential Enquiry Into Patient Outcome and Death*. London: National Confidential Enquiry into Patient Outcome and Death.

NICE (2007). *Acutely Ill Patients in Hospital*. London: National Institute for Health and Clinical Excellence.

NPSA (2007). *Safer Care for the Acutely Ill Patient: Learning from Serious Incidents*. London: National Patient Safety Agency.

Resuscitation Council UK (2006). *Medical Emergencies and Resuscitation*. London: Resuscitation Council.

MALNUTRITION UNIVERSAL SCREENING TOOL (MUST)

This is a five-step screening tool to identify adult patients who are malnourished or at risk of malnutrition. It has been developed by the British Association for Parenteral and Enteral Nutrition.

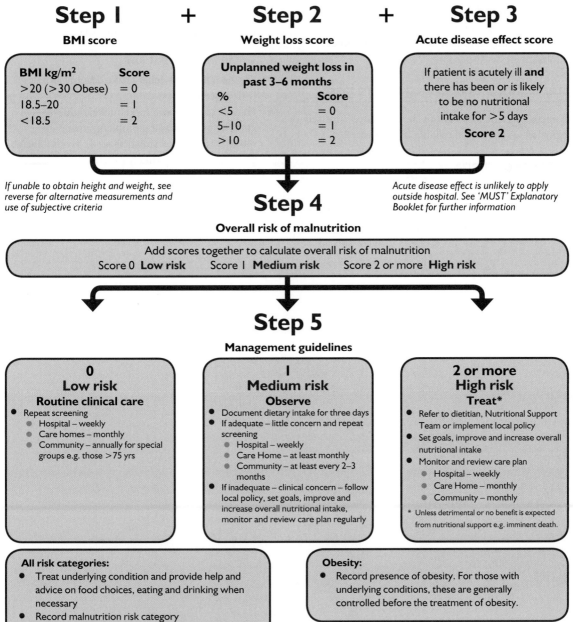

Step 1 + Step 2 + Step 3

BMI score

BMI kg/m²	Score
>20 (>30 Obese)	= 0
18.5–20	= 1
<18.5	= 2

If unable to obtain height and weight, see reverse for alternative measurements and use of subjective criteria

Weight loss score

Unplanned weight loss in past 3–6 months	
%	Score
<5	= 0
5–10	= 1
>10	= 2

Acute disease effect score

If patient is acutely ill **and** there has been or is likely to be no nutritional intake for >5 days

Score 2

Acute disease effect is unlikely to apply outside hospital. See 'MUST' Explanatory Booklet for further information

Step 4

Overall risk of malnutrition

Add scores together to calculate overall risk of malnutrition

Score 0 **Low risk**   Score 1 **Medium risk**   Score 2 or more **High risk**

Step 5

Management guidelines

0 Low risk	1 Medium risk	2 or more High risk
Routine clinical care	**Observe**	**Treat***
• Repeat screening	• Document dietary intake for three days	• Refer to dietitian, Nutritional Support Team or implement local policy
• Hospital – weekly	• If adequate – little concern and repeat screening	• Set goals, improve and increase overall nutritional intake
• Care homes – monthly	• Hospital – weekly	• Monitor and review care plan
• Community – annually for special groups e.g. those >75 yrs	• Care Home – at least monthly	• Hospital – weekly
	• Community – at least every 2–3 months	• Care Home – monthly
	• If inadequate – clinical concern – follow local policy, set goals, improve and increase overall nutritional intake, monitor and review care plan regularly	• Community – monthly

* Unless detrimental or no benefit is expected from nutritional support e.g. imminent death.

All risk categories:
- Treat underlying condition and provide help and advice on food choices, eating and drinking when necessary
- Record malnutrition risk category
- Record need for special diets and follow local policy

Obesity:
- Record presence of obesity. For those with underlying conditions, these are generally controlled before the treatment of obesity.

Re-assess subjects identified at risk as they move through care settings

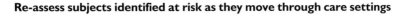

Alternative measurement and considerations

Step 1: BMI (body mass index)

If height cannot be measured

- Use recently documented or self-reported height (if reliable and realistic).
- If the subject does not know or is unable to report their height, use one of the alternative measurements to estimate height (ulna, knee height or demispan).

Step 2: Recent unplanned weight loss

If recent weight loss cannot be calculated, use self-reported weight loss (if reliable and realistic).

Subjective criteria

If height, weight or BMI cannot be obtained, the following criteria which relate to them can assist your professional judgement of the subject's nutritional risk category. Please note, these criteria should be used collectively not separately as alternatives to steps 1 and 2 of 'MUST' and are not designed to assign a score. Mid upper arm circumference (MUAC) may be used to estimate BMI category in order to support your overall impression of the subject's nutritional risk.

1. BMI

- Clinical impression – thin, acceptable weight, overweight. Obvious wasting (very thin) and obesity (very overweight) can also be noted.

2. Unplanned weight loss

- Clothes and/or jewellery have become loose fitting (weight loss).
- History of decreased food intake, reduced appetite or swallowing problems over 3–6 months and underlying disease or psycho-social/physical disabilities likely to cause weight loss.

3. Acute disease effect

- Acutely ill and no nutritional intake or likelihood of no intake for more than 5 days.

INDEX